The Botanical Pharmacy

The Pharmacology of 47 Common Herbs

QUARRY HEALTH BOOKS

The Fundamentals of Naturopathic Medicine
by Dr Fraser Smith

Naturopathic First Aid
by Dr Karen Barnes

A Call to Women: The Healthy Breast Program
by Dr Sat Dharam Kaur

Hoffer's Laws of Natural Nutrition
by Dr Abram Hoffer

Dr Hoffer's ABC of Natural Nutrition for Children
by Dr Abram Hoffer

Vitamin B-3 & Schizophrenia
by Dr Abram Hoffer

Vitamin C & Cancer
by Dr Abram Hoffer & Linus Pauling

Masks of Madness: Science of Healing
by Dr Abram Hoffer & Margot Kidder

The Botanical Pharmacy

The Pharmacology of 47 Common Herbs

Heather Boon
BScPhm, PhD
&
Michael Smith
MRPharmS, ND

QUARRY HEALTH BOOKS

in cooperation with

The Canadian College of Naturopathic Medicine

The publisher gratefully acknowledges the support of
The Canada Council for the Arts and the Department of Canadian Heritage
for the arts of writing and publishing in Canada.

The Canada Council for the Arts since 1957 | Le Conseil des Arts du Canada depuis 1957

Canada

The nutritional, medical, and health information presented in this book is based on the research, training, and professional experience of the authors, and is true and complete to the best of their knowledge. However, this book is intended only as an informative guide for those wishing to know more about health, nutrition, and medicine; it is not intended to replace or countermand the advice given by the reader's personal physician. Because each person and situation is unique, the authors and the publisher urge the reader to check with a qualified health professional before using any procedure where there is a question as to its appropriateness. The authors and the publisher are not responsible for any adverse effects or consequences resulting from the use of the information in this book. It is the responsibility of the reader to consult a physician or other qualified health care professional regarding his or her personal care.

ISBN 1-55082-230-6 HC
1-55082-252-7 PB

Design by Susan Hannah.

Printed and bound in Canada by AGMV Marquis,
Cap-Saint-Ignace, Quebec.

Published by Quarry Press Inc., P.O. Box 1061,
Kingston, Ontario K7L 4Y5 Canada,
www.quarrypress.com

CONTENTS

To my parents, Shirley and Glenn Boon,
who encouraged me to pursue my academic dreams
and to my husband,
Dr. Albert H.C. Wong,
who challenged me in lively debates
regarding the art and science of healing.
— *Heather Boon*

To my parents, Anne and Jack Smith,
for their love, support
and frequent and much needed counsel.
— *Michael Smith*

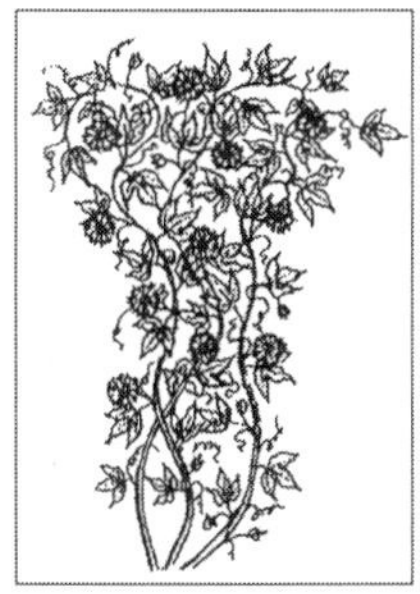

FOREWORD

Everyone involved in the delivery of health care is now aware of the increased interest in complementary and alternative medicine (CAM). While this has been described as a revolution in modern health-care, it is more accurate to describe it as a dynamic evolution. While questions about echinacea and Asian ginseng could once be ignored as a passing trend, now physicians and pharmacists are expected to be knowledgeable about many common herbs. This book was written in response to these changes in modern health-care.

This project was planned as a correspondence course with the objective of training pharmacists about botanical medicine. After much deliberation, it was decided that the best approach would be to prepare a series of monographs reviewing the herbal medicines most often seen by pharmacists in clinical practice. A very special team had to be created to make sure this project was a success. As the one of the primary sites of training in CAM in Canada, the Canadian College of Naturopathic Medicine (CCNM) agreed to manage the day-to-day running of the program. In order, to ensure that the information was correct and balanced, an advisory board of experts was established to review all the material. The majority of the monographs were also submitted to the Canadian Council on Continuing Education in Pharmacy (CCCEP) for its approval. After almost a year of work, the first fifteen monographs were sent out in the fall of 1997 and the project was completed in the summer of 1998.

In reading these monographs, not only is it important to realize what they are but also what they are not. Herbal medicine is a complex subject. It is both a science and an art. No book could cover all the subtle nuances of this fascinating therapy. We have intentionally concentrated on the published 'scientific' material, but attempted to incorporate empirical information wherever possible. While many conventional practitioners are not familiar with the traditional elements of herbalism, this empirical knowledge plays a pivotal role in the practice of botanical medicine.

It is important to establish the parameters we used in obtaining the information. An extensive search was done of MEDLINE and the Complementary Medicine Index (CMI). In addition, a manual search of the journals, periodicals and texts held in the Learning Resource Center at CCNM was commissioned. Given that much of the information available on the subject is published in a language other than English (notably German), a selection of articles was translated for this project.

A challenge we faced was to organize the monographs using a common format despite the fact that the nature and quantity of information varied so much from herb to herb. Consequently, while each monograph has common major headings (e.g., Thumbnail Sketch, Introduction, Therapeutic

Uses & Relevant Pharmacology), the arrangement of information within these headings is herb specific. A list of terms commonly used in herbal medicine which may not be familiar to most members of the conventional health-care team may be found in the introduction.

Many people need to be thanked for their help with this project: David Schleich (President, CCNM) and Colleen Mahy (Continuing Education, CCNM) for their enthusiasm; Dr Cory Ross (Vice President Academic, CCNM), 'troubleshooter extraordinaire' for his continued support and advice; Dr Robin Marles (Dept. of Botany, University of Brandon) for guiding us through the complex world of medical botany; Sharon McKinnon (Dept. of Pharmaceutical Sciences, University of British Columbia) and Dr. Ruth Ann Baron (Vice Chair of the Board, CCNM) for keeping us on the straight and narrow and ensuring the information was relevant; Dr. Albert Wong (Centre for Addiction and Mental Health, Toronto) for his candor and critiques; Kim Pietraczk, Tasleem Kassam and Sean Wharton without whose hard work and diligence this project would never have been possible.

While this book will not answer all your questions about botanical medicine, we hope that it will be a useful resource for understanding the safe use of these herbs.

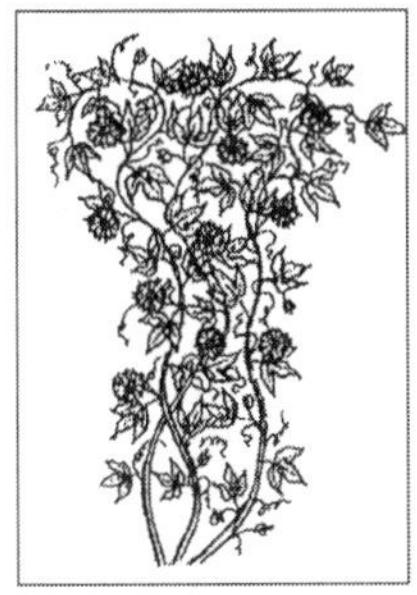

INTRODUCTION

Pharmacists are often asked for advice regarding a wide range of botanical products. This may be because of the accessibility of pharmacists to the general public, but is also influenced by the fact that many community pharmacies now sell a variety of botanical products. A brief introduction to the field of Botanical Medicine will help to contextualize the following modules.

DEMOGRAPHICS

According to several recent Canadian surveys, 15 to 25 per cent of the population use some form of alternative or complementary medicine.[1,2] This is comparable to a much-quoted American survey which reported that 34 per cent of the respondents had used at least one unconventional therapy in the past year.[3] Only one third of those who reported use of complementary health care products in the US study reported seeing a complementary health care provider, which indicates a high level of self-medication.[3]

Botanical medicine is becoming big business for pharmacists. *Pharmacy Post*'s 1996 Trends Report indicates that three out of every four Canadian community pharmacies now sell herbal and/or homeopathic products and that approximately half of those surveyed intended to increase these sections.[4] Another report suggests that the average "medium sized" community pharmacy in Canada sells at least 35 plant-derived products (including natural source vitamins), marketed by at least 8 phyto-pharmaceutical manufacturers.[5] In addition, a recent issue of *Pharmacy Practice* reports that Canadians spent $175 million on herbal products in 1996, which is an increase from the $150 million spent in 1995.[6] Although some see botanical medicine as a new "niche" for pharmacy,[7] the debate about whether botanical medicine belongs in pharmacies or in health food stores is becoming heated.[8] The opponents of the sale of botanical products in pharmacies emphasize the fact that most pharmacists have little or no training in this field.

LEGISLATION

Canada

The Drugs Directorate has published Canadian guidelines regarding the manufacture and sale of botanical products.[9-12] Canadian botanical products currently fall into one of three categories.

1) Food Supplements:
do not require Drug Identification Numbers (DIN);
cannot make therapeutic claims;
recommended dosage must not exceed 25% of therapeutic dosage levels;
do not require cautions, contraindications, or possible side effect information

2) Phyto-pharmaceuticals with full drug status:
compliance with Health Protection Branch (HPB) regulations
approved therapeutic indications
approved dosage
efficacy supported by scientific evidence
DINs

3) Traditional Herbal Medicines (THMs):[11]
intended for self-medication only
all active constituents are herbal ingredients
little or no scientific evidence required
efficacy supported solely (but is well-documented) in herbal references
(acceptable references are specified in the regulations[12])
approved therapeutic indications
approved dosage

DINs

Drug Identification Numbers (DINs) for products in the second category are obtained by submitting a regular application and products derived from botanical sources are given no special consideration. However, applications for DINs in the Traditional Herbal Medicines (THMs) category are based not on scientific evidence; rather, the application must be supported by a minimum of two acceptable herbal references[12]. A specific list of herbs have been identified as unacceptable as medicinal components of THMs. These include: Arnica (not permitted for internal use), Comfrey, Gelsemium, Germander, Goldenseal (not permitted as a single ingredient and not over 300 mg/day in a multi-ingredient THM), Gotu kola, and Mistletoe.[12]

Herbal products in the latter two categories must meet the following labeling standards:[11]

1) each herbal ingredient must be identified by both its common name and Latin binomial
2) the part of the plant used must be identified
3) the dosage form must be specified (e.g., powdered extract, tincture, etc.)
4) the quantity of each medicinal ingredient in each dosage unit must be listed
5) indications for use must be listed

In addition, Traditional Herbal Medicines must:[11]

1) be identified as Traditional Herbal Medicines on the label
2) contain a caution that they are for use by adults (those 12 years and older) and that they should not be used in pregnancy or lactation (unless use in these populations is supported by the herbal literature)
3) the term "natural" may only be used to describe a product sold in its original state (i.e., without processing or refinement)

4) the term "natural source" may be used only when the product has undergone a minimum of processing (e.g., drying)

Good Manufacturing Practice Guidelines for the manufacture of herbal medicine products are also available from the Drugs Directorate.[9]

The United States of America

Herbal products in the United States are regulated as "dietary supplements," as defined by The Dietary Supplement Heath and Education Act of 1994 (DSHEA). This definition also encompasses nutritional supplements such as vitamins, minerals and amino acids. Companies marketing "dietary supplements" cannot make specific medical claims regarding their products; however, they make make "statements of nutritional support" or "structure and function claims" (statements explaining how the product may affect the structure or function of the body). Under the DSHEA regulations, manufacturing companies may also indicate to customers possible areas of concern such as potential side-effects and contraindications.

Despite the fact that most herbal products are regulated as "dietary supplements," pharmaceutical companies have the option to apply for regulation for herbal products via the same system as applies to conventional non-prescription drugs. However, the lack of patent protection for these products and the time (average of 15 years) and money (average US $500 million) needed to submit a New Drug Application (NDA) make this an unpopular option.

In order to address growing public and professional discontent with the current regulatory situation, President Clinton appointed a seven person review body known as the Commission on Dietary Supplement Labels (CDSL) in 1995. In 1997, the CDSL released a report recommending that an expert review panel be convened. The CDSL suggested that this review panel should make herbal products with strong scientific merit their priority. Further changes to the regulation of herbal products in the United States may be expected based on new recommendations from the CDSL and the review panel. For example, the CDSL has recommended that manufacturers who wish to make therapeutic claims for dietary supplements, including herbal products, must meet a standard of "significant scientific agreement" (the standard that is currently set in the Nutrition Labeling and Education Act of 1990).

BOTANICAL DOSAGE FORMS[13-16]

Herbal Teas

A time-honored method of taking herbal medicines is in the form of a tea. There are primarily two kinds: decoctions and infusions. A decoction is normally reserved for fibrous plant material such as stems, bark, roots and rhizomes. It is made by boiling the plant material until it is reduced to a specific volume. Steeping the more delicate plant parts (flowers, leaves) in either hot or cold water makes an infusion. The temperature of the water will influence the constituent(s) extracted.

The use of these dosage forms is often limited by poor palatability and the fact that only water-soluble constituents are extracted.

Liquid Dosage Forms: Tincture/Fluid (liquid) Extracts

A tincture is made by macerating /percolating the plant material in a mixture of water and alcohol. The components extracted are determined by the alcohol/water ratio used in the solvent. While the percentage of alcohol can be as high as 90%, it is more commonly in the range of 25%

to 60%. The strength of the tincture is usually given as the ratio of solid herbal product used compared to the total volume of the solution. The commonest range is between 1:3 to 1:5 (plant: total solution).

A fluid (liquid) extract is also an hydroalcoholic product; however in these products one unit of the preparation is equivalent to one unit of the original plant product (i.e., they are more concentrated than tinctures). While this increased potency definitely has its advantages, questions have been raised about the way in which some commercial products are manufactured. Many of the commercially available fluid-extracts are made by simply evaporating the solvent from a tincture and then reconstituting the residue to the appropriate volume. This method can cause degradation of the more unstable constituents. Unfortunately, in practice, the terms tincture and fluid extract are often used interchangeably. In addition, it is uncommon for liquid dosage forms to indicate either alcohol content or strength on the label.

Tincture and fluid (liquid) extracts are usually ingested in a little water. Using warm water allows the evaporation of most of the alcohol present, reducing its undesirable effects. These dosage forms have advantages of: 1) containing both alcohol and aqueous soluble components; and 2) allowing prescribers to combine herbs. As with herbal teas, poor palatability is often a problem.

A glycerite is a 'tincture-like' product in which glycerin is used as a solvent. They appear particularly useful in the management of pediatric conditions or where alcohol is strictly contraindicated.

Solid Dosage Forms

Herbal medicines are available in a range of solid doses, including capsules, tablets, freeze-dried products and lozenges. While capsules usually simply contain the dried herbs, tablets are often made from concentrates. Concerns have been raised regarding the small quantity of herbs often present in these dosage forms.

Standardized Extract

A standardized extract is a product in which a specific concentration of a particular constituent or group of constituents is guaranteed. While all the original constituents may still be present, they are often not in the proportions found in the original herb. While this approach is attractive to the conventional medical model, it is dependent on the existence, extraction and identification of a discrete single (or group of) active constituent(s). The effect of this approach to the synergy, which is reputed by herbalists to exist between components, has yet to be clarified.

In order to assure quality, some preparations may be standardized to a 'marker' component guaranteeing that the correct plant was harvested and used. This 'marker' agent need not necessarily be the active constituent.

Dosage Considerations

Botanical medicine is not practiced in a homogenous manner. Different groups follow distinct philosophies which favor specific dosage systems. Suggested dose regimens may come from herbal traditions (Chinese, Ayurvedic), established European pharmacopoeias or as a result of clinical and pharmacological evaluation. This situation presents the practitioner or consumer with a dilemma regarding a standard dosing regimen for any given herb. As a general rule, doses used by practitioners trained in North America are usually lower than those used by their European counterparts. For this project, the authors have attempted to include a variety of dosage regimens commonly seen in Canada.

SAFETY ISSUES

A misconception often shared by practitioners and the public alike is that complementary therapies are completely safe. Unfortunately, this is not the case. Adverse effects from a number of complementary therapies, including botanical medicine, have been noted. O'Neill classifies the dangers of complementary medicine as falling into one of the following four categories:

1. *Sins of omission* are those in which the patient deteriorates because the CAM practitioner does not recognize the seriousness of his/her condition and does not refer him/her to appropriate medical care.[17] The quality of education and the professional character of the complementary health-care provider play a role in determining both their safety and competence.[18] While many "professional" associations of Canadian herbal practitioners do exist, none have the authority to regulate the practice. With the exception of the practice of naturopathic medicine in Ontario, Manitoba, Saskatchewan, and British Columbia, no federal or provincial regulations exist regarding the practice of herbal medicine. This results in little uniformity between herbal practitioners. Cases in which a patient self-medicates inappropriately would also fall in this category.

2. *Intrinsic procedural risks* are those arising as a direct result of the administration of the therapy.[17] Examples of adverse reactions which result directly from the use of a specific herbal product, including allergic responses, have been noted.[19-26] Complications and ill effects have also been noted due to: misidentification of the herbal content,[26-28] intentional/unintentional adulteration of the product with heavy metals or pharmaceuticals,[26, 29-32] and suspected interactions with conventional medication.[33, 34]

3. *Situational amplifications* occur in cases where CAM therapy aggravates an existing condition.[17] The use of some herbs, especially as part of a 'detoxifying' protocol, may exacerbate a patient's condition at the onset of treatment.[13] Also, critical and objective evidence regarding the use of herbal medicines in certain scenarios such as pregnancy is lacking. Most information in this area comes from anecdotal and historical sources, the importance of which has yet to be investigated.[35]

4. The final category O'Neill identifies is the delivery of worthless procedures for financial or other gains on part of the practitioner.[17] Unfortunately, as the popularity of 'natural' medicine increases, so does the opportunity for misrepresentation of their use. This is especially a concern when effective treatment (either conventional or unconventional) exists for the condition.[36]

IMPLICATIONS FOR PHARMACY PRACTICE

Most practising pharmacists have very little knowledge about botanical medicine. With the exception of several new elective courses being offered at a handful of faculties of pharmacy, pharmacists receive no formal training in botanical medicine. This situation is particularily distressing because the rate at which botanical products are being placed on community pharmacy shelves far exceeds the rate at which community pharmacists are being educated about those products. This situation may be slowly changing. Continuing education seminars are providing instruction on topics of botanical medicine are becoming available. Articles with titles such as "What Pharmacists Should Know About Herbal Remedies"[37] and "Herbal Medicine"[38] are becoming more common in the pharmacy literature. The *Canadian Pharmaceutical Journal* has been publishing high-quality reviews of specific botanical products for several years. However, more in-depth courses for pharmacists are still required.

One of the cornerstones of pharmaceutical care is helping patients to make informed decisions about their health-care. As patients' options expand to include options such as botanical medicine, pharmacists are being asked to wade through large amounts of (mis)information to help patients make the most informed choices possible.

When patients choose to make use of botanical products, it is important for pharmacists to provide monitoring and report adverse effects and herb-drug or herb-herb interactions when necessary. This potential new role requires a pharmacist who has a good working knowledge of botanical medicine and can apply problem-solving skills to "fill in the gaps" of our current knowledge of these products. The authors hope that this book will provide pharmacists with a foundation of knowledge from which they can counsel patients about the use of botanical products with confidence.

PATIENT COUNSELING TIPS

1. Is the herbal product being used to treat a self-limiting condition?
2. Is a herbal therapy appropriate?
3. Is the patient currently taking any other medications (conventional or unconventional)?
4. Do you know that the herbal products available to you are of good quality?
5. Is the patient currently under the care of a complementary health-care provider?
6. Are there any other factors you must consider (e.g., pregnancy, heart condition, diabetes etc.)?

FORMAT OF REVIEWS

The reviews of each herb follow a basic outline: Thumbnail Sketch; Introduction (family; synonyms; history/background; constituents); Therapeutic Uses and Relevant Pharmacology; Adverse Effects; Cautions/Contraindications; Drug Interactions; and Dosage Regimens. However, given the different types of information available for each herb (scientific, anecdotal, cross-cultural), as well as the quality and quantity of the available information, the Therapeutic Uses and Relevant Pharmacology section may be organized in different ways.

GLOSSARY OF BOTANICAL MEDICINE TERMS

Adaptogen An agent that supports the body's ability to accommodate varying physical and emotional stresses.

Alterative An agent with the ability to restore normal body function(s) from an initial unhealthy state. This includes a variety of herbal medicine categories, including: antimicrobials, digestive or hepatic tonics.

Astringent An agent, normally rich in tannins, that can precipitate proteins resulting in a contraction of tissues.

Bitter An agent that aids and supports the digestive process, promoting salivation and the secretion of stomach acid and digestive enzymes.

Carminative A primarily digestive agent that supports and soothes the digestive system relieving gas, spasm and distention.

Cathartic An agent with a pronounced laxative effect, resulting in dramatic evacuation of the bowels.

Cholagogue An agent that promotes secretion of bile by causing contraction of the gall-bladder.

Choleretic An agent that promotes the production and secretion of bile.

Demulcent A normally mucilaginous agent that soothes irritated tissues, notably mucous membranes.

Diaphoretic An agent that promotes detoxification by promotion of perspiration.

Emmenagogue An agent that stimulates or harmonizes menstrual flow.

Febrifuge A fever lowering agent

Galactagogue An agent that promotes lactation.

Glycoside Botanical constituent consisting of sugar and non-sugar (aglycone) components.

Hepatic General term used to describe an agent that supports healthy liver function.

Nervine An agent that affects the nervous system, either tonifying, sedating or stimulating.

Phytoestrogen Compounds, usually flavonoids, which have a weak affinity for estrogen receptors.

Stomachic An agent that supports gastric functions and promotes appetite.

Tonic A nurturing agent that invigorates either specific organ(s) or the entire individual.

Vulnerary An agent that supports wound healing.

REFERENCES

1. Northcott H, Bachynsky J. Concurrent Use of Chiropractic, Prescription Medicines, Nonprescription Medicines and Alternative Health Care. *Social Science and Medicine.* 1993; 37(3): 431-5.
2. Canada Health Monitor. Highlights Report. Survey #9. March 1993. Toronto: Price Waterhouse, Suite 3300, Box 190, 1 First Canadian Place, Toronto, Ontario, M5X 1H7.; 1993.
3. Eisenberg DM, Kessler RC, Foster C, Norlock FE, Calkins DR, Delbanco TL. Unconventional medicine in the United States: Prevalence, costs and patterns of use. *The New England Journal of Medicine.* 1993; 328 (4): 246-52.
4. Clarke K. Herbs, homeopathy rising stars. *Pharmacy Post.* 1996; November 17.
5. Health Management Institute. Plant derived pharmaceuticals — A renewed direction. Reference HMI 960201 White Paper. Fredericton, New Brunswick: Health Management Institute (HMI): 1996.
6. Anonymous. Pharmacy Trends. *Pharmacy Practice.* 1997; 13(6): 48-50.
7. Dundass H. The Herbal Niche. *The Canadian Pharmaceutical Journal.* 1993; 125(6): 292-5.
8. Howden KM, Sheard LM, Christensen IP, *et al*. Counter prescribing of herbal remedies: A comparative study of pharmacies and health food shops. *The Pharmaceutical Journal.* 1989; Sepember 30: R28.
9. Drugs Directorate. Good Manufacturing Guidelines for the Manufacture of Herbal Medicinal Products. Final Version. Ottawa: Drugs Directorate; 1996.
10. Drugs Directorate (Bureau of Nonprescription Drugs). Herbs Used as Non-medicinal Ingredients in Nonprescription Drugs for Human Use. Ottawa: Drugs Directorate (Bureau of Nonprescription Drugs); 1995.
11. Drugs Directorate. Drugs Directorate Guideline. Traditional Herbal Medicines (Revised). Ottawa; 1995.
12. Drugs Directorate (Bureau of Nonprescription Drugs). Medicinal Herbs in Traditional Herbal Medicines. Ottawa: Drugs Directorate (Bureau of Nonprescription Drugs); 1995.
13. Mills S. *The Essential Book of Herbal Medicine*. London: Penguin; 1991: 677.
14. Bone K. Dosage considerations in herbal medicine. *The British Journal of Phytotherapy.* 1993-4; 3(3): 128-37.
15. Werback M, Murray M. *Botanical Influences on Illness.* Tarzana, CA: Third Line Press; 1994: 344.
16. Chevalier A. *The Encyclopedia of Medicinal Plants*. London: Readers Digest: 1996: 336.
17. O'Neill A. Danger and safety in medicines. *Social Science and Medicine.* 1994; 38(4): 497-507.
18. Mills S. Safety awareness in complementary medicine. *Complementary Therapies in Medicine.* 1996; 4: 48-51.
19. Coremans P, Lambrecht G, Schepens P *et al.* Anti-cholinergic intoxication with commercially available thornapple tea. *Journal of Toxicology: Clinical Toxicology.* 1994; 32: 589-92.
20. Tennekoon K, Jeevathayaparan S, Angunawala P *et al.* Effect of *Momordica charantia* on key hepatic enzymes. *Journal of Ethnopharmacology.* 1994; 44: 93-7.
21. D'Arcy P. Adverse reactions and interactions and herbal medicine. Part 1 Adverse reactions. *Adverse Drug React. Toxicol. Rev.* 1991; 10(4): 189-208.
22. Smith A, Feddersen R, Gardner K *et al.* Cystic renal cell carcinoma and acquired renal cystic disease associated with consumption of chaparral tea: A case report. *Journal of Urology.* 1994; 152: 2089-91.
23. Atherton D. Towards the safer use of traditional remedies. *British Medical Journal.* 1994; 308: 673-4.
24. Itami N, *et al.* Herbal medicine can induce hypertension. *Nephron.* 1991; 59: 339-40.
25. Hogan R. Hemorrhagic diathesis caused by drinking an herbal tea. *Journal of the American Medical Association.* 1983; 249(19): 2679-80.
26. Perharic L, Shaw D, Colbridge M *et al*. Toxicological problems resulting from exposure to traditional remedies and food supplements. *Drug Safety.* 1994;11(4): 284-94.
27. Vanhaelen M, Vanhaelen-Fastre R, But P *et al.* Identification of aristocholic acid in Chinese herbs. *Lancet.* 1994: 174.
28. Bryson P, Watanabe A, Rumack B *et al.* Burdock root tea poisoning. *Journal of the American Medical Association.* 1978; 239(20): 2157.
29. Raman A, Jamal J. 'Herbal' hayfever remedy found to contain conventional drugs. *The Pharmaceutical Journal.* 1997; 258: 105-6.
30. Hughes J, Higguis E, Pembroke A *et al*. Oral dexamethasone masquerading as a Chinese herbal remedy. *British Journal of Dermatology.* 1994; 130: 261.
31. Markowitz S, Nuuez C, Klitzman S *et al.* Lead poisoning due to hai ge fen. *Journal of the American Medical Association*. 1994; 271: 932-4.
32. Stricht B. Remedies may contain cocktail of active drugs. *British Medical Journal.* 1994; 308: 1162.
33. Mcrae S. Elevated serum digoxin levels in a patient taking digozin and siberian ginseng. *Canadian Medical Association Journal.* 1996; 155(3): 293-5.

34. Jones, B, Runikis A. Interaction of ginseng with phenelzine. *Journal of Clinical Psychopharmacology*. 1987; 7(3): 201-2.
35. Lepik K. Safety of herbal medicines in pregnancy. *Canadian Pharmaceutical Journal.* 1997; May: 29-33.
36. Jonas W. Safety in complementary medicine. In: Ernst E, ed. *Complementary Medicine, An Objective Appraisal.* Oxford: Butterworth-Heinermann; 1996: 127-49.
37. Tyler VE. What pharmacists should know about herbal remedies. *Journal of the American Pharmaceutical Association.* 1996; NS36: 29-37.
38. Kyriakos T. Herbal Medicine. *Canadian Pharmaceutical Journal.* 1996; September: 46-50.

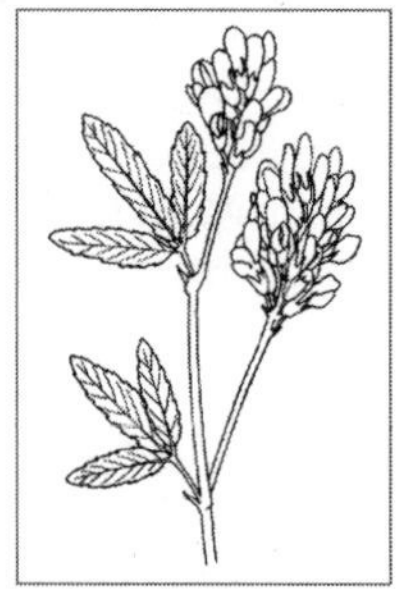

ALFALFA

Medicago sativa L.

THUMBNAIL SKETCH

Active Constituents
- Saponins
- Triterpenoidal glycosides

Common Uses
- Hypercholesterolemia
- May be used for problems related to menstruation and menopause

Adverse Effects
- Rare diarrhea and stomach upset
- Theoretically photosensitivity may occur
- Reactivation of systemic lupus erythematosus (SLE) has been reported

Cautions/Contraindications
- Systemic lupus erythematosus (SLE)
- Pregnancy and lactation (seeds only)

Drug Interactions
- Possible interactions with anticoagulants, hormone replacement therapy, birth control pills

Doses
- 5-10 g dried herb three times daily
- 5-10 mL liquid extraxt (1:1; 25% alcohol) three times daily

INTRODUCTION

Family: Fabaceae (also known as Leguminosae)

Synonyms: Lucerne, Buffalo herb, Chilean clover, Purple medick[1]

Alfalfa was originally cultivated by the Greeks and Romans and is currently produced primarily as a fodder crop in North America. Although alfalfa has been used medicinally in traditional Chinese medicine (to treat digestive disorders) and Ayurvedic medicine (for digestive conditions, as a diuretic and in the treatment of arthritis), it is not often mentioned in North American textbooks of herbal medicine.[1] Modern day herbalists consider alfalfa to be a good general tonic, due largely to its reputation as an excellent source of vitamins, minerals and protein.

This perennial herb with clover-like leaves and spiralling seed pods grows to approximately 1 m. Its flowers range in colour from purplish-blue to yellow. Alfalfa is native to Eastern Mediterranean Europe and the Middle East, but now can be found throughout the world.[2, 3]

Constituents[4-8]

- Amino acids: canavanine
- Saponins with the aglycone medicagenic acid
- Isoflavone flavonoids: genistein, daidzein, formononetin
- Coumarins: coumestans, medicagol
- Alkaloids
- Miscellaneous: carbohydrates, peptides, pigments, acids, vitamins (esp. vitamins A, B1, B6, B12, C, E, K)

THERAPEUTIC USES & RELEVANT PHARMACOLOGY

EFFECTS ON CHOLESTEROL

Several studies have demonstrated that the addition of alfalfa meal to cholesterol-containing diets prevented hypercholesterolemia in rats;[9, 10] and prevented hypercholesterolemia, decreased hypertriglyceridemia and prevented atherosclerosis in rabbits and monkeys.[9, 11-16] In addition, it has been shown that alfalfa decreased cholesterolemia, decreased plasma phospholipids, normalized plasma lipoproteins and reduced the extent of aortic and coronary atherosclerosis in monkeys when added to their high-cholesterol diet.[17, 18]

Two human trials have been published.[19, 20] One clinical trial was an uncontrolled, non-blinded trial with 11 patients diagnosed with type II and 4 patients diagnosed with type IV hyperlipoproteinemia who were given 40 g of heat prepared alfalfa seeds 3 times daily at mealtimes for 8 weeks (remainder of diet unchanged). Of the patients with type II hyperlipoproteinemia, 9 showed significantly lowered total plasma cholesterol, low density lipoprotein (LDL), and apolipoprotein B, while apolipoprotein A-1 did not change. The 4 patients with type IV did not appear to have the same beneficial effects; however, the small number made it difficult to detect statistically significant effects.[20]

Several researchers have suggested that the alfalfa saponins are the active component of the plant. Rat experiments have indicated that saponins from alfalfa decrease the absorption of cholesterol from the intestine.[9, 10, 21] This is partially supported by the finding that alfalfa increases the excretion of fecal neutral steroids in rabbits and monkeys, which implies that alfalfa interferes with the absorption of cholesterol.[16, 22, 23] In addition, *in vitro* experiments showed that alfalfa plant saponins bound significant amounts of cholesterol from both ethanol solution and from micellar suspension. The amount of cholesterol bound was significantly decreased with the removal of saponins from alfalfa; however, the ability to absorb bile acid was unaffected. The hypocholesterolemic action of alfalfa was thought to be a combination of the saponin-cholesterol interaction and an interaction with bile acids.[24]

MISCELLANEOUS

Cardiovascular Effects

Alfalfa has been used in the management of clotting disorders, primarily due to its high vitamin K content. The clinical relevance of this indication is questionable. It may be of use in situations arising from vitamin K deficiency.[1]

Women's Health Care

The isoflavones found in alfalfa (genistein, daidzein) have also been extracted from other plants and shown to have phytoestrogenic properties. [1, 2] Consequently, alfalfa has been suggested by many complementary practitioners to be useful in the management of menopause and menstrual discomfort.

Immune System Effects

A Chinese study suggests that polysaccharides isolated from alfalfa may have immunopotentiating effects.[25] This has yet to be confirmed.

ADVERSE EFFECTS

Allergic reactions to alfalfa powder have been reported. In addition, diarrhea and stomach upset may occur occasionally.[1] Photosensitivity reactions have been noted in animals and very rarely skin reactions in humans are seen.[26]

Early animal studies found no toxicity associated with alfalfa or alfalfa saponins; [18, 27] however, there was some evidence of growth inhibition in studies where alfalfa was ingested without the addition of cholesterol to the diet.[28-30] Ames mutagenicity testing was negative for a variety of extracts from alfalfa.[31]

Alfalfa may have more severe adverse effects as was noted in a 1981 case study in which a man who ingested 80-160 g alfalfa seeds daily on eight occasions for up to 6 weeks at a time (as part of a study) developed pancytopenia.[32] This letter was followed by a report of systemic lupus erythematosus (SLE)-like syndrome in monkeys fed alfalfa sprouts[33] and a letter reporting two cases in which patients with SLE, which was clinically and serologically in remission, had reactivations of their disease in association with the ingestion of alfalfa tablets.[34] L- Canavanine is the component of alfalfa which appears to be responsible for these unwanted effects (not the saponins which are considered to be the active ingredient needed for positive cholesterol-lowering effects).[33, 35, 36]

Ingestion of a diet consisting 1.0 to 1.2% of alfalfa saponins by monkeys and rabbits is considered to be harmless.[15, 18] Humans currently ingest saponins from a variety of sources, including alfalfa sprouts, soybeans, chick peas, spinach, asparagus and sunflower seeds, without any ill effects.[37]

CAUTIONS/CONTRAINDICATIONS

- Patients with a history of systemic lupus erythematosus (SLE).[34]
- Seeds should be avoided during pregnancy and lactation.[8]

DRUG INTERACTIONS

Given the possible anti-coagulant action of the vitamin K and the coumarins (e.g., medicagol) found in alfalfa, excessive doses may interfere with concomitant anti-coagulant therapy.[8] However, simple coumarins have more toxicity to rodents and dogs than humans. A more significant risk occurs when the plant becomes infected with mold and the coumarin is converted to the more potent anti-coagulant dicoumarol. Thus quality control for mold-free products is a significant issue here.[38]

In addition, the estrogenic nature of the isoflavones present may interfere with hormone replacement therapy and birth control pills if taken in excessive doses.[8]

DOSAGE REGIMENS

- 5-10 g dried herb three times daily[8]
- 5-10 mL liquid extraxt (1:1; 25% alcohol) three times daily[8]

REFERENCES

1. Briggs C. Alfalfa. *Canadian Pharmaceutical Journal*. 1994;March:84-6.
2. Leung AY, Foster S. *Encyclopedia of Common Natural Ingredients Used in Food, Drugs, and Cosmetics*. 2nd ed. New York: John Wiley and Sons Inc; 1996:649.
3. Chevallier A. *The Encyclopedia of Medicinal Plants.* London: Readers Digest; 1996:336.
4. Natelson S. Canavanine to arginine ratio in alfalfa (*Medicago sativa*), clover (*Trifolium*), and the jack bean (*Canavalia ensiformis*). *Journal of Agriculture and Food Chemistry*. 1985;33:413-419.
5. Natelson S. Canavanine in alfalfa (*Medicago sativa*). *Experentia*. 1985;41:257-259.
6. Polachek I, Zehavi V, Naim M, *et al*. Activity of compound G2 isolated from alfalfa roots against medically important yeasts. *Antimicrobial Agents and Chemotherapy*. 1986;30:290-294.
7. Berrang B, Davis KHJ, Wall ME, Hanson CH, Pedersen ME. Saponins of two alfalfa cultivars. *Phytochemistry*. 1974;13:2253-60.
8. Newall CA, Anderson LA, Phillipson JD. *Herbal Medicines: A Guide for Health Care Professionals.* London: The Pharmaceutical Press; 1996:296.
9. Malinow MR, McLaughlin P, Kohler GO, Livingston AL. Prevention of elevated cholesterolemia in monkeys by alfalfa saponins. *Steroids*. 1977;29:105-110.
10. Malinow MR, McLaughlin P, Papworth L, *et al*. Effect of alfalfa saponins on intestinal cholesterol absorption in rats. *American Journal of Clinical Nutrition*. 1977;30(12):2061-2067.
11. Cookson FB, Altschul R, Federoff S. The effects of alfalfa on serum cholesterol and in modifying or preventing cholesterol induced atherosclerosis in rabbits. *Journal of Atherosclerosis Research.* 1967;7:69.
12. Cookson FB, Fedoroff, S. Quantitative relationships between administered cholesterol and alfalfa required to prevent hypercholesterolaemia in rabbits. *British Journal of Experimental Pathology*. 1968;49:348.
13. Kritchevsky D, Tepper SA, Story JA. Isocaloric, isogravic diets in rats, Part 3 (Effect of non-nutritive fibre (alfalfa or cellulose) on cholesterol metabolism). *Nutrition Reports International*. 1974;9:301.
14. Yanaura S, Sakamoto M. Influence of alfalfa meal on experimental hyperlipidemia. *Nippon Yakurigaku Zasshi – Folia Pharmacologica Japonica.* 1975;71:387.
15. Malinow MR, McLaughlin P, Stafford C, Livingstone AL, Kohler GO. Alfalfa saponins and alfalfa seeds: Dietary effects on cholesterol-fed rabbits. *Atherosclerosis*. 1980;37:433-38.

16. Malinow MR, Connor WE, Mclaughlin P, *et al.* Cholesterol and bile acid balance in *Macaca fascicularis*: Effects of alfalfa saponins. *Journal of Clinical Investigation*. 1981;67:156-62.
17. Malinow MR, McLaughlin P, Naito HK, *et al.* Effect of alfalfa meal on shrinkage (regression) of atherosclerotic plaques during cholesterol feeding in monkeys. *Atherosclerosis*. 1978;30(1):27-43.
18. Malinow MR, McNulty, WP, Houghton, DC, *et al*. Lack of toxicity of alfalfa saponins on cynomolgus macaques. *Journal of Medical Primatology.* 1982;11(106-118).
19. Malinow MR, McLaughlin P, Stafford C. Alfalfa seeds: Effects on cholesterol metabolism. *Experimentia*. 1980;36:562-3.
20. Molgaard J, von Schenck H, Olsson AG. Alfalfa seeds lower low density lipoprotein cholesterol and apolipoprotein B concentrations in patients with type II hyperlipoproteinemia. *Atherosclerosis*. 1987; 65: 173-9.
21. Malinow MR, McLaughlin P, Stafford C, *et al.* Comparative effects of alfalfa saponins and alfalfa fiber on cholesterol absorption in rats. *American Journal of Clinical Nutrition*. 1979; 32(9): 1810-1812.
22. Barichello AW, Federoff S. Effect of ileal bypass and alfalfa on hypercholesterolemia. *British Journal of Experimental Pathology*. 1971;52:81.
23. Hornick B, Cookson FB, Federoff S. Effect of alfalfa feeding on the excretion of fecal neutral sterols in the rabbit. *Circulation*. 1967;36 (Suppl. II):II-18.
24. Story JA, LePage SL, Petro MS, *et al.* Interactions of alfalfa plant and sprout saponins with cholesterol in vitro and in cholesterol-fed rats. *American Journal of Clinical Nutrition*. 1984; 39: 917-929.
25. Zhao WS, Zhang YQ, Ren LJ, Zhang L, Yang J. Immunopotentiating effects of polysaccharides isolated from *Medicago sativa* L. (Chinese; English abstract). *Acta Pharmacologica Sinica*. 1993; 14(3): 273-6.
26. De Smet PA, *et al*. Adverse Effects of Herbal Drugs. 2nd ed. Verlag: Springer; 1992.
27. Malinow MR, McNulty WP, McLaughlin P, *et al*. The toxicity of alfalfa saponins in rats. *Food and Cosmetics Toxicology*. 1981;19:443-445.
28. Anderson JO. Effect of alfalfa saponin on the performance of chicks and laying hens. *Poultry Science*. 1957;36:873-6.
29. Reshef G, Gestetner B, Birk Y. Effect of alfalfa saponins on the growth and some aspects of lipid metabolism of mice and quails. *Journal of the Science of Food and Agriculture.* 1976;27:63-72.
30. Wilcox EB, Galloway LS. Serum and liver cholesterol, total lipids and lipid phosphorus levels of rats under various dietary regimes. *American Journal of Clinical Nutrition*. 1961;9:236-43.
31. White RD, Kauperman PH, Cheeke PR, Buhler DR. An evaluation of acetone extracts from six plants in the Ames mutagenicity test. *Toxicology Letters*. 1983;15:25-31.
32. Malinow MR, Bardana EJ, Goodnight SH. Pancytopenia during ingestion of alfalfa seeds. *Lancet*. 1981:i:615.
33. Malinow MR, Bardana EJ, Pirofsky B, *et al.* Systemic lupus erythematosus-like syndrome in monkeys fed alfalfa sprouts: Role of a non-protein amino acid. *Science*. 1982;216:415-417.
34. Roberts JL, Hayashi JA. Exacerbation of SLE associated with alfalfa ingestion. [Letter]. *New England Journal of Medicine*. 1983;308(22):1361.
35. Rosenthal GA. The biological effects and mode of action of L-canavanine, a structural analogue of L-arginine. *Quarterly Review of Biology.* 1977;52:155-78.
36. Alcocer-Varela J, Iglesias A, llorente L, Alarcon-Segovia D. Effects of L-canavanine on T cells may explain the induction of systemic lupus erythematosus by alfalfa. *Arthritis and Rheumatology*. 1985;28(1):52-57.
37. Oakenfull D. Saponins in food. *Food Chemistry*. 1980;6:19-40.
38. Marles RJ, Associate Professor, Department of Botany, Brandon University, Brandon, Manitoba. Review of Medicinal Plant Modules for CCNM; 1997.

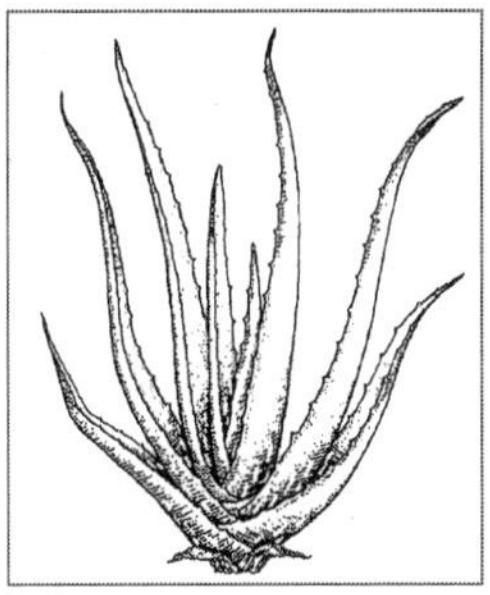

ALOE VERA

A. vera (L.) Burm.f.

THUMBNAIL SKETCH

Active Constituents

- Aloe vera gel: polysaccharides including acemannan
- Aloes: anthraquinones

Common Uses

- Aloe vera gel: treatment of skin irritation, wounds, burns, etc.
- Aloes: laxative

Adverse Effects

- Aloe vera gel: rare 'allergic-type' reactions
- Aloes: severe abdominal cramping is common; reversible pigmentation of the colonic mucosa; discoloration of the urine; nephritis, gastritis, vomiting, bloody diarrhea, and watery diarrhea have been reported

Cautions/Contraindications

- Aloe vera gel:
  External: known allergy
  Internal: trace anthraquinone glycosides may be of concern in pregnancy and lactation
- Aloes: Contraindicated in pregnancy and menstruation; as well as appendicitis and abdominal pain of unknown origin. Not recommended for treatment of chronic constipation, or in the presence of hemorrhoids

Drug Interactions

- Aloe vera gel: none known
- Aloes: possible interaction with cardiac glycosides

Doses

- Aloe vera gel:
  - *Externally*: vehicle must contain a minimum of 70% concentration of aloe vera; pure aloe vera gel is also available
  - *Internally*: no standard dosing

- Aloes: 50-200 mg aloe (dried sap) three times daily

INTRODUCTION

Family: Aloeaceae (formerly Aloe was included in the Liliaceae family)[1]

Synonyms: Curacao aloe; *A. barbadensis* P. Miller; *A. vulgaris* Lam.[1, 2]

Aloe vera gel has been widely used in the treatment of wounds since before 550 B.C. [3] For example, the Greek physician Dioscorides claimed that aloe vera gel could be used to heal skin infections, chapping and hemorrhoids. [4, 5] There are many legends about the powers of aloe vera, including that it was the secret of Cleopatra's beauty,[6] which may account for its use in a variety of health and beauty aids. Aloe vera has been widely used in India as a cathartic, stomachic and anthelminthic;[7, 8] in China as a common dermatological remedy;[9] and in Mexico to treat minor skin irritations.[6] It is also a common folk remedy in most of America and the West Indies.[10]

There are actually more than 300 species of Aloe plants; [11, 12] however, the species used primarily for medicinal purposes is now known as *A. vera* (L.) Burm.f.[1] Previously it was identified as *A. barbadensis* P. Miller or *A. vulgaris* Lam.[2, 3, 13] The aloe vera plant grows in a rosette from a base which reaches 8 cm or more in diameter at maturity. The leaves, which protrude from the base, are long and spear-like with thorny ridges. They can reach 0.5 m in length and 8 to 10 cm across at the base, tapering to a point.[6] The clear mucilaginous gel from the cells in the inner portion of the leaves (parenchyma) is the part of the plant used medicinally for skin abrasions and infections.[2, 3] This gel (often referred to simply as aloe gel) is distinct from the bitter, yellow juice found in the rind of the leaves (just beneath the epidermis), which is a potent laxative.[2] Aloe vera has been cultivated since the 1950s for this bitter yellow juice, which was an important source of drug aloes or 'aloin', known for its purgative effects.[14, 15] Its use as a laxative has been all but discontinued in North America; however, the plant continues to be cultivated for the gel, which is primarily used externally to treat a variety of skin conditions. Although these two products (aloes and aloe vera gel) are obtained from the leaves of the same plant, their chemistry, pharmacology and uses are very different and thus they will be described separately.

Aloes (or aloe) is the dried exudate ('latex' or 'juice') collected from freshly cut leaves. Aloes is often sold as a reddish-black or dark-brown solid mass, which tastes bitter and has a characteristic unpleasant odor. Originally this concentrated form was produced by boiling the 'latex' in a copper kettle until it reached the required consistency and then it was left to harden. Today, the liquid is more often vacuum-dried, which produces a powdered product.[16]

In contrast, the colorless aloe vera gel is collected from the center of the leaf. It is very sensitive to light and heat, and thus is removed from the leaf mechanically and preserved, buffered and stabilized immediately. This process may differ from manufacturer to manufacturer, which means that the quality of aloe vera gel is highly variable.[16]

Constituents[3, 4, 16-26]

Aloe Vera Gel

- Polysaccharides: celluolose, glucose, mannose, L-rhamnose, aldopentose, acemannan
- Enzymes: oxidase, amylase, catalase, lipase, alkaline phosphatase, glutathione peroxidase; cyclooxygenase
- Vitamins: B1, B2, B6, choline, folic acid, C, alpha-tocopherol, beta-carotene,
- Essential amino acids: lysine, threonine, valine, methionine, leucine, isoleucine, phenylalanine
- Inorganic: calcium, sodium, chlorine, manganese, magnesium, zinc, copper, chromium, potassium sorbate
- Aloinosides including barbaloin (aloins A and B) emodin, aloe-emodin (trace amounts only)

Aloes

- Aloinosides including barbaloin (aloins A and B), aloe-emodin, emodin, chrysophanol
- Chromone derivatives: aloeresin A, B, C

THERAPEUTIC USES & RELEVANT PHARMACOLOGY

Aloe Vera Gel

WOUND HEALING

Most of the medicinal use of aloe vera gel centers around claims that it increases wound healing. In North America, where it is a common household plant, many individuals apply the gel obtained by breaking the leaves to minor cuts, abrasions and burns. However, there is some controversy surrounding its effectiveness and mechanism of action. The first case report of the use of aloe vera for wound healing was published in 1935.[27] Fresh aloe vera gel provided rapid relief from the itching and burning of a woman's acute radiodermatitis (caused by a depilatory X-ray dose to her scalp 8 months earlier). Three similar cases have been reported in the literature.[28, 29] Studies of the effects of aloe vera on wound healing since the 1930s abound. For example, researchers using the fresh leaf demonstrated effective treatment of palmar eczema and puritus vulvae.[30] In addition, a controlled, unblinded study (n=12) found that finger abrasions treated with 50% fresh aloe vera gel in petroleum jelly healed faster than those treated with petroleum jelly alone.[31] Most of these early studies were not blinded or controlled and involved only very small numbers of participants.

Early studies also demonstrated that aloe vera gel was an effective treatment of thermal burns.[32, 33] This finding is supported by a recent study which found aloe cream to be more effective than fresh aloe vera gel in the treatment of first degree thermal burns, but that both dosage forms were equally effective in second degree thermal burns. Assessment of effectiveness in the treatment of third degree burns was not possible due to high rates of infection.[34]

However, not all the published studies are positive. Some studies have found that aloe vera gel actually hinders the healing process.[35] Several controlled (but unblinded) studies funded by the US army found no difference in experiments comparing the effects of aloe gel and no treatment on rates of wound healing (in rats and rabbits).[36] A similar study in humans (n=6) with second- and third-degree thermal burns also found no improvement with aloe vera treatment.[36] Unfortunately, these researchers did not use the fresh herb and they do not identify the commercial preparations used.

In addition, studies into the effects of aloe vera on the healing of full-thickness wounds have found either insignificant or negative results.[37, 38] The most well-known of these involved the treatment of 21 women with wound complications after cesarian delivery or laparotomy for gynecologic surgery. In this non-blinded study, wounds treated with standard management healed significantly faster than those treated with aloe vera.[38] In contrast, a recent controlled study assessing the effect of a commercial preparation of aloe vera on partial-thickness wounds showed a significant increase in healing.[39] It has been suggested that aloe vera should not be used to treat full-thickness wounds because it causes the dermal layer to fuse too quickly, inhibiting the wound from healing properly; however, its use in partial-thickness wounds continues to be supported by many authors.

Several mechanisms of action for the wound healing properties of aloe vera gel have been suggested. The first is that aloe vera is occlusive and may simply act as a protective barrier.[40, 41] Several early non-blinded and/or uncontrolled studies, which found that the application of aloe vera gel increased the healing rate of frostbite injuries, provide some support for this hypothesis (because no vehicle control was used).[42-44] In another example, guinea pig thermal wounds treated with aloe vera healed faster than those treated with silver sulfadiazine, but again, there was no vehicle control.[45] Other researchers have demonstrated increased capillary perfusion after the application of aloe vera topically and suggest that this may provide further insight into the mechanism of action of aloe vera.[46, 47]

Effects on the Immune System

The most recently suggested mechanism of action is that aloe vera gel may directly stimulate the immune system.[48] Most of these studies involve the oral ingestion or im/sc injection of acemannan, an active ingredient isolated from aloe vera gel. Acemannan has been shown to enhance phagocytosis in a dose-dependent fashion;[49] increase numbers of circulating monocytes and macrophages;[50, 51] permit monoctye driven signals to enhance T-cell response to lectin;[48] increase lymphocyte response to alloantigen; [48] enhance the release of cytokines, including interleukin-1, interleukin-6, interferon and tumor necrosis factor *in vitro*;[52-54] and activate macrophages.[54, 55] One study demonstrated that the immune response of chickens to Newcastle disease virus was increased by adding acemannan to a Newcastle vaccine. [56] A study of avian polyomavirus in birds with similar results has also been published.[57] Acemannan has also been shown to have anti-viral activity.[58, 59] Although most of these experiments have been *in vitro* studies, the concentrations of acemannan used appear to be achievable *in vivo*.[60]

Antibacterial Activity

In the early 1950s, it was suggested that aloe vera gel had an antibiotic action.[61] Early studies found that aloe vera gel inhibited *Myobacterium tuberculosis* and *Bacillus subtilis in vitro*.[62, 63] In addition, aloe vera juice was shown to be bacteriostatic to *Staphylococcus aureus, Streptococcus pyogenes,* and *Salmonella paratyphi*; however, the juice was also reported to be unstable.[64] More recent studies provide similar results. Different concentrations of aloe vera extracts have been found to be bactericidal to a variety of bacteria including: 1) *Streptococcus agalctiae, Enterobacter cloacae, Citrobacter species, Serratia marcescens, Klebsiella pneumoniae, Pseudomonas aeruginosa* (at a concentration of 60%); 2) *Staphylococcus aureus* (at a concentration of 70%); 3) *Escherichia coli* (at a concentration of 80%); and 4) *Streptococcus faecali,* a yeast — *Candida albicans* (at a concentration of 90%).[19, 65] Other studies have not found any antibacterial activity against *Staphylococcus aureus* or *Escherichia coli.*[66]

Anti-inflammatory Activity

Many studies have demonstrated the anti-inflammatory properties of aloe vera and other *Aloe* species.[19, 26, 67-74] For example, researchers have shown that aloe vera gel and hydrocortisone decrease inflammation in an additive, dose-related manner when they are used concurrently.[75] Another study found direct anti-inflammatory activity which could be attributed to known sterols isolated from aloe vera gel (e.g., lupeol, campesterol). In this study, aloe vera gel also appeared to block hydrocortisone's inhibitory effects on wound healing.[73] Another research team demonstrated that constituents of an aqueous gel-extract of aloe vera inhibited the release of reactive oxygen species by human PMNs, reducing the harmful effects of this release at the site of inflammation.[76]

Three primary mechanisms of action for the anti-inflammatory effects of aloe vera have been postulated: 1) anti-bradykinin activity has been found in some *Aloe* species (e.g., *A. arborescens, A. saponaria*);[26, 68] 2) emodin, aloe-emodin and aloin were shown to produce salicylates when metabolized, which appear to inhibit thromboxane production by competitive inhibition through stereochemical means;[19, 77] and 3) magnesium lactate, a constituent of aloe vera, is a known inhibitor of histidine decarboxylase and thus may prevent the formation of histamine in mast cells.[11, 19] The first hypothesis has been demonstrated in other *Aloe* species,[26, 68, 78] but there is little evidence of such action in studies with aloe vera. The second hypothesis has more support in the literature. A clinical case report in which a commercial preparation of aloe vera was applied to a monkey who was accidentally scalded provides some support because the amount of thromboxane A_2 produced by the monkey was decreased.[79] Other studies also provide support for this finding.[19, 43, 47, 77, 80] However, one researcher noted that many of the vehicles used in commercial aloe vera preparations (e.g., petrolatum, mineral oil, and aquaphor) are inhibitors of prostaglandin production themselves.[80] This emphasizes the need for well-designed (i.e., vehicle-controlled) studies of aloe vera.

It has been reported that decolorized (anthraquinone-free) aloe vera gel is a more potent inhibitor of inflammation than the colorized form.[81] One study in support of this hypothesis found that high concentrations of anthraquinones increased the production of prostaglandins, while trace amounts appeared to decrease the inflammatory response.[6] However, another study found that an aloe vera gel extract containing anthraquinone was more effective than an anthraquinone-free product.[82] In addition, one researcher demonstrated that anthraquinone is necessary for the absorption of aloe vera given orally.[70]

Protection Against Radiation

Investigation of the effectiveness of aloe vera gel in the treatment of radiation burns began in the late 1930s when radiation-induced burns or ulcers were a common model to test the ability of aloe vera to increase wound healing. Several early studies demonstrated an increased rate of healing.[33, 83-86] One of the best was a study with 20 albino rabbits in which 4 different treatments (fresh aloe vera gel, commercial aloe vera ointment, dry gauze bandage and nothing) were applied to the four quadrants of a wound caused by beta radiation. Visual assessment over a period of 58 days led to the findings that both aloe vera treatments resulted in statistically significant accelerated healing.[85] A more recent double-blind, placebo-controlled study in 194 women receiving breast or chest wall irradiation found no difference between the 98% pure aloe vera gel and a placebo.[87]

Use in Diabetes

Aloe vera has been used in diabetes for its enhancement of wound healing. Researchers have demonstrated in a controlled (unblinded) study of mice that aloe vera increases the rate of healing, provides pain relief, and decreases edema as compared to a saline control in both normal mice and those with streptozotocin-induced diabetes.[88]

MISCELLANEOUS

Anti-cancer

Acemannan, a compound isolated from aloe vera, has been reported to have anti-tumor activity.[89-91] For example, it has been used to in the treatment of fibrosarcomas in dogs and cats.[92] In addition, Roidex (a formulation of squalene, vitamin A, vitamin E and aloe vera) demonstrated more chemopreventive and curative properties than squalene alone in the prevention and treatment of mouse skin tumors.[93] Aloe juice has also been reported to have antimetastatic activity and to enhance the activity of 6-fluorouracil and cyclophosphamide.[94]

Anti-viral

Acemannan has also been reported to have anti-viral activity,[58, 59, 95, 96] and it has been suggested that it may play a role as an adjuvant treatment in HIV/AIDS[50, 58, 97, 98]

Psoriasis

A recent double-blind, placebo-controlled clinical study of 60 patients diagnosed with psoriasis vulgaris found that treatment with 0.5% aloe vera extract (without occlusion) was a significantly better treatment than placebo.[99]

Peptic Ulcer

Aloe vera gel has been taken internally for the treatment of peptic ulcers.[40] One group of authors claim several complete cures among 12 patients diagnosed with duodenal lesions (X-ray confirmation). However, no follow up studies appear to have been performed.[40]

Dental Conditions

Several studies report the effectiveness of aloe vera gel in increasing the rate of healing after dental procedures.[100, 101]

Veterinary Use

Effective use of aloe vera in animals has been reported for the treatment of ringworm, allergies, abscesses, fungal infections and different types of inflammation.[102] Although aloe vera as a 'panacea' in veterinary medicine has been questioned,[103] a detailed investigation of 2 cases using the commercial preparation (Dermaide Aloe®) to treat the severe accidental thermal burns of 2 dogs showed that aloe vera accelerated the rate of healing, decreased the production of prostaglandins and inhibited infection by *Pseudomonas aeruginosa*.[77] Its use was also reported to be beneficial in the treatment of a monkey who was accidentally scalded.[79]

FINAL NOTES

Variation in the quality of aloe vera has been documented and may account for some of the negative or inconclusive studies.[6, 104, 105] In addition, aloe vera has been reported to be biochemically unstable and may deteriorate in a short time period, [6, 106] which may also explain some of the conflicting study results.

More good-quality, clinical trials are needed to provide conclusive evidence of aloe vera's effectiveness in the management of skin conditions.

Aloes

LAXATIVE

The anthraquinone glycosides are responsible for the well-documented laxative effect of aloes.[16] They induce the intestinal secretion of water and electrolytes and modify intestinal motility. Laxative effects occur approximately 8 hours after the ingestion of aloes, which is metabolized by intestinal bacteria to form the active compound, aloe-emodin-9-anthrone.[107, 108] This substance has been shown to inhibit rat colonic Na+, K+-ATPase *in vitro*, and *in vivo* to increase the paracellular permeability of rat colonic mucosa.[109] Due to its strong purgative effect, aloes is not commonly recommended for use as a routine laxative (see adverse effects).

USE IN DIABETES

Aloes' use as a hypoglycemic agent has been demonstrated in 5 non-insulin dependent patients and in an animal model (mice) of diabetes.[110, 111] The mechanism of action for this effect has yet to be determined, although it is hypothesized that it may be mediated through stimulation of the synthesis and/or release of insulin from the beta-cells of the Islets of Langerhans.[111]

MISCELLANEOUS

Aloes has been used to flavor products used to discourage nail biting (it has a very bitter taste).[16] Several hydroxyanthracene derivatives have been shown to inhibit a variety of viruses *in vitro*, including herpes simplex (types 1 and 2), varicella-zoster, pseudo-rabies and influenza. It was not active against adenovirus or rhinovirus.[112]

ADVERSE EFFECTS

Aloe Vera Gel

Adverse effects associated with the external application of aloe vera gel have been very rarely reported in the literature. Contact dermatitis, possibly due to an allergic reaction, has been reported in several cases.[80, 113-116] There is one report of wide-spread dermatitis after the topical application of aloe vera gel to stasis dermatitis[117] and one report of an acute bullous allergic reaction.[118] One case of cathartic effects after topical application of aloe vera gel to the mucosal surface has also been reported.[80]

Aloes

Adverse effects are most common with chronic use, which tends to result in tolerance. In addition, chronic use may lead to a reversible pigmentation of the colonic mucosa. After aloes use is discontinued, the pigmentation disappears in 4 to 12 months. Urine may become orange (if pH is acidic) or reddish purple (if pH is alkaline). This is caused by the renal elimination of the hydroxyanthracene derivatives. Severe abdominal cramping is common.[119] Nephritis, gastritis, vomiting, bloody diarrhea with mucous, and watery diarrhea leading to osmotic imbalances have been reported.[16]

CAUTIONS/CONTRAINDICATIONS

Aloe Vera Gel

External: known allergies

Internal: trace anthraquinone glycosides may be of concern in pregnancy and lactation[119]

Aloes

Contraindicated in pregnancy, lactation and menstruation; appendicitis and abdominal pain of unknown origin; spasmodic obstipation. Not recommended for treatment of chronic constipation, in the presence of hemorrhoids or chronic renal disease.[16, 119]

DRUG INTERACTIONS

Aloe Vera Gel: none known

Aloes: Although no clinical examples appear to have been published, the anthraquinone glycosides have been known to induce hypokalemia which may interfere with the action of cardiac glycosides.

DOSAGE REGIMENS

Aloe Vera Gel

Externally: A minimum of 70% concentration of aloe vera is necessary for wound healing and anti-inflammatory effects.[120] Pure aloe vera gel is also available

Internally: no standard dosing

Antiviral: oral doses of 800 to 1600 mg of acemannan [50, 121]

Aloes

Laxative: 50-200 mg aloe (dried sap) three times daily

Hypoglycemic agent: 2.5 mL (1/2 tsp) of the dried sap (aloes) daily[110]

REFERENCES

1. Marles RJ, Associate Professor, Department of Botany, Brandon University, Brandon, Manitoba. Review of Medicinal Plant Modules for CCNM; 1997.
2. Tyler VE. *Herbs of Choice. The Therapeutic Use of Phytomedicinals.* Binghamton, NY: Pharmaceutical Products Press; 1994:209.
3. Shelton RW. Aloe vera, its chemical and therapeutic properties. *International Journal of Dermatology.* 1991;30(10):679-683.
4. Coats BC, Ahola R. *Aloe Vera the Silent Healer. A Modern Study of Aloe Vera.* Dallas: Bill C. Coats; 1979.
5. Gunther RT. *The Greek Herbal of Dioscorides.* Oxford: Oxford University Press; 1934.
6. Grindlay D, Reynolds T. The aloe vera leaf phenomena: A review of the properties and modern use of the leaf parenchyma gel. *Journal of Ethnopharmacology.* 1986;16:117-151.
7. Chopra RN, Nayar SL. *Glossary of Indian Medicinal Plants.* New Delhi: Council of Scientific and Industrial Research; 1956.
8. Dastur JF. *Aloe barbadensis* Mill. *Medicinal Plants of India and Pakistan.* Bombay: D.B. Taraporevala Sons and Co. Private Ltd.; 1962:16-17.
9. Cole HN, Chen KK. Aloe vera in oriental dermatology. *Archives of Dermatology and Syphilology.* 1943;47:250.
10. Morton JF. *Atlas of Medicinal plants of Middle America: Bahamas to Yucatan.* Springfield, Illinois: Charles C. Thomas; 1981.

11. Klein SD, Penneys NS. Aloe vera. *Journal of the American Academy of Dermatology*. 1988;18:714-719.
12. Harding TBC. Aloes of the world: A checklist, index and code. *Excelsa*. 1979;9:57-94.
13. Budavari SE. *An Encyclopedia of Chemicals, Drugs, and Biologicals.* Rahway, NJ: Merck and Co.; 1989.
14. Mapp RK, McCarthy TJ. The assessment of purgative principles in Aloes. *Planta Medica*. 1970;18:361-5.
15. Morton JF. Aloe. *Major Medicinal Plants — Botany, Culture and Uses.* Springfield, Illinois: Charles C. Thomas; 1977:46-50.
16. Canigueral S, Vila R. Aloe. *British Journal of Phytotherapy*. 1994;3(2):67-75.
17. Rowe TD, Parks LM. A phytochemical study of aloe vera leaf. *Journal of the American Pharmaceutical Association*. 1941;30:262-5.
18. Tyler VE, Brady LR, Roberts JE. *Pharmacognosy*. Philadelphia: Lea and Febiger; 1976:4-62
19. Robson MC, Heggers JP, Hagstrom WJ. Myth, magic, witchcraft or fact? Aloe vera revisited. *Journal of Burn Care and Rehabilitation*. 1982;3:157-62.
20. Bruce WGG. Medicinal properties in the Aloe. *Excelsa*. 1975;5:57-68.
21. Suga T, Hirata T. The efficacy of the Aloe plant chemical constituents and biological activities. *Cosmetics and Toiletries*. 1983;98:105-8.
22. Reynolds T. The compounds in Aloe leaf exudates: a Review. *Botanical Journal of the Linnean Society*. 1985;90:157-77.
23. Sabeh F, Wright T, Norton SJ. Purification and characterization of a glutathione peroxidase from the Aloe vera plant. *Enzyme Protein*. 1993;47:92-98.
24. Yamaguchi I, Mega N, Sanada H. Components of the gel of Aloe vera (L.) Burm. f. *Bioscience Biotechnology and Biochemistry.* 1993;57(8):1350-2.
25. Afzal M, Ali M, Hassan RAH, Sweedan N, Dhami MSI. Identification of some prostanoids in Aloe vera extracts. *Planta Medica*. 1991;57:38-40.
26. Fujita K, Shasike I, Teradaira R, *et al*. Properties of a carboxypeptidase from aloe. *Biochemical Pharmacology*. 1979;28:1261-2.
27. Collins CE, Collins C. Roentgen dermatitis treated with fresh whole leaf of aloe vera. *American Journal of Roentgenology*. 1935;33:396.
28. Wright CS. Aloe vera in treatment of roentgen ulcers and telangiectasis. *Journal of the American Medical Association*. 1936;106:1363-4.
29. Loveman AB. Leaf of aloe vera in treatment of roentgen ray ulcers. *Archives of Dermatology Syphilol*. 1937;36:838-43.
30. Crewe JE. The external use of aloes. *Minnesota Medicine*. 1937;20:670-3.
31. Barnes TC. The healing action of extracts of aloe vera leaf on abrasions of human skin. *American Journal of Botany*. 1947;34:597.
32. Crewe JE. Aloes in the treatment of burns and scalds. *Minnesota Medicine.* 1939;2:538-9.
33. Tchou MT. Aloe vera (jelly leeks). *Archives of Dermatology and Syphilol*. 1943;47:249.
34. Bunyapraphatsara N, Jirakulchaiwong S, Thirawarapan S, Manonukul J. The efficacy of Aloe vera cream in the treatment of first, second and third degree burns in mice. *Phytomedicine*. 1996;2(3):247-51.
35. Kaufman T, Kalderon N, Ullman Y, *et al.* Aloe vera gel hindered wound healing of experimental second-degree burns: A quantitative controlled study. *Journal of Burn Care and Rehabilitation*. 1988;9:156.
36. Ashley FL, O'Loughlin BJ, Peterson BJ, *et al.* The use of aloe vera in the treatment of thermal and irradiation burns in laboratory animals and humans. *Plastic and Reconstructive Surgery*. 1957;20:383-96.
37. Watcher MA, Wheeland RG. The role of topical agents in the healing of full-thickness wounds. *Journal of Dermatologic Surgery and Oncology.* 1989;15:1188-95.
38. Schmidt JM, Greenspoon JS. Aloe vera dermal wound gel is associated with a delay in healing. *Obstetrics and Gynecology*. 1991;78(1):115-117.
39. Fulton JE. The stimulation of post dermabrasion wound healing with stabilized aloe vera gel-polyethylene oxide dressing. *Journal of Dermatologic Surgery and Oncology*. 1990;16:460-7.
40. Blitz J, Smith JW, Gerard JR. Aloe vera gel in peptic ulcer therapy: Preliminary report. *Journal of the American Osteopathic Association.* 1963;63:731-5.
41. Ship AG. Is topical aloe vera plant mucus helpful in burn treatment? *Journal of the American Medical Association*. 1977;238:1770.
42. Sjostrom B, Weatherly-White RCA, Paton BC. Experimental studies in cold injury. *Journal of Surgical Research.* 1964;4:12-16.

43. Raine TJ, London MD, Golouch K, *et al.* Antiprostaglandins and antithromboxanes for treatment of frostbite. *Surgical Forum*. 1980;31:557-9.
44. McCauley RL, Hing DN, Robson MC, *et al*. Frostbite injuries: A rational approach based on pathophysiology. *Journal of Trauma*. 1983;23:143-7.
45. Rodriguez-Bigas M, Cruz NI, Suarez A. Comparative evaluation of aloe vera in the management of burn wounds in guinea pigs. *Plastic and Reconstructive Surgery*. 1988;81:386-9.
46. Zawacki BE. Reversal of capillary stasis and prevention of burns. *Annals of Surgery*. 1974;180:98-102.
47. El Zawahry M, Hegazy MR, Helal M. Use of aloe in treating leg ulcers and dermatoses. *International Journal of Dermatology*. 1973;12:68-73.
48. Womble D, Helderman JH. Enhancement of allo-responsiveness of human lymphocytes by acemannan (Carrisyn). *International Journal of Immunopharmacology*. 1988;10(8):967-974.
49. Shida T, Yogi A, Nishimura H, Nishioka I. Effect of aloe extract on peripheral phagocytosis in adult bronchial asthma. *Planta Medica*. 1985;51:273-275.
50. McDaniel HR, *et al.* An increase in circulating monocyte/macrophages (MM) is induced by oral acemannan (ACE-M) in HIV-1 patients. *American Journal of Clinical Pathology*. 1990;94:516-517.
51. Egger SF, Brown GS, Kelsey LS, *et al*, Talmadge JE. Studies on optimal dose and administration schedule of a hematopietic stimulatory b-(1,4)-linked mannan. *International Journal of Immunopharmacology*. 1996;18(2):113-26.
52. Marshall GD, Gibbons AS, Parnell LS. Human cytokines induces by acemannan. *Journal of Allergy and Clinical Immunology.* 1991;91:295.
53. Ramamoorthy L, Kemp MC, Tizard IR. Effects of acemannan on the production of cytokine in a macrophage cell line RAW264.7. *Joint Meeting of the European Tissue Repair Society and Wound Healing Society*. Amsterdam, The Netherlands; 1993.
54. Zhang L, Tizard IR. Activation of a mouse macrophage cell line by acemannan: The major carbohydrate fraction from Aloe vera gel. *Immunopharmacology*. 1996;35:119-28.
55. Karaca K, Sharma JM, Nordgren R. Nitric oxide production by chicken macrophages activated by acemannan, a complex carbohydrate extracted from Aloe vera. *International Journal of Immunopharmacology*. 1995;17(3):183-8.
56. Chinnah AD, Baig M, Tizard IR, Kemp MC. Antigen dependent adjuvant activity of a polydispersed B-(1-4)-linked acetylated mannan (acemannan). *Vaccine*. 1992;10:551-7.
57. Ritchie BW, Niagro FD, Latimer KS, *et al.* Antibody response and local reactions to adjuvant avian polyomavirus vaccines in psittacine birds. *Journal of the Association of Avian. Veterinarians* 1994;8:21-6.
58. Kahlon JB, Kemp, MC, Yawei N, *et al.* In vitro evaluation of the synergistic anti-viral effects of acemannan in combination with azidothymidine and acyclovir. *Molecular Biotherapy.* 1991;3:214-223.
59. Kahlon JB, Kemp MC, Carpenter RH, *et al*. Inhibition of AIDS virus replication by acemannan *in vitro*. *Molecular Biotherapy*. 1991;3:127-135.
60. Fogelman RW, Chapdelaine JM, Carpenter RH, McAnalley BH. Toxicologic evaluation of injectible acemannan in the mouse, rat, and dog. *Veterinary and Human Toxicology.* 1992;34:201-5.
61. Benigni R. Substances with antibiotic action contained in anthraquinonic drugs. *Chemical Abstracts.* 1950;44:11036.
62. Gottshall RY, Jennings JC, Weller LE, *et al*. Antibacterial substances in seed plants active against tubercle bacilli. *American Review of Tuberculosis*. 1950;62:475-80.
63. Bruce WG. Investigations of antibacterial activity in the aloe. *South African Medical Journal*. 1967;51:984.
64. Lorenzetti LJ, Salisbury R, Beal JL, *et al.* Bacteriostatic property of aloe vera. *Journal of Pharmaceutical Sciences.* 1964;53:1287.
65. Heggers JP, Pineless GR, Robson MC. Dermaide/Aloe vera gel comparison of the antimicrobial effects. *Journal of the American Medical Technologist*. 1979;41:293-4.
66. Fly LB, Kiem I. Test of Aloe vera for antibiotic activity. *Economic Botany*. 1963;17:46-9.
67. Hanley DC, Solomon WAB, Saffran B, *et al*. The evaluation of natural substances in the treatment of adjuvant arthritis. *Journal of the American Podiatric Medical Association.* 1982;72:275-84.
68. Fujita K, Teradaira R. Bradykininase activity of aloe extract. *Biochemical Pharmacology*. 1976;25:205.
69. Rubel BL. Possible mechanisms of the healing actions of Aloe gel. *Cosmetics and Toiletries*. 1983;98:109-14.
70. Davis RH, Leitner MG, Russo JM, *et al.* Antiinflammatory activity of aloe vera against a spectrum of irritants. *Journal of the American Podiatric Medical Association*. 1989;79:263-76.

71. Parish LC, Witkoski JA, Millikan LE. Aloe vera: its chemical and therapeutic properties. *International Journal of Dermatology*. 1991;30:679.
72. Davis RH, Leitner MG, Russo, *et al.* Wound healing: oral and topical activity of Aloe vera. *Journal of the American Podiatric Medical Association*. 1989;79:559.
73. Davis RH, DiDonato JJ, Johnson RWS, Stewart CB. Aloe vera, hydrocortisone, and sterol influence on wound tensile strength and anti-inflammation. *Journal of the American Podiatric Medical Association*. 1994;84(12):614-21.
74. Davis RH, Di Donato JJ, Hartman GM, Haas RC. Anti-inflammatory and wound healing activity of a growth substance in aloe vera. *Journal of the American Podiatric Medical Association*. 1994;84(2):77-81.
75. Davis RH, Parker WL, Murdoch DP. Aloe vera as a biological active vehicle for hydrocortisone acetate. *Journal of the American Podiatric Medical Association*. 1991;81:1.
76. Hart LA, Nibbering PH, van den Barselaar MT, *et al*. Effects of low molecular constituents from aloe vera gel on oxidative metabolism and cytotoxic and bactericidal activities of human neutraphils. *International Journal of Immunopharmacology*. 1990;12(4):427-34.
77. Cera LM, Heggers JP, Robson MC, Hagstrom WJ. The therapeutic efficacy of aloe vera cream (dermaide aloe) in thermal injuries:Two case reports. *Journal of the American Animal Hospital Association*. 1980;16:768-72.
78. Yagi A, Harada N, Yamada H, Iwadare S, Nishioka I. Antibradykinin active material in *Aloe saponaria*. *Journal of Pharmaceutical Sciences*. 1982;71:1172-4.
79. Cera LM, Heggers JP, Hagstrom WJ, *et al.* Therapeutic protocol for thermally injured animals and its successful use in an extensively burned rhesus monkey. *Journal of the American Animal Hospital Association*. 1982;18:633-8.
80. Penneys NS. Inhibition of arachidonic acid oxidation *in vitro* by vehicle components. *Acta Dermato Venereologica*. 1982;62:59-61.
81. Davis RH, Kabbani JM, Maro NP. Wound healing and antiinflammatory activity of aloe vera. *Proc Pa Acad Sci*. 1986;60:79.
82. Davis RH, Agnew PS, Shapiro E. Antiarthritic activity of anthaquinones found in aloe for podiatric medicine. *Journal of the American Podiatric Medical Association*. 1986;76:61-2.
83. Mandeville FB. Aloe vera in the treatment of radiation ulcers of mucous membranes. *Radiology*. 1939;32:598-9.
84. Rowe TD, Lovell BK, Parks LM. Further observations on the use of aloe vera leaf in the treatment of third degree x-ray reactions. *Journal of the American Pharmaceutical Association*. 1941;30:265-9.
85. Lushbaugh CC, Hale DB. Experimental acute radiodermatitis following beta irradiation: V. Histopathological study of the mode of action of therapy with Aloe vera. *Cancer*. 1953;6:690-7.
86. Rowe TD. Effect of fresh Aloe vera jell in the treatment of third-degree Roentgen reactions on white rats. *Journal of the American Pharmaceutical Association*. 1940;30:262-6.
87. Williams MS, Burk M, Loprinzi CL, *et al.* Phase III double-blind evaluation of an aloe vera gel as a prophylactic agent for radiation-induced skin toxicity. *International Journal of Radiation Oncology, Biology and Physiology*. 1996;36(2):345-9.
88. Davis RH, Leitner MG, Russo JM. Aloe vera, a natural approach for treating wounds, edema, and pain in diabetes. *Journal of the American Podiatric Medical Association*. 1988;78:60-68.
89. Peng SY, Norman J, Curtin G, *et al.* Decreased mortality of Norman murine sarcoma in mice treated with the immunomodulator, acemannan. *Molecular Biotherapy*. 1991;3(2):79-87.
90. Harris C, Pierce K, King G, *et al*. Efficacy of acemannan in treatment of canine and feline spontaneous neo plasms. *Molecular Biotherapy*. 1991;3(4):207-213.
91. King GK, Yates KM, Greenlee PG, *et al*. The effect of Acemannan immunostimulant, surgery and radiation on spontaneous canine and feline fibrosarcoma. *Journal of the American Animal Hospital Association*. 1995;31:439-47.
92. Manna S, McAnalley BH. Determination of the position of the O-acetyl group is a B-(1,4)-mannan (acemannan) from *Aloe barbadensis* Miller. *Carbohydrate Research*. 1993;241:317-9.
93. Desai KN. The preventive and therapeutic potential of the squalene-containing compound, Roidex, on tumor promotion and regression. *Cancer Letters*. 1996;101(1):93-6.
94. Gribel NV, Pashinskii VG. Protivometastaticheskie svoistva soka aloe. *Voprosy Onkologii*. 1986;32:38-40.
95. McDaniel HR, McNalley BH, White A. *In vitro* studies on acemannan (Carrisyn™) for antiviral effect. *ASCP/CAP*. 1987;69:(abstract).
96. McDaniel HR, Perkins S, McAnalley BH. A clinical pilot study using acemannan (Carrisyn™) in the treatment of acquired immunodeficiency syndrome (AIDS). *ASCP/CAP*. 1987;68:(abstract).
97. McDaniel HR, Rosenberg LJ, McAnalley BH. CD4 and CD8 lymphocyte levels in acemannan (ACM) -treated

HIV1 infected long-term survivors. *International Conference on AIDS*. 1993;9(1):498: abstract no. PO B29-2179.
98. McDaniel HR, *et al*. Extended survival and prognostic criteria for acemannan (ACE-M) treated HIV-1 patients. *Antiviral Research*. 1990;13 (Supp.1):117.
99. Syed TA, Ahmed SA, Holt AH, *et al*. Management of psoriasis with aloe vera extract in a hydrophillic cream: a placebo-controlled, double-blind study. *Tropical Medicine and International Health*. 1996;1(4):505-9.
100. Bovik EG. Aloe vera. Panacea or old wives' tale? *Texas Dental Journal*. 1966;84:13-6.
101. Payne JM. Tissue response to aloe vera gel following peridontal surgery. *Dentistry*: Baylor University; 1970.
102. Northway RB. Experimental use of Aloe vera extract in clinical practice. *Veterinary Medicine/Small Animal Clinician*. 1975;70:89.
103. Anderson BC. Aloe vera juice: A veterinary medicament? *The Compendium on Continuing Education for Practising Veterinarian*. 1983;5:S364-8.
104. Leung AY. Aloe vera in cosmetics. *Drugs and Cosmetic Industry*. 1977;120:34-5; 154-5.
105. Madis Laboratories. Aloe vera L. and its products, applications and nomenclature. *Cosmetics and Toiletries*. 1983;98:99-104.
106. Madis Laboratories. *Aloe Vera Gel. The Ageless Beauty Ingredient*. 9th ed. South Hackensack, NJ: Madis Laboratories Inc; 1984.
107. Hattori M, Kanda T, Shu YZ, Akao T, Kobashi K, Namba T. Aloe vera. *Chemical and Pharmaceutical Bulletin. (Toyko)*, 1988; 36: 4462-66.
108. Che QM, Akao T, Hattori M, Kobashi K, Namba T. Isolation of human intestinal bacterium capable of transforming barbaloin to aloe-emodin anthrone. *Planta Medica*. 1991;57:15-19.
109. Ishii Y, Tanizawa H, Takino Y. Studies on Aloe. III Mechanism of cathartic effect. *Chemical and Pharmaceutical Bulletin(Tokyo)*. 1990;38:197-200.
110. Ghannam N. The antidiabetic effect of aloes: Preliminary clinical and experimental observations. *Hormone Research*. 1986;24:288-294.
111. Ajabnoor MA. Effect of aloes on blood glucose levels in normal and alloxan diabetic mice. *Journal of Ethnopharmacology*. 1990;28:215-220.
112. Sydiskis RJ, Owen DG, Lohr JL, Rosler KH, Blomster RN. Inactivation of enveloped viruses by anthraquinones extracted from plants. *Antimicrobial Agents and Chemotherapy*. 1991;35:2463-6.
113. Shoji A. Contact dermatitis to Aloe arborescens *Chemical and Pharmaceutical Bulletin(Tokyo)*. 1988;36:4462-66. *Contact Dermatitis*. 1982;8:164-7.
114. Nakamura T, Kotajima S. Contact dermatitis from *aloe arborescens*. *Contact Dermatitis*. 1984;11:51.
115. Hunter D, Frumkin A. Adverse reactions to vitamin E and aloe vera preparations after dermabrasion and chemical peel. *Cutis*. 1991;47:193-96.
116. Dominguez-Soto L. Photodermatitis to aloe vera. *International Journal of Dermatology*. 1992;31:372.
117. Hogan DJ. Widespread dermatitis after topical treatment of chronic leg ulcers and stasis dermatitis. *Canadian Medical Association Journal*. 1988;138:336-8.
118. Morrow DM, Rappaport MJ, Strick RA. Hypersensitivity to aloe. *Archives of Dermatology*. 1980;116:1064-5.
119. Newall CA, Anderson LA, Phillipson JD. *Herbal Medicines. A Guide For Health Care Professionals.* London: The Pharmaceutical Press; 1996:296.
120. Gottlieb K. *Aloe Vera Heals: The Scientific Facts.* Denver, CO: Royal Publications; 1980.
121. Murray MT. *Natural Alternatives to Over-the-Counter and Prescription Drugs.* New York: William Morrow and Company, Inc; 1994:383.

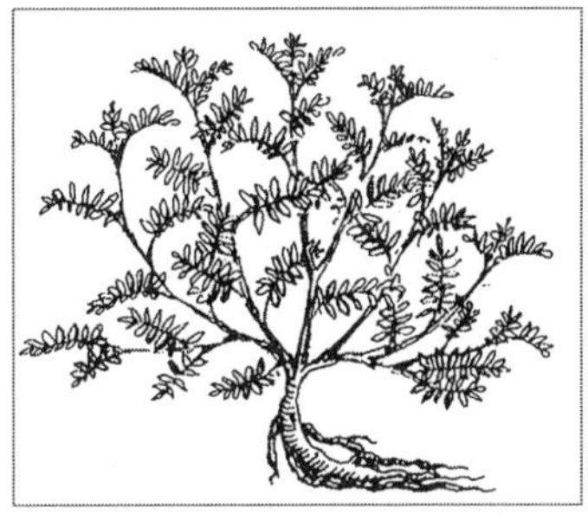

ASTRAGALUS

Astragalus membranaceus Moench

THUMBNAIL SKETCH

Active Constituents

- Astragalan
- Astragalosides

Common Uses

- Strengthening the body's resistance to disease
- Ailments due to stress including viral infections and fatigue
- Adjunctive therapy to chemotherapy and radiation treatment

Adverse Effects

- None known

Cautions/Contraindications:

- None known

Drug Interactions:

- None known

Doses:

- Adult dose: Dried root (or as tea): normally 9-15 g daily in divided doses
- Tincture (1:5): 2-6 mL three times daily
- Powdered solid extract (2:1): 250-500 mg three times daily

INTRODUCTION

Family: Fabaceae (also known as Leguminosae)

Synonyms: Milk-vetch root; Membranous vetch; Yellow vetch; Huang qi (Chinese)[1,2]

Astragalus has a long history of medicinal use in China, where it is one of the most widely used herbs in Fu-zheng therapy — the use of herbs to augment the host defense mechanisms.[2-5] The species of Astragalus which has been used for medicinal purposes, *Astragalus membranaceus* Moench (and its variety *mongholicus*), has been extensively studied in the Orient. In the Orient, the seeds of *Astragalus complanatus* R.Br. have also been used medicinally.[6]

Astragalus is a herbaceous perennial that grows up to 1m in height.[7] It is native to northern China and Tibet, growing both in the grassland and in the lightly forested areas which are well drained.[2,7] The part of the plant used medicinally is the root, which is harvested from 4-7 year old plants.[7]

Astragalus has long been a part of Traditional Chinese Medicine. In fact, it was included in the classic *Shen Nong Ben Cao Jing* which was written 2000 years ago.[2] It is thought to strengthen the body's 'vital energy' or qi and was often used in conditions of physical weakness and during chronic illness. It was believed to both strengthen and invigorate.[2] Astragalus is considered a sweet and warming tonic which is used to increase stamina, endurance and resistance to disease.[8] As a classic tonic it is considered superior to Asian ginseng in young adults.[8] It is interesting to note that many of the traditional uses coincide with the current indications for astragalus. For example, astragalus is currently used as an immune stimulant and thought to be helpful for the common cold.[8]

Constituents[7-11]

- Triterpene glycosides (saponins): astragalosides, acetylastragalosides, isoastragalosides, astramembrannins
- Polysaccharides: astragalans
- Flavonoids: kaempferol, quercetin, isorhamnetin, astragalin γ-aminobutyric acid
- Miscellaneous: free amino acids (including arginine, glutamic acid, canavanine, alanine), trace minerals (including zinc, manganese, magnesium), sterols

THERAPEUTIC USES & RELEVANT PHARMACOLOGY

EFFECTS ON THE IMMUNE SYSTEM

The immune effects of astragulus have been investigated in a multitude of *in vitro* and *in vivo* studies. Astragulus has been shown to: significantly increase the spontaneous incorporation of [3H]thymidine in mononuclear cells;[4] increase the proliferation of lymphocytes;[4,12] potentiate IL-2 production and activity;[13-15] activate T cell blastogenesis;[16] increase T cell cytotoxicity;[3,16] enhance the secretion of tumor necrosis factor (TNF);[9] potentiate the phagocytic function of the reticuloendothelial system (RES);[17] increase natural killer (NK) cells' cytoxicity;[16,18] and increase the activity of peritoneal macrophages.[17] Astragalus has also been shown to augment the interferon response of mice who are exposed to viruses.[19]

In addition, many studies have investigated the effects of astragalus when it is given in situations of immunosuppression.[5,12,15,16,20] For example, in a large clinical study, 572 cancer patients were given Fu-zheng therapy (which included astragalus) in combination with standard medical treatment for 2 months. The study results suggested that patients experienced protection of adrenal cortical function during radiation and chemotherapy treatment, and reduced bone marrow depression and gastrointestinal effects.[5] This is supported by a controlled study in which mice were given astragalus concurrently with mitomycin C. In this study, astragalus showed protective effects against immunosuppression in the mice. The authors of the study hypothesized that this resistance to immunosuppression may be correlated with the observed stimulation of the reticuloendothethial system (RES), activation of T cell blastogenesis and increased NK cell cytotoxicity.[16] In addition, a randomized, controlled, clinical trial of 115 patients with leukopenia who were treated with two concentrations of astragalus preparation (15 g twice daily (BID) vs. 5 g BID) for 8 weeks found that there was an obvious rise in the white blood cell counts (WBC) of both groups, but that the group with the larger dose had a significantly greater increase, suggesting a dose-dependent effect.[12] However not all studies were positive. In another controlled study an extract of astragalus in combination with the herb *Ligustrum lucidum* W.T. Aiton (Oleaceae) did not prevent cyclophosphamide-induced myelosuppression in mice.[20]

CARDIAC EFFECTS

A variety of trials have investigated the effect of astragalus in patients (or animal models) with Coxsackie B virus (CBV) myocarditis. One controlled clinical trial of patients (10 in the treatment group; 8 controls) with CBV myocarditis who were treated with Astragalus i.m. (8g/day) for 3-4 months or given conventional treatment only, found that the clinical condition of those treated with astragalus was improved in comparison to the control group.[18] Another study found that astragalus treatment increased the survival rate and decreased the percentage of abnormal action potential in mice infected with coxsackie B-3 virus when compared with controls.[21] In searching for the mechanism of action of these effects, researchers have found that astragalus: significantly enhanced the OKT3, OKT4 and OKT4/OKT8 ratio in patients with viral myocarditis;[22] and appeared to inhibit the replication of coxsackie B-3 virus RNA in the myocardial tissue of mice *in vivo*[23] and *in vitro*[24] and significantly inhibited the Ca^{2+} influx across the myocardial plasma membrane *in vitro.*[24] Several researchers have suggested that astragalus is a rational treatment choice for patients with viral myocarditis.[24]

In other studies of cardiac effects, components of astragalus have been shown to be effective as positive inotropes, which can improve the condition of patients with congestive heart failure. In one uncontrolled study, 19 patients were given i.v. astragaloside IV (an 'active' component of astragalus) for 2 weeks at which point their symptoms of chest distress, and dyspnea were relieved and their capacity for exercise was increased.[10] In another study, 22 patients with positive ventricular late potentials were treated with a 24 g iv drip of astragalus (control group were given lidocaine) for 2 weeks. The researchers reported that treatment with astragalus successfully shortened the duration of late potentials (significantly more than lidocaine).[25] Astragalus treatment has also been shown to be more effective than nifedipine (a calcium channel antagonist) in the treatment of 92 patients suffering from ischemic heart disease,[26] and also effective in increasing cardiac output in 20 patients with angina pectoris.[27] One team of researchers suggested that the cardiotonic action of astragalus may be partially due to its anti-oxygen free radical action. This was based on their study of 43 patients suffering from their first acute myocardial infarction.[28]

MISCELLANEOUS

Antiviral Effects

Several researchers have reported that astragalus has an antiviral effect.[29-32]

Anti-Cancer

An *in vitro* study showed that astragalus increased the secretion of both Tumor Necrosis Factor-α and Tumor Necrosis Factor -β.[9] A clinical study of 54 consecutive cases of small cell lung cancer treated with both standard medical treatment and Traditional Chinese Medicine (including astragalus) reported increased survival when compared to average survival statistics of conventional medical treatment alone.[33] This is supported by a controlled *in vivo* study of mice with renal cell carcinoma. The group receiving 500 mcg each of astragalus and *Ligustrum lucidum* intra-peritoneally daily for 10 days had a significantly higher cure rate than saline controls.[34] It has been hypothesized that the antitumor effects of astragalus are the result of an augmentation of phagocyte and LAK cell activities.[34, 35]

Prevention of Ototoxicity

A study in guinea pigs found that a mixture of astragalus and *Pyrola rotundifolia* L.(Pyrolaceae) significantly reduced the ototoxicity and nephrotoxicity of gentamicin.[36] The ototoxic effects of aminoglycoside antibiotics are thought to be related to a decrease of cAMP, and astragalus has been shown by other researchers to increase cAMP.

Miscellaneous

One study demonstrated that an aqueous solution of astragalus was able to significantly increase the motility to human sperm *in vitro.* The active constituents responsible for this effect are as yet unknown.[37]

ADVERSE EFFECTS

None known.

CAUTIONS/CONTRAINDICATIONS

Since astragalus has been reported to increase tumor necrosis factor, theoretically its use may be of concern in the management of HIV. Clarification of this potential effect is necessary.

DRUG INTERACTIONS

None known.

DOSAGE REGIMENS

- Adult dose: Dried root (or as tea): normally 9 to 15 g daily in divided doses; however, doses from 30 to 60 g daily are also seen occasionally.[2, 7, 38]

- Tincture (1:5): 2 to 6 mL three times daily[38]
- Powdered solid extract (2:1): 250 to 500 mg three times daily[38]

Astragalus is often seen in combination formulas with other similar herbs such as Chinese privet (*Ligustrum lucidum* Ait. Oleaceae), codonopsis (*Codonopsis pilosula* (Franch) Nannf., Campanulaceae) and Asian ginseng (*Panax ginseng* C.A. Meyer., Araliaceae).[2] It is also often mixed with Chinese licorice.[39]

REFERENCES

1. Scalzo R. Botanical materia medica for sinusitis. *The Protocol Journal of Botanical Medicine.* 1997;2(2):147-62.
2. Foster S, Chongxi Y. *Herbal Emissaries. Bringing Chinese Herbs to the West.* Rochester, VT: Healing Arts Press; 1992:356.
3. Zhao KS, Mancini C, Doria G. Enhancement of the immune response in mice by *Astragalus membranaceus* extracts. *Immunopharmacology.* 1990;20(3):225-233.
4. Sun Y, *et al.* Preliminary observations on the effects of the Chinese medicinal herbs Astragalus membranaceus and Ligustrum lucidum on lymphocyte blastogenic responses. *Journal of Biological Response Modifiers.* 1983;2:227-237.
5. Sun Y, Chang YH, Yu GQ, *et al.* Effect of Fu-zheng therapy in the management of malignant diseases. *Chinese Med. Journal.* 1981;61:97-101.
6. Marles RJ, Associate Professor, Department of Botany, Brandon University, Brandon, Manitoba. Review of Medicinal Plant Modules for CCNM. ; 1997.
7. Leung AY, Foster S. *Encyclopedia of Common Natural Ingredients Used in Food, Drugs, and Cosmetics.* 2nd ed. Toronto/New York: John Wiley and Sons Inc; 1996:649.
8. Chevallier A. *The Encyclopedia of Medicinal Plants*. London: Readers Digest; 1996:336.
9. Zhao KW, Kong HY. Effect of Astragalan on secretion of tumour necrosis factor in human peripheral blood mononuclear cells. *Chung-Kuo Chung Hsi i Chieh, Ho Tsa Chih*. 1993;13(5):263-5.
10. Luo HM, Dai RH, Li Y. Nuclear cardiology study on effective ingredients of *Astragalus membranaceus* in treating heart failure. *Chung-Kuo Chung Hsi i Chieh, Ho Tsa Chih.* 1995;15(12):709-9.
11. Hirotani M, Zhou Y, Rui H, Furuya T. Cycloartane triterpene glycosides from the hairy root cultures of *Astragalus membranaceus*. *Phytochemistry*. 1994;37(5):1403-7.
12. Weng XS. Treatment of leucopenia with pure astragalus preparation — an analysis of 115 leucopenic cases [Chinese]. *Chung-Kuo Chung Hsi i Chieh, Ho Tsa Chih*. 1995;15(8):462-4.
13. Chu DT, *et al.* Immunotherapy with Chinese medicinal herbs. II. Reversal of cyclophosphamide-induced immune suppression by administration of fractionated *Astragalus membranaceus in vivo*. *Journal of Clinical Laboratory Immunology*. 1988;25:125-129.
14. Chen YC. Experimental studies on the effects of danggui buxue decoction on IL-2 production of blood-deficient mice [Chinese]. *Chung-Kuo Chung Hsi i Chieh*. 1994;19(12):739-41, 763.
15. Liang H, Zhang Y, Geng B. The effect of astragalus polysaccharides (APS) on cell medicated immunity (CMI) in burned mice. *Chung-Hua Cheng Hsing Shao Shang Wai Ko Tsa Chih*. 1994;10(2):138-41.
16. Jin R, Wan LL, Mitsuishi T. Effects of shi-ka-ron and Chinese herbs in mice treated with anti-tumor agent mito mycin C [Chinese]. *Chung-Kuo Chung Hsi i Chieh, Ho Tsa Chih*. 1995;15(2):101-3.
17. Sugiura H, Nishida H, Indaba R, Iwata H. Effects of exercise in the growing stage in mice and of Astragalus membranaceus on immune functions [Japanese]. *Nippon Eiseigaku Zasshi* — Japanese Journal of Hygiene. 1993;47(6):1021-31.
18. Yang YZ, Jin PY, Guo Q, *et al.* Effect of *Astragalus membranaceus* on natural killer cell activity and induction of a- and g- interferon in patients with coxsackie B viral myocarditis. *Chinese Medical Journal.* 1990;103(4):304-307.
19. Hou YD, Ma GL, Wu SH, Li HT. Effect of radix Astrageli seu Hedysari on the interferon system. *Chinese Medical Journal.* 1981;94:35-40.
20. Khoo KS, Ang PT. Extract of *Astragalus membranaceus* and *Ligustrum lucidum* does not prevent cyclophosphamide-induced myelosuppression. *Singapore Medical Journal.* 1995;36(4):387-90.
21. Rui T, Yang Y, Zhou T, *et al*. Effect of *Astragalus membranaceus* on electrophysiological activities of acute experimental Coxsackie B-3 viral myocarditis in mice. *Chinese Medical Sciences Journal.* 1993;8(4):203-6.

22. Huang Z, Qin NP, Ye W. Effect of *Astragalus membranaceus* on T-lymphocyte subsets in patients with viral myocarditis [Chinese]. *Chung-Kuo Chung Hsi i Chieh, Ho Tsa Chih*. 1995;15(6):328-30.
23. Peng T, Yang Y, Riesemann H, Kandolf R. The inhibitory effect of *astragalus membranaceus* on coxsackie B-3 virus RNA replication. *Chinese Medical Sciences Journal*. 1995;10(3):146-50.
24. Guo Q, Peng TQ, Yang YZ. Effect of *Astragalus membranaceus* on Ca2+ influx and coxsackie virus B3 RNA replication in cultured neonatal rat heart cells [Chinese]. *Chung-Kuo Chung Hsi i Chieh, Ho Tsa Chih*. 1995;15(8):483-5.
25. Shi HM, Dai RH, Fan WH. Intervention of lidocaine and *Astragalus membranaceus* on ventricular late potentials [Chinese]. *Chung-Kuo Chung Hsi i Chieh, Ho Tsa Chih*. 1994;14(10):598-600.
26. Li SQ, Yuan RX, Gao H. Clinical observation of the treatment of ischemic heart disease with *Astragalus membranaceus* [Chinese]. *Chung-Kuo Chung Hsi i Chieh, Ho Tsa Chih*. 1995;15(2):77-80.
27. Lei ZY, Qin H, Liao JZ. Action of *Astragalus membranaceus* on left ventricular function of angina pectoris [Chinese]. *Chung-Kuo Chung Hsi i Chieh, Ho Tsa Chih*. 1994;14(4):199-202.
28. Chen LK, Liao JZ, Guo WQ. Effects of *Astragalus membranaceus* on left ventricular function and oxygen free radical in acute myocardial infarction patients and mechanism of its cardiotonic action [Chinese]. *Chung-Kuo Chung hsi i Chieh, Ho Tsa Chih*. 1995;15(3):141-3.
29. Yang YZ, Guo Q, Jin PY, *et al*. Effect of *Astragalus membranaceus* injecta on Coxsackie B-2 virus infected rat beating heart cell culture. *Chinese Medical Journal*. 1987;100:595.
30. Hou YD. Study on the biological active ingredients of *Astragalus membranaceus*. *Chung His i Chieh Ho Tsa Chih*. 1984;4:420.
31. Zhang XQ, *et al*. Studies of *Astragalus membranaceus* on antiinfluenza virus activity, interferon induction and immunostiluation in mice. *Chinese Journal of Microbiology and Immunology*. 1984;4:92.
32. Research Group of Common Cold and Bronchitis. Investigation into *Astragalus membranaceus*. II. A research on some of its mechanism of reinforcing the Qi (vital energy). *Journal of Traditional Chinese Medicine*. 1980;3:67.
33. Cha RJ, Zeng DW, Chang QS. Non-surgical treatment of small cell lung cancer with chemo-radio-immunotherapy and traditional Chinese medicine [Chinese]. *Chung-Hua Nei Ko Tsa Chih* — Chinese Journal of Internal Medicine. 1994;33(7):462-6.
34. Lau BH, Ruckle HC, Botolazzo T, Lui PD. Chinese medicinal herbs inhibit growth of murine renal cell carcinoma. *Cancer Biotherapy*. 1994;9(2):153-61.
35. Chu DT, Lin JR, Wong W. The *in vitro* potentiation of LAK cell cytotoxicity in cancer and AIDS patients indiced by F3 — a fractionated extract of *Astragalus membranaceus* [Chinese]. *Chung-Hua Chung Liu Tsa Chih* — Chinese Journal of Onocology. 1994;16(3):167-71.
36. Xuan W, Dong M, Dong M. Effects of compound injection of *Pyrola rotunifolia* L. and *Astragalus membranaceus* BGE on experimental guinea pigs' gentamicin ototoxicity. *Annals of Otology Rhinology and Laryngology*. 1996;194:374-80.
37. Hong C, Ku J, *et al*. *Astragalus membranaceus* stimulates human sperm motility *in vitro*. *American Journal of Chinese Medicine*. 1992;20:289-94.
38. Murray MT. *The Healing Power of Herbs*. Rocklin, CA: Prima Publishing; 1992:246.
39. Teegarden R. *Chinese Tonic Herbs*. New York: Japan Publishing Inc; 1985:197.

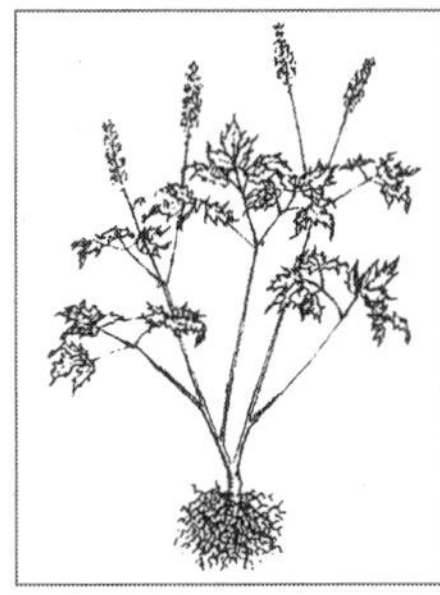

BLACK COHOSH

Cimicifuga racemosa (L.) Nutt.

THUMBNAIL SKETCH

Active Constituents

- Terpenoids
- Formononetin

Common Uses

- Symptoms of menopause (hot flashes, anxiety, depression)
- Premenstrual syndrome and dysmenorrhea
- Uterine spasm

Adverse Effects

- Rare, limited to gastric upset.
- Historical evidence suggests throbbing headaches, nervous and cardiovascular depression can occur at high doses.

Cautions/Contraindications

- Pregnancy and lactation

Drug Interactions

- None known

Doses

- 0.3-2g of dried herb in decoction three times daily
- 40mg of herb contained in 40-60% alcoholic liquid daily

INTRODUCTION

Family: Ranunculaceae

Synonyms: Bugbane, Rattleroot, Rattletop, Richweed, Rattlesnakeroot, Rattleweed, Bugwort, Macrotys, Squaw root, Papoose root, Christopher weed, Cimicifuga, *Actaea racemosa* L., *Macrotys actaeoides*[1-3]

Black cohosh is an upright perennial, native to the temperate climates of the Northern Hemisphere, including North America where it is found from Maine to Ontario and south to Georgia and Missouri.[4] It grows up to 2 meters high, producing numerous small white flowers on a wand-like raceme. The plant grows from a thick fibrous root stock, which is the part used medicinally.[5]

Black cohosh has long been used for its medicinal properties, especially by peoples of the First Nations. The Cherokee and the Iroquois used a tea made from the root to alleviate rheumatic pains, promote lactation and promote menses. Its use was commonly accepted into the eclectic medical movement in the early to mid 19th century where it was prized as an antispasmodic, analgesic and gynecological agent.[1] Its name comes from the latin *cimex* meaning bug and *fuga* meaning to repel, referring to the fact that it appears to act as an effective insect repellent.[4] Even though black cohosh is especially popular in Germany for its medicinal properties, all commercial stocks come from the United States and Canada.[2]

Constituents [6-12]

- Triterpenoids: a complex mixture including actein, cimigoside, 12-acetylactein, cimifugoside, 27-deoxyacetylacteol.
- Flavonoids: formononetin
- Acids: isoferulic, salicylic, acetic, butyric, palmitic.
- Miscellaneous: phytosterols, hydrolysable tannins, cimicifugin, resinous material referred to as acteina.

THERAPEUTIC USES & RELEVANT PHARMACOLOGY

ENDOCRINE

It has long been known that *Cimicifuga racemosa* contained agents that possess 'hormone-like' characteristics. Using ovariectomized rats, Jarry *et al.* demonstrated that the administration of an extract of *Cimifuga racemosa* caused a selective reduction in serum concentrations of luteinizing hormone (LH).[6, 7] They also noted that three 'endocrine active' agents could be identified in a methanolic extract of this plant. One of these three constituents was identified as formononetin. While formononetin was seen to bind with estrogen receptors, it failed to reduce LH levels, leading to the conclusion that other agents present in the methanolic extract were responsible for this action.[7] Duker *et al.* demonstrated similar findings during a placebo controlled trial in humans. A group of menopausal women (n=110, mean age 52) were divided into equal groups, one received a placebo and the other 8mg (4mg twice daily) of a commercially available dried hydroalcoholic extract, Remifemin®. After 8 weeks, a selective and significant decrease was seen in LH levels but not follicle stimulating hormone (FSH) levels. In an attempt to determine the 'active constituents' a lipophilic extract was prepared and subjected to sephadex chromatography. It was discovered that there were in fact three groups of active components:

Group 1	Non-estrogen ligands which decreased LH secretion on chronic administration
Group 2	Estrogen ligands which also suppressed LH release
Group 3	Constituents which showed an affinity for estrogen receptors but failed to decrease LH release

The authors hypothesized that the agents in group 1 could be exerting their effects on LH release by acting at a central site (similar to clonidine). They also suggested that the agents in group 3 failed to exert an action on LH levels because they may be rapidly metabolized. The authors also go on to suggest that since pulsatile LH secretion is associated with the presentation of many of the unpleasant consequences of menopause, this may explain the therapeutic action of *Cimicifuga racemosa*.[13]

The vast majority of clinical investigations regarding this plant's medicinal action have been carried out in Europe, notably Germany. In a randomized study conducted over 6 months with women (n=60, age < 40yrs) who had ovarian insufficiency following hysterectomy but with at least one functioning ovary, investigators compared the effectiveness of a commercial product of *Cimicifuga racemosa* (Remifemin®) and conventional hormone based therapies. At a dose of 2 tablets twice daily, Remifemin® was shown to decrease menopausal symptoms (measured using Kupperman Menopausal Index) comparable to the three conventional therapy groups (estriol 1mg daily; conjugated estrogen 1.25mg; combined estrogen/gestagen therapy).[14] In addition, Warnecke demonstrated that Remifemin® (40 drops twice daily) given over 12 weeks showed estrogen-like stimulation of the vaginal mucosa similar to conjugated estrogens (0.625mg daily) and an improvement in neurovegatitive symptoms comparable to diazepam 2mg daily.[15] Another randomized placebo controlled double-blind study conducted over 12 weeks on women (n=80) suffering from the unpleasant consequences of menopause also noted positive results. Remifemin® (2 tabs twice daily) was shown to increase proliferation of vaginal epithelium and decrease physical and mental symptoms (Kuppermann menopausal index and Hamilton Anxiety Index) in a fashion superior to both placebo and conjugated estrogen.[16] Similar results have been noted in other clinical studies of Remifemin® including: effectiveness in cases where conventional therapy is contraindicated[17], refused[18] and in a protocol removing conventional treatment.[19]

In a review article, Beuscher comments on a study using a combination product containing both black cohosh and an extract of St John's Wort (*Hypericum perforatum* L., Clusiaceae). In this multi-center trial conducted over 12 weeks on women (n=812) suffering from psychovegetative symptoms of menopause (including irritability, poor concentration, fear, insomnia, depression), 90% of patients noted an improvement.[2] It should be noted that standardized extracts of St. John's Wort have now been shown to be effective in the management of mild-moderate depression when given as a single agent.[20, 21]

It should also be noted that the vast majority of the clinical trials described above have been carried out with one specific proprietary product. Remifemin® tablets are standardized to 27-deoxyactein content (1mg/unit dose).

Commission E, a German regulatory agency, considers black cohosh useful in the management of premenstrual syndrome, dysmenorrhoea and nervous conditions associated with menopause.[22]

A recent Danish study conducted on immature rats and ovariectomized rats failed to demonstrate any 'traditional' estrogenic effect.[23]

MISCELLANEOUS

Cardiovascular

The administration of the resinous material, acteina, has been shown to exert a hypotensive action in various animal models and cause peripheral vasodilation and increased blood flow in humans.[24] Triterpene compounds extracted from a plant described as "Japanese Cimicifuga" showed hypocholesterolemic activity *in vivo*.[25]

Antimicrobial

Extracts of a related species, *Cimicifuga dahurica* (Turcz. Ex Fisch. & C.A. Meyer) Maxim, have been shown to possess antimicrobial activity towards both gram+ and gram– bacteria *in vitro*.[26]

ADVERSE EFFECTS

Adverse effects appear rare, usually being limited to occasional stomach pains.[22] The consumption of large doses (amounts not specified) were noted by early eclectic physicians to cause: severe 'bursting' frontal headaches, sensory and circulatory depression.[1]

Given the lack of long-term toxicity studies, treatment should be limited to 6 months.[22]

CAUTIONS/CONTRAINDICATIONS

Cimicifuga racemosa should be avoided in pregnancy and lactation. [12, 27]

DRUG INTERACTIONS

No cases of drug interactions could be found for this plant.[22]

DOSAGE REGIMENS

- Dried root: 40-200 mg taken by decoction or as a solid dose daily[27]
- Alcoholic extract equivalent to 40mg of herb (40 to 60% alcohol) daily[22]
- 0.4-2mL daily of tincture of the root daily (1:10, 60% ethanol)[27]

It should be noted that in the case of menopause treatment, the onset of action of this plant can take up to 2 weeks to occur.

REFERENCES

1. Brinker F. A comparative review of eclectic female regulators. *British Journal of Phytotherapy*.1997;4(3):123-142.
2. Beuscher N. *Cimicifuga racemosa* L.-Black Cohosh. *Zeitschrift fur Phytotherapie.* 1995;16:301-310. (English translation in *Quarterly Review of Natural Medicine*).
3. Chevallier A. *The Encyclopedia of Medicinal Plants*. London: Reader's Digest; 1996:336.

4. Marie Snow J. *Cimicifuga racemosa* (L) Nutt. (Ranunculaceae). *The Protocol Journal of Botanical Medicine*. 1996;1(4):17-19.
5. Leung A, Foster S. *Encyclopedia of Common Natural Ingredient Used in Food, Drugs and Cosmetics*. 2nd ed. New York, NY: John Wiley and Sons; 1996:649.
6. Jarry H, Harnischfeger G. Untersuchungen zur endokrinen wirksamkeit von inhaltsstoffen aus *Cimicifuga racemosa*. Einfluss auf die serumspiegel von hypophysenhormonen ovariektomieter ratten. *Planta Medica*. 1985;51:46-49.
7. Jarry H, Harnischfeger G, Duker E. Untersuchungen zur endokrinen wirksamkeit von inhaltsstoffen aus *Cimicifuga racemosa*. In vitro-bindung von inhaltsstoffen an ostrogenrezeptoren ratten. *Planta Medica*. 1985;51:316-319.
8. Linde H. Die inhaltsstoffe von *Cimicifuga racemosa*. Mitt: zur struktur des acteins. *Archiv der Pharmazie*. 1967;300:885-892.
9. Linde H. Die inhaltsstoffe von *Cimifuga racemosa*. Mitt: uber die konstitution der ringe A,B, und C des acteins. *Archiv der Pharmazie*. 1967;300:982-992.
10. Linde H. Die inhaltsstoffe von *Cimicifuga racemosa*. Mitt: actein: der ring D und seitenkette. *Archiv der Pharmazie*.1968;301:120-138.
11. Linde H. Die inhaltsstoffe von Cimicifuga racemosa. Mitt: 27-desoxyacetylacteol. *Archiv der Pharmazie*. 1968;301:335-341.
12. Newall C, Anderson L, David Phillipson J. *Herbal Medicines: A Guide for Health Care Professionals*. London: The Pharmaceutical Press; 1996:296.
13. Duker E-M, Kopanski L, Jarry H, Wuttke W. Effects of Extracts from *Cimicifuga racemosa* on Gonadotropin Release in Menopausal Women and Ovariectomized Rats. *Plant Medica*. 1991;57:420-424.
14. Lehmann-Willenbrock E, Riedel H. Klinische und endokrinologische untersuchungen zur therapie ovarieller aus fallserscheinungen nach hysterekomie unter belassung der adnexe. *Zentralblatt fur Gynakologie*. 1988;110:611-618.
15. Warnecke G. Beeinflussung klimakterisch Beschwerden durch ein Phytotherapeutikum. *Die Medizinische Welt*. 1985;36:871-874.
16. Stoll W. Phytotherapeutikum beeinflust atrophisches Vaginalepithel. *Therapeutikon*. 1987;1:23-31.
17. Daiber W. Menopause symptoms: Success without hormones. *Arztliche Praxis*. 1983;35:1946-47.
18. Vorberg G. Treatment of menopause symptoms. *Zeitschrift Fuer Alternsforshung*. 1984;60:626-29.
19. Petho A. Menopause symptoms: is it possible to switch from hormone treatment to a botanical gynecologicum? *Arztliche Praxis*. 1987;47:1551-53.
20. Linde K, Ramirez G, Mulrow C, *et al*. St John's Wort for depression — an overview and meta-analysis of randomized clinical trials. *British Medical Journal*. 1996;313:253-258.
21. Ernst E. St John's Wort, an anti-depressant? A systematic, criteria-based review. *Phytomedicine*. 1995;2(1):67-71.
22. Blumenthal M, Brusse WR, Goldberg A, *et al*. *The Complete Commission E Monographs*. Austin, TX: American Botanical Council; 1998: 685.
23. Einer-Jensen N, Zhao J, Andersen K, Kristoffersen K. *Cimicifuga* and *Melbrosia* lack estrogenic effects in mice and rats. *Maturitas*. 1996;25(2):149-53.
24. Genazzani E, Sorrentino L. Vascular action of acteina: active constituents of *Actea racemosa* L. *Nature*. 1962;194:544-5.
25. Resing K, Fitzgerald A. Crystal data for 15-o-acetylacerinol and two related triterpenes isolated from Japanese *Cimicifuga* plants. *J.Appl.Cryst*. 1978;11:58.
26. Moskalenko S. Preliminary screening of Far-Eastern ethnomedicinal plants for antibacterial activity. *Journal of Ethnopharmacology*. 1986;15:231-59.
27. Bradley P. *British Herbal Compendium*. Bournemouth: BHMA; 1992:239.

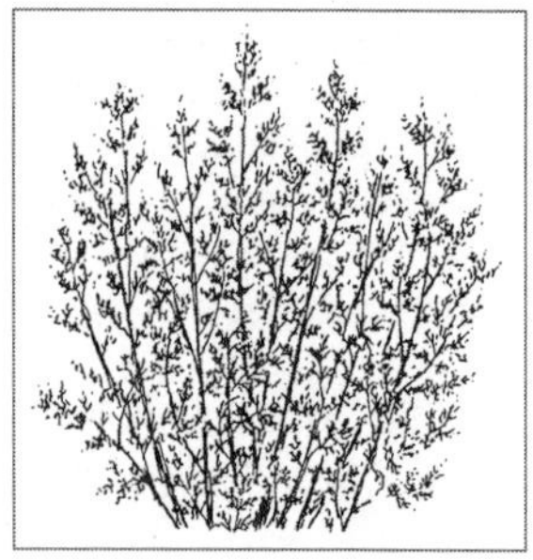

BURDOCK

Arctium lappa L.

THUMBNAIL SKETCH

Active Constituents
- Inulin
- Polyacetylenes
- Volatile oil
- Arctiopicrin

Common Uses
- *Internal:* skin conditions and rheumatic conditions resulting from 'toxins'
- *External:* eczema and skin ulcers

Adverse Effects
- Temporary worsening of symptoms

Cautions/Contraindications
- Pregnancy, diabetes

Drug Interactions
- Possible interaction with oral hypoglycemic agents

Doses
- 2-6g dried root three times daily
- 8-12mL of tincture (1:10 in 45% alcohol) three times daily
- 2-6mL of liquid extract (1:1 in 25% alcohol) three times daily

INTRODUCTION

Family: Asteraceae (also known as Compositae)

Synonyms: Great burdock, Bardane, Begger's buttons, Thorny burr, Bardana, Gobo, Lappa, Edible burdock[1-3]

Burdock is a biennial or perennial plant, native to both Asia and Europe, and naturalized across North America.[4] While the root is the primary part used therapeutically, the leaves and seeds are also said to have medicinal properties. The roots are more favored in the Western herbal tradition, but the seeds are often used in traditional Asian medicine.[2] Within Western herbalism, burdock is considered an important alterative herb (an agent capable of favorably altering unhealthy conditions of the body and tending to restore normal function). It was used to 'cleanse' the blood, removing toxins from the body. Consequently, it was used for many conditions of the skin and situations of chronic inflammation.[2]

Constituents

Root[2-7]

- Carbohydrates: inulin (up to 50%), mucilage, and pectin
- Polyacetylenes, notably sulfur containing thiophenes
- Volatile acids: including acetic acid, propionic acid, butyric acids, and isovaleric acids.
- Polyphenolic acids: caffeic acid, chlorogenic acid
- Aldehydes: including acetaldhyde, benzaldehyde, and valeraldehyde
- Miscellaneous: arctiopicrin (sesquiterpene lactone), tannin, 'bitters' (lappatin), quercetin (flavonoid), kaempferol (flavonoid).

Leaves[3, 4, 7]

- Terpenoids including arctiopicrin, sterols and triterpenols
- Miscellaneous: mucilage, essential oil, tannins, inulin

Seeds[2, 3]

- Flavonoids, essential oil, fixed oils

THERAPEUTIC USES & RELEVANT PHARMACOLOGY

COMMON USES

Burdock root is reputed to be alterative,[1-3, 8] diaphoretic,[3, 8, 9] diuretic,[1-3, 8, 9] antimicrobial,[1, 3, 8] antipyretic,[3] anti-tumor,[3] and a mild laxative.[2] Oral consumption is considered useful in the management of many conditions including chronic skin diseases,[2, 3, 8] rheumatic conditions,[1-3, 8] and infections.[2, 3, 8] Externally, it is used in the treatment of skin conditions such as eczema and skin ulcers.[3]

Anti-bacterial Effects

Extracts of the leaves, flowers and roots have all been shown to possess antibacterial activity. The leaves are reported to be active against both gram negative and positive bacteria, while the flowers and roots are active only against gram negative bacteria.[10] In addition, arctiopicrin has been shown to have an antimicrobial action against gram negative bacteria.[6, 11] The clinical relevance of this antimicrobial action is questionable since the constituents thought to be responsible for this action are not normally found in the dried commercial herb.[5]

Miscellaneous

Bever *et al.* demonstrated that extracts of *Arctium lappa* root could produce a "pronounced and long lasting decrease in blood sugar" when administered to rats. It also improved carbohydrate tolerance with negligible toxicity. The constituent(s) responsible for this action is/are unknown.[6]

Dietary fiber extracted from the traditional Japanese food "gobo" (burdock root) and added to the basal diet of rats (5%) was shown to protect against the toxic effects of various food colorings (erthrosine, tartrazine, indigo carmine, new coccine, and brilliant blue).[12]

A desmutagenic factor has been isolated from burdock juice.[13] Other investigators have also noted this antimutagenic potential.[3, 5]

ADVERSE EFFECTS

A well-publicized instance of poisoning in a 26-year-old woman has been reported. She consumed 'burdock tea' purchased in local health-food store and presented to the emergency room suffering from symptoms characteristic of atropine poisoning (i.e., blurred vision, inability to void, rapid pulse, dry mouth and 'bizarre' behavior). Since tropane alkaloids (like atropine) are not normally found in burdock root, the product was analyzed and was found to contain an atropine concentration of 300mg/g. It was assumed that the plant had been adulterated with a member of the Nightshade family, probably deadly nightshade (*Atropa belladonna* L. Solanaceae).[5, 14, 15] Unfortunately, this appears not to be an isolated example, with other instances of probable atropine adulteration being noted.[16, 17] This is often cited as a example of the poor quality control surrounding herbal medicines and the need for stricter guidelines.[3, 5]

Three cases of contact irritation (1 adolescent and 2 adults) have been noted following the application of medicinal plasters containing burdock root.[18] There is no clinical evidence to suggest that the preparation made from the leaves will cause a similar problem.[3] However, some sesquiterpene lactones are known to be allergenic and some polyacetylenes and thiophenes are known to be photosensitizers. Thus there is a potential for skin irritation with plant parts containing these compounds, especially in the case of presensitized individuals or with inappropriate use (e.g., too concentrated, too long, too frequent exposure or sun exposure soon after use).[19]

While little information is available, concerns have been raised regarding burdock's pronounced 'detoxifying' action. It has been noted that by treating these 'toxic' states, the symptoms of the conditions being treated may worsen temporarily causing undue distress to the patient.[2]

Burdock root has been shown to possess no carcinogenic potential in mice even when given for a prolonged time at a high dose.[20]

CAUTIONS/CONTRAINDICATIONS

Given the hypoglycemic nature shown in animal studies,[6] caution should be used in cases of diabetes.[5]

An extensive review article suggested that burdock possesses uterine stimulant properties,[21] and thus it should be contraindicated during pregnancy and lactation.[3, 5]

DRUG INTERACTIONS

While no instance of a drug interaction could be found, given this plant's influence on blood sugar levels concerns have been raised over concomitant use with oral hypoglycemic agents.[5]

DOSAGE REGIMENS [3, 5, 7]

Internal

- 2-6g of dried root, or decoction, three times daily
- 2-6mL of liquid extract (1:1 in 25% alcohol) three times daily
- 8-12mL of tincture (1:10 in 45% alcohol) three times daily
- Decoction of 1 part in 20, 500mL per day

External

- An infusion or tincture (1:5, 25% alcohol) of the leaf can be used externally as a poultice.

REFERENCES

1. Wren R. *Potter's New Encyclopedia of Botanical Drugs and Preparations.* Saffron Walden: C.W. Daniel Company; 1988:362.
2. Mills S. *The Essential Book of Herbal Medicine.* 2nd ed. London: Penguin; 1991:677.
3. Chandler F, Osborne F. Burdock. *Canadian Pharmaceutical Journal*. 1997;130(5):46-49.
4. Leung A, Foster S. *Encyclopedia of Common Natural Ingredient Used in Food, Drugs and Cosmetics*. 2nd ed. New York, NY: John Wiley and Sons; 1996:649.
5. Newall C, Anderson L, David Phillipson J. *Herbal Medicines: A Guide for Health Care Professionals.* London: The Pharmaceutical Press; 1996:296.
6. Bever B, Zahnd G. Plants with oral hypoglyceamic action. *Quarterly Journal of Crude Drug Research*. 1979;17:139-196.
7. Bradley P. British *Herbal Compendium.* Bournemouth: BHMA; 1992:239.
8. Chevallier A. *The Encyclopedia of Medicinal Plants.* London: Reader's Digest; 1996:336.
9. Weiss R. *Herbal Medicine.* Beaconsfield: Beaconsfield Publishers;1988:362.
10. Moskalenko S. Preliminary screening of Far-Eastern ethnomedicinal plants for antibacterial activity. *Journal of Ethnopharmacology*. 1986;15:231-59.
11. Cappalletti E, Trevisan R, Caniato R. External antirheumatic and antineuralgic herbal remedies in the traditional medicine of North-eastern Italy. *Journal of Ethnopharmacology*. 1982;6:161-190.
12. Tsujita J, Takeda H, Ebihara K, Kiriyama S. Comparison of protective activity of dietary fiber against the toxicities of various food colours in rats. *Nutrition Reports International*. 1979;20:635-642.
13. Morita K, Kada T, Namiki M. Desmutagenic factor isolated from burdock (*Arctium Lappa* L.). *Mutation Research*. 1986;129:25-31.
14. Bryson P, Watanabe A, Rumack B, Murphy R. Burdock root tea poisoning. *Journal of the American Medical Association*. 1978;239(20):2157.
15. Bryson P. Burdock root tea poisoning. *Journal of the American Medical Association*. 1978;240:1586.
16. Tyler V. *The Honest Herbal.* 3rd ed. Binghamton, NY: Pharmaceutical Products Press; 1993:375.
17. Rhoads P, Tong T, Banner W, Anderson R. Anticholinergic poisonings associated with commercial burdock root tea. *Journal of Toxicology-Clinical Toxicology*. 1985;22(6):581-584.
18. Rodriguez P, Blanco S, Juste S, *et al*. Allergic contact dermatitis due to burdock (*Arctium Lappa*). *Contact Dermatitis*. 1995;33:134-135.
19. Marles RJ, Associate Professor, Department of Botany, Brandon University, Brandon, Manitoba. Review of

Medicinal Plant Modules for CCNM; 1997.
20. Hirono I, Mori H, Kato K, Ushimaru Y. Safety examination of some edible plants. Part 2. *Journal of Environmental Pathology Toxicology and Oncology*. 1977;1:72-74.
21. Farnsworth N, Bingel A, Cordell G, *et al*. Potential value of plants as sources of new antifertility agents I. *Journal of Pharmaceutical Sciences*. 1975;64(4):535-98.

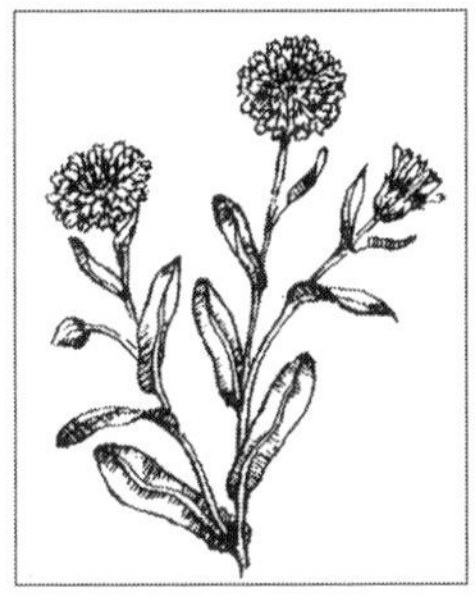

CALENDULA

Calendula officinalis L.

THUMBNAIL SKETCH

Active Constituents
- Flavonoids
- Volatile oil
- Terpenoids

Common Uses
- *External*: Skin abrasions, minor burns and to promote wound healing
- *Internal*: Minor digestive irritation.

Adverse Effects
- None

Cautions/Contraindications
- Caution in pregnancy

Drug Interactions
- None noted

Doses
- *Internal*
  - 1-4g of dried florets three times daily
  - 0.5-1mL of liquid extract (1:1 in 40% alcohol) three times daily
  - 0.3-1.2mL of tincture (1:5; 90% alcohol) three times daily
- *External*
  - See monograph for details

INTRODUCTION

Family: Asteraceae (also known as Compositae)

Synonyms: Gold-bloom, Marigold, Marybud, Pot marigold, Holigold, Mary bud[1-5]

Calendula is a hairy annual which stands 30-60cm high and is easily recognizable by its brilliant orange single flowers.[4, 6] While native to Egypt, the Middle East and Mediterranean Europe, it can now be found throughout the world[1, 6] because the attractive flowers are highly prized by horticulturists and landscapers and often form the center piece in ornamental gardens.[6] Since the flowers are edible, it is also often found in culinary gardens.[1] It is important to note that this plant is distinct from members of the *Tagetes* genus which are also commonly referred to as Marigolds.[4]

Calendula has enjoyed a long medicinal history dating back to the early cultures of the Middle-east and Indian sub-continent. Its colorful flowers were thought to lift spirits and encourage cheerfulness.[7] Creams, salves and plasters were and are still used to treat skin conditions and promote wound healing. The flowers are edible and are often added to salads or made into teas and cordials.[1] While the leaves and whole aerial part of the plant can be used medicinally,[1] the whole flowers and petals (actually florets) are most commonly used.[6]

Constituents[2-5, 8-10]

- Terpenoids: lupeol, taraxerol, taraxasterol, faradiol, saponins, volatile oil component, campesterol, stigmasterol
- Flavonoids: rutinoside, rutin, isoquercetin, narcissin, neohesperoside
- Polysaccharides: rhamnoarabinogalactan, arabinogalactans
- Miscellaneous: bitter priniciple called loiliolide (calendin), carotenoid pigments (beta carotene, lycopene, violaxanthin)

THERAPEUTIC USES & RELEVANT PHARMACOLOGY

ANTI-INFLAMMATORY EFFECTS

Calendula has been reported to have anti-inflammatory properties.[8, 11-14] Following topical application both the triterpene[8, 12] and flavonoid[13] fractions have been shown to possess an anti-inflammatory action *in vivo*. The most pronounced effect has been noted with the faridol esters extracted from the essential oil.[12] In addition, it has been suggested that the anti-inflammatory action of the isorhamnetin flavonoid glycosides is due to an inhibition of lipoxygenase activity.[13]

Physiological regeneration and epithelization have been noted following topical application of calendula to surgically induced wounds in an animal study. It is thought to act by increasing the metabolism of various proteins during the regenerative phase.[2]

MISCELLANEOUS EFFECTS

As has been seen in other plants, the high-density polysaccharides are reported to have immunostimulant properties *in vitro*.[15] The clinical relevance of the consumption of high alcohol content calendula products has been questioned, since these constituents are predominately water soluble.[1] In addition, calendula has been reported to have antibacterial[1, 14, 16] and antiviral activity.[14]

Calendula extracts have a reputation in France of having antineoplastic effects. Calendula extracts (made from various parts of *Calendula off.*) have been shown to possess *in vitro* cytotoxicity and *in vivo* antitumoral activity. These actions appear not to be parallel since the saponin rich extract which exerted the most pronounced antitumor activity showed only weak cytotoxic potential.[14]

A related species, *Calendula arvensis* L., has been shown to have molluscicidal activity[17,18] and is suggested to be potentially useful in killing the snail vector of schistosomiasis.[17]

COMMON USES

External

Salves or diluted tincture are reported to be useful in the management of superficial wounds, minor scalds and skin abrasions.[6, 7, 19-21] Calendula is also used as a gargle or mouthwash for mouth sores and mucosal irritation.[6, 19] Due to its astringent properties calendula has been used to stop bleeding and 'dry' discharges.[6] Calendula has also been suggested in the treatment of fungal vaginal infections.[6, 20]

No information could be found regarding attempts at clinical evaluation of these indications. In one case, the addition of a compound herbal product to 0.5% hydrocortisone decreased the healing times of abraded skin when compared to hydrocortisone alone. The clinical relevance of this with regard to calendula in particular is slight since the compound product used contained other phytomedicines with known vulnerary properties.[5]

The product Unguentum lymphaticum®, regarded as being useful in the management of lymphedema, was evaluated for efficacy in rats with induced acute lymphedema. Moderate relief was noted only in edema occurring in the animal's legs.[22] Again since this is a combination herbal product, clinical relevance to the specific action of calendula is unknown.

Internal

Calendula has been used in the management of indigestion and in the treatment of gastritis and other situations of digestive irritation.[6, 7, 20] Calendula is also considered to be an emmenagogue and is used in the treatment of delayed menstruation and dysmenorrhea.[7, 20] However, no evidence could be found to support these claims.

ADVERSE EFFECTS

None reported.

CAUTIONS/CONTRAINDICATIONS

While no instances of allergic reactions could be found, it should be noted that other members of the Asteraceae family (e.g., German chamomile, feverfew) have been shown to have allergic potential.

Calendula should be used with caution in pregnancy due to a reputed action on the menstrual cycle.[2]

DRUG INTERACTIONS

None reported; however, calendula has been noted to extend the duration of action of hexobarbitol in rats.[1] The implication to pharmacy practice is unknown.

DOSAGE REGIMEN

Internal

- Dried florets 1-4g (infusion) three times daily [2]
- 0.3-1.2mL of tincture (1:5, 90% alcohol) three times daily [2]
- 0.5-1.0mL of liquid extract (1:1 in 40% alcohol) three times daily [2]

External

- 1 to 2 teaspoonfuls of dried florets steeped in 240mL of boiling water for 10 minutes and allowed to cool can be used as a gargle or used to treat skin conditions[19]
- Calendula is often combined with other vulnerary herbs such as *Symphytum officinale* L., Boraginaceae (Comfrey), *Matricaria recutita* L., Asteraceae (German Chamomile) or *Echinacea* spp., Asteaceae (Coneflower).
- It may also be used in combination with phytomedicines with a reported antimicrobial action such as *Hydrastis canadensis* L., Ranunculaceae (Goldenseal).
- Calendula is available, either alone or in combination, as many different dosage forms, including vaginal suppositories, creams, salves, tooth pastes and cosmetics.

REFERENCES

1. Aldstat E. *Calendula off. Eclectic Dispensatory of Botanical Therapeutics* Portland: Eclectic Medical Publishers; 1989.
2. Newall C, Anderson L, David Phillipson J. *Herbal Medicine: A Guide for Health Care Professionals*. London: The Pharmaceutical Press; 1996:296.
3. Wren R. *Potter's New Encyclopedia of Botanical Drugs and Preparations*. Saffron Walden: C.W. Daniel Company; 1988:362.
4. Leung A, Foster S. *Encyclopedia of Common Natural Ingredient Used in Food, Drugs and Cosmetics.* 2nd ed. New York, NY: John Wiley and Sons; 1996:649.
5. Fleischener A. Plant extracts: to accelerate healing and reduce inflammation. *Cosmetics and Toiletries*. 1985; 100(10): 45-58.
6. Mills S. *The Essential Book of Herbal Medicine.* 2nd ed. London: Penguin; 1991:677.
7. Chevallier A. *The Encyclopedia of Medicinal Plants.* London: Reader's Digest; 1996:336.
8. Akihisa T, Yasukawa K, Oinuma H, *et al.* Triterpene Alcohols from the Flowers of Compositae and their Anti-inflammatory effects. *Phytochemistry*. 1996; 43(6):1255-1260.
9. Willuhn G, Westhaus R. Loliolide (Calendin) from *Calendula officianalis*. *Planta Medica*. 1987; 53: 304.
10. Vidal-Olivier E, Elias R, Faure F, *et al.* Flavonol Glycosides from *Calendula officianalis* flowers. *Planta Medica*. 1989;55(73-74).
11. Mascolo N, *et al.* Biological screening of Italian medicinal plants for anti-inflammatory activity. *Phytotherapy Research*. 1987;1(28).
12. Della Loggia R, Tubaro A, Becker H, *et al.* The role of Triterpenoids in the topical anti-inflammatory activity of *Calendula officinalis* flowers. *Planta Medica*. 1994;60:516-520.
13. Bezakova L, Masterova I, Paulikova I, Psenak M. Inhibitory activity of isorhamnetin glycosides from *Calendula*

officinalis L. on the activity of lipoxygenase. *Pharmazie*. 1996;51(2):126-7.

14. Boucaud-Maitre Y, Algernon O, Raynaud J. Cytotoxic and antihumoral activity of *Calendula officinalis* extracts. *Pharmazie*. 1988; 43:221-222.
15. Wagner H. The immune stimulating polysaccharides and heteroglycans of higher plants. A preliminary communication. *Arzneimittelforschung*. 1984;34(6):659-661.
16. Dumenil G, Chemli R, Balansard G, Guirand H, Lallemand M. Evaluation of antibacterial properties of marigold flowers and homeopathic mother tincture of *Calendula off. Annales Pharmaceutiques Francaises*. 1980;36(6):493-9.
17. Rawi S, El-Gindy H, Abd El Kader A. New possible molluscicides from *Calendula micrantha officinalis* and *Ammi majus*. *Ecotoxicology and Environmental Safety*. 1996;35:261-267.
18. Hammouda O, Borbely G. Alterations in protein synthesis in the *Cyanobacetrium Synechococcus* sp. Strain PCC 6301 in response to *Calendula micrantha* extract with molluscicidal activity. *Ecotoxicology and Environmental Safety*. 1995;31:201-204.
19. Tyler V. *Herbs of Choice. The Therapeutic Use of Phytomedicinals.* Binghamton, NY: Pharmaceutical Products Press; 1994:209.
20. Hoffman D. *Holistic Herbal.* Rockport,MA: Element Books; 1996:256.
21. Weiss R. *Herbal Medicine*. Beaconsfield: Beaconsfield Publishers;1988:362.
22. Casley-Smith J, Casley -Smith J. The effect of "Unguentum Lymphaticum' on acute experimental lymphedema and other high-protein edemas. *Lymphology*. 1983;16:150-156.

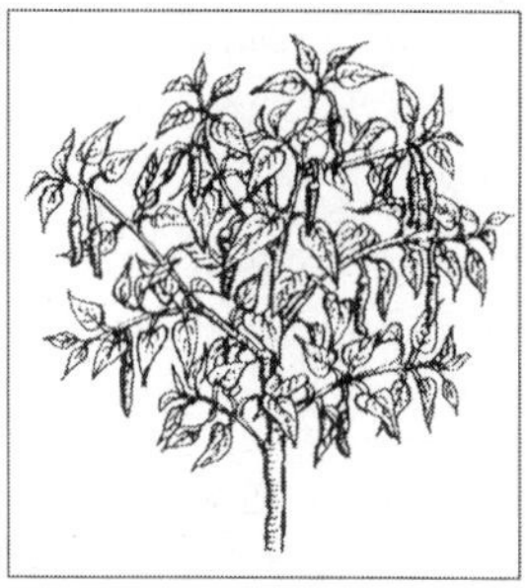

CAPSICUM

Capsicum annuum L.

THUMBNAIL SKETCH

Active Constituents

- Capsaicinoids, especially capsaicin

Common Uses

External:

- diabetic neuropathy
- post-herpetic neuralgia
- other painful conditions

Internal:

- digestive tonic
- cardiovascular tonic

Adverse Effects

- Redness and burning sensation at site of application
- Rare allergy

Cautions/Contraindications

- *External:* known allergy
- *Internal:* severe hypertension, acute gastric irritation, pregnancy and lactation

Drug Interactions

- May influence the hepatic metabolism of some drugs
- Caution in concomitant use of MAOIs and antihypertensives

Doses

External:

- Diabetic Neuropathy: 0.075% capsaicin cream/ointment applied 4 times daily
- Post-herpetic Neuralgia: 0.025% capsaicin cream/ointment applied 4 times daily

Internal:

- 30-120 mg three times daily
- Capsicum tincture: 0.3 to 1 mL daily

INTRODUCTION

Family: Solanaceae

Synonyms: Chili pepper, Red pepper, Cayenne pepper, Tobasco pepper, Hot pepper[1-3]

Capsicum is one the oldest and most widely used spices in the world. One author estimates that approximately 25% of the world's population use capsicum on a daily basis.[4] Recognized world wide for its pungency, capsicum may have been cultivated as early as 7000 BC in Mexico and Peru.[5] While there are over 50 species of capsicum, the common sweet red, green, yellow, and orange peppers, as well as paprika and numerous types of chili peppers are all now considered to be varieties of the same species.[6] The fruit is oblong in shape and approximately 1.5 to 2.5 cm in length.

The spice itself has enjoyed a long history in many healing disciplines. Historically, it was used as a stimulant to the whole body, and thought to aid digestion, the nervous system and circulation.[7, 8] During the early part of the last century, it was a key herbal remedy used by the Thomsonian practitioners of North America. Within this 'heroic' school of medicine, the aim was to stimulate the "vital energy" and expel pathogenic factors by inducing a 'therapeutic' fever.[7] In addition, capsaicin, the main active ingredient in capsicum, has been used for a variety of medicinal purposes, most often pain relief. Govindarajan *et al.* have produced a number of excellent reviews on capsicum.[9-13]

The nomenclature associated with capsicum is somewhat confusing. Capsicum is generally defined as the dried, ripe fruit of *Capsicum annuum* L. and a large number of varieties and hybrids of this.[1, 4] In contrast, capsaicin is a compound purified from these species (Chemical Abstracts (CAS) registry #404-86-4, under the name: N-[(4-hydroxy-3-methoxyphenyl)-methyl]-8-methyl-(E)-6-nonenamide). There are two possible stereoisomers of capsaicin, but only the *trans* isomer exists in nature. The *cis* isomer, civamide, is assigned a separate CAS registry number. To complicate matters even further, a third compound often called "synthetic capsaicin" has been synthesized and is often found as an adulterant in products labelled capsaicin. "Synthetic capsaicin" does not have the same chemical formula as either capsaicin or civamide and should not be used in their place. The official name of this adulterant is nonivamide, but it has also been called pelargonic acid vanillylamide. Nonivamide has never been found in capsicum fruit extracts.[4] Because of wide-spread misrepresentation and adulteration of capsaicin products with nonivamide, efficient analytic systems have now been developed to distinguish unambiguously between the two.[14-20]

Constituents[2, 3, 21, 22]

- Capsaicinoids: capsaicin, dihydrocapsaicin, nordihydrocapsaicin, homocapsaicin, homodihydrocapsaicin
- Carotenoids: lutein, carotein, capsanthin
- Vitamins: A and C

The active constituents of capsicum are considered to be the capsaicinoids.[21, 22] Of these, capsaicin is by far the most important.

THERAPEUTIC USES & RELEVANT PHARMACOLOGY

ANALGESIC ACTIVITY

Diabetic Neuropathy

The use of topical applications of capsaicin for the relief of diabetic neuropathy has been extensively studied.[23-29] The formation of The Capsaicin Study Group has resulted in numerous high-quality clinical trials.[24, 26] Most studies have employed topical capsaicin 0.075% in a cream base and have concluded that capsaicin is a safe and effective treatment for painful diabetic neuropathy. For example, one 8-week, double-blind, vehicle-controlled study of 0.075% capsaicin cream (Axsain®) applied four times daily by 54 patients with moderate to severe diabetic neuropathy, showed symptom improvement in 90% of capsaicin-treated patients, which was significantly better than the control group.[27] A variety of other trials using the same protocol (0.075% capsaicin cream applied 4 times daily) have confirmed that capsaicin 0.075% cream was more effective than a vehicle control.[24-26, 28-30] This literature review found only one published negative trial with capsaicin.[31]

Post-herpetic Neuralgia

A lower strength (0.025%) of capsaicin is used for the treatment of post-herpetic neuralgia than for diabetic neuropathy (0.075%). In an uncontrolled study of 33 patients, 55% of the patients completing the study reported good or excellent pain relief; however, burning sensation after the application of capsaicin was so severe in one-third of the patients that the trial was discontinued prematurely.[32] A large (n=208) open-labelled, uncontrolled trial concluded that topical capsaicin was a promising new treatment for post-herpetic neuralgia.[33] This supports the conclusions of several earlier studies.[34-37] However, the percentage of patients with substantial pain relief varied from 39% to 75%.[32,35] This variation may be due to different treatment schedules: Watson *et al.*, used capsaicin 0.025% 4 times daily, while Bernstein *et al.* asked patients to apply capsaicin 0.025% 5 times daily for 1 week, followed by 3 times daily for an additional 3 weeks. Another study using a 5 times daily treatment regimen, but a 0.001% capsaicin cream reported moderate pain relief in 62% of patients with post-herpetic neuralgia.[38] In addition, a case report suggests the use of topical capsaicin (0.025% — Zostrix ®) in the mouth may be an effective treatment for post-herpetic vesicles in the oral cavity. One episode of xerostomia (dry mouth) forced the discontinuation of therapy for one day only.[39] The signature burning sensation of capsaicin makes it very difficult to maintain a blinded trial; thus to date, these findings have not been confirmed by a randomized, double-blind, controlled trial.

Miscellaneous Pain Indications

Capsaicin cream has reportedly been effective in the treatment of Post-mastectomy Pain Syndrome;[40, 41] rheumatoid arthritis;[42] osteoarthritis;[42, 43] cluster headaches;[44, 45] reflex sympathetic dystrophy;[46] relief of local stump pain;[47] idiopathic trigeminal neuralgia;[48] relief of sores of oral mucositis caused by chemotherapy or radiation;[49] pain caused by Guillain-Barre syndrome;[50] and painful psoriasis vulgaris.[51]

Mechanism of Action

Capsaicin depletes substance P (SP), a substance that mediates pain transmission from the peripheral nerves to the spinal cord. [1, 52] It does this via four stages: 1) SP is immediately released from both central and peripheral terminals; 2) SP fibres are functionally impaired; 3) the axoplasmic transport of SP is inhibited; and 4) SP is depleted (this starts after 1 day and may last for weeks).[53] Although generally believed to be specific for type C nociceptive neurons (i.e., unmyelinated, slow-conducting fibres that transmit cutaneous pain information to the central nervous system),[54, 55] other research suggests that capsaicin causes damage to all unmyelinated sensory fibres.[56] Myelinated fibres of the A delta category may also be damaged with high doses of capsaicin.[56] It has been suggested that capsaicin may be a useful neurochemical tool for research into the interaction of sensory neurons with other neuronal systems. Excellent reviews of capsaicin's action on a variety of systems including the gastro-intestinal, thermoregulatory, cardiovascular, respiratory and nervous systems have been published.[57-68]

MISCELLANEOUS

Oral administration of capsicum has been shown to inhibit the rise of cholesterol in the liver and increase the fecal excretion of both cholesterol and bile acids in rats.[69] Administration of capsaicin did not effect serum levels of cholesterol; however, it did appear to stimulate lipid mobilization from adipose tissue and it lowered the serum trigylceride concentration in lard-fed rats.[70]

ADVERSE EFFECTS

Capsicum

- *Topical:* Allergic contact dermatitis has been reported[71, 72]
- *Internal:* Sweating (generally confined to the head and neck), flushing of the face and upper body, salivation, lacrimation, and nasal secretion[52] have been reported. In addition, the principle agents in capsicum can be very irritating to the mucosal membranes.[3] A toxicity study of chronic administration of capsicum extract to hamsters reported decreased vitamin A levels in liver tissue and eye toxicity including: a focal increase in corneal epithelial cells, and hyalinisation and thickening of the substantia propria in the eyeballs.[73] No similar effects have ever been reported in humans. Other effects which have been reported in humans include: increased fibrinolytic activity and hypocoagulability of blood.[74] However, these effects have been reported after ingestion of capsicum in the diet, as opposed to medicinal effects.

Capsaicin

- *Topical:* erythema; burning and stinging sensations (no vesication) are common at both the 0.025%[32] and 0.075% concentrations when applied topically, but the intensity is diminished for most patients with continued use (i.e. after 2 weeks). Some dry skin has been reported.[24-28, 32, 34, 35, 57, 75, 76] Also, inhalation reactions (coughing, sneezing) occurred occasionally.[24, 27] Capsaicin is generally considered to be safe. No changes in cutaneous sensation of temperature or vibration were noted after administration of 0.075% capsaicin four times daily for up to 32 weeks continuously.[25, 77, 78]
- *Internal:* increased gastric acid concentration is possible;[79] however, two other studies found no increase in gastric acid secretion.[80, 81] *In vitro* experiments suggest that capsaicin is a potent inhibitor of platelet aggregation.[82] Ingestion of large doses has been associated with necrosis, ulceration and even carcinogenesis; however, small amounts appear to have few deleterious effects.[83]

CAUTIONS/CONTRAINDICATIONS

Topical: Known allergy.
Internal: Contraindicated in cases of severe hypertension,[7] and caution should be used in situations of acute gastric irritation.[3, 7] During pregnancy capsicum should not be used at doses exceeding normal dietary levels.[3] Although not used medicinally, the leaves and stems of capsicum have been shown to be uterine stimulants in animal studies.[84] In addition, caution is recommended during lactation (due to the pungency of capsicum).[3]

DRUG INTERACTIONS

No specific drug interactions appear to have been reported in the literature; however, since high doses of capsicum have been shown to increase the activity of two hepatic enzymes in rats (glucose-6-phosphate dehydrogenase and adipose lipoprotein lipase),[70] the hepatic metabolism of some drugs may be affected.[3] In addition, since catecholamine amine secretion is increased, caution is suggested with concommitant use of monoamine oxidase inhibitors (MAOIs) and antihypertensives.[3]

DOSAGE REGIMENS

External: Found in a variety of external analgesic preparations including: Heet lotion, InfraRub ointment, Sloan's liniment, Zostrix, Zostrix-HP and Axsain

- Diabetic Neuropathy: 0.075% capsaicin cream/ointment applied 4 times daily
- Post-herpetic Neuralgia: 0.025% capsaicin cream/ointment applied 4 times daily

Internal: 30-120 mg of the fruit three times daily[3]

- Capsicum tincture (BPC 1986) 0.3 to 1 mL daily[3]

REFERENCES

1. Tyler VE. *Herbs of Choice: The Therapeutic Use of Phytomedicinals*. Binghamton, NY: Pharmaceutical Products Press; 1994:209.
2. Leung AY, Foster S. *Encyclopedia of Common Natural Ingredients Used in Food, Drugs, and Cosmetics*. 2nd ed. New York: John Wiley and Sons Inc; 1996:649.
3. Newall CA, Anderson LA, Phillipson JD. *Herbal Medicine: A Guide for Health Care Professionals*. London: The Pharmaceutical Press; 1996:296.
4. Cordell GA, Araujo OE. Capsaicin: Identification, nomenclature, and pharmacotherapy. *Annals of Pharmacotherapy*. 1993;27:330-336.
5. Pickersgill B. The domestication of chilli peppers. In: B.J. U, Dimbleby GW, eds. *The Domestication and Exploitation of Plants and Animals:* London: Gerald Duckworth; 1969.
6. Marles RJ, Associate Professor, Department of Botany, Brandon University, Brandon, Manitoba. Review of Medicinal Plant Modules for CCNM; 1997.
7. Mills S. *Essential Book of Herbal Medicine*. London: Penguin; 1991:677.
8. Chevallier A. *The Encyclopedia of Medicinal Plants.* London: Readers Digest; 1996:336.
9. Govindarajan VS. Capsicum — production, technology, chemistry, and quality. I. History, botany, cultivation and primary processing. *CRC Critical Reviews in Food Science and Nutrition*. 1985;22:109-76.
10. Govindarajan VS. Capsicum — production, technology, chemistry, and quality. II. Processed products, standards, world production, and trade. *CRC Critical Reviews in Food Science and Nutrition*. 1986;23:207-88.
11. Govindarajan VS. Capsicum — production, technology, chemistry, and quality. III. Chemistry of the color, aroma and pungency stimuli. *CRC Critical Reviews in Food Science and Nutrition.* 1986;24:245-355.
12. Govindarajan VS, Rajalakshmi D, Chand N. Capsicum — production, technology, chemistry, and quality. IV.

Evaluation of quality. *CRC Critical Reviews in Food Science and Nutrition.* 1987;25:185-283.

13. Govindarajan VS, Sathyanarayana MN. Capsicum — production, technology, chemistry, and quality. V. Impact on physiology, pharmacology, nutrition, and metabolism; structure, pungency, pain and desentization sequences. *CRC Critical Reviews in Food Science and Nutrition.* 1991;29:435-73.
14. Kosuge S, Furata M. Studies on the pungent principles of Capsicum XIV. Chemical constitution of the pungent principles. *Agric Biol Chem.* 1970;34:248-56.
15. Muller-Stock A, Joshi RK, Buchi J. Components of capsaicinoids: quantitative gas chromatographic determination of individual homologs and analogs of capsaicin in mixtures from a natural source and of vanillylpelargonic amide as an adulteration. *Journal of Chromatography.* 1971;63:281-7.
16. Muller-Stock A, Joshi RK, Buchi J. Thin-layer and column chromatographic separation of capsaicinoids: Study of the constituents of capsicum. *Journal of Chromatography.* 1973;79:229-41.
17. Todd P, Bensinger M, Biftu T. TLC screening techniques for the qualitative determination of natural and synthetic capsaicinoids. *Journal of Chromatographic Science.* 1975;13:577-9.
18. Jurenitsch J, Kubelka W, Jentzsch K. Gas chromatographic determination of the content of individual and total capsaicinoids in Capsicum fruits after thin-layer chromatographic separation. *Sci Pharm.* 1978;46:307-18.
19. Heresch F, Jurenitsch J. Off-line mass spectrometric monitoring of HPLC effluents — an improved identification and quantitation method for mixtures of similar compounds. Natural Capsaicinoids. *Chromatographia.* 1979;12:647-50.
20. Jurenitsch J, Leinmuller R. Quantification of nonylic acid vanillylamide and other capsaicinoids in the pungent principle of Capsicum fruits and preparation by gas-liquid chromatography on glass capillary columns. *Journal of Chromatography.* 1980;189:389-97.
21. Bennett DJ, Kirby GW. Constitution and biosynthesis of capsaicin. *Journal of Chemical Society, Chemical Communications.* 1968:442-6.
22. Jentzsch K, Pock H, Kubelka W. Isolation of dihydrocapsaicin and homodihydrocapsaicin form Capsicum fruits. *Monatsch Chem.* 1968;99:661-3.
23. Ross DR, Varipapa RJ. Treatment of painful diabetic neuropathy with topical capsaicin [Letter]. *New England Journal of Medicine.* 1989;321(7):474-475.
24. Donofrio PD, Walker F, Hunt V, *et al.* Treatment of painful diabetic neuropathy with topical capsaicin: a multicentre, double-blind, vehicle-controlled study. *Archives of Internal Medicine.* 1991;151:2225-9.
25. Tandan R, Lewis GA, Krusinski PB, *et al.* Topical capsaicin in painful diabetic neuropathy. Controlled study with long term follow-up. *Diabetes Care.* 1992;15(1):8-14.
26. Dailey GE. Effect of treatment with capsaicin on daily activities of patients with diabetic neuropathy. *Diabetes Care.* 1992;15(2):159-65.
27. Scheffler NM, *et al.* Treatment of painful diabetic neuropathy with capsaicin 0.075%. *Journal of the American Podiatric Medical Association.* 1991;81(6):288-293.
28. Basha KM, Whitehouse FW. Capsaicin: a therapeutic option for painful diabetic neuropathy. *Henry Ford Hospital Medical Journal.* 1991;39(2):138-140.
29. Pfeifer MA, *et al.* A highly successful and novel model for treatment of chronic painful diabetic peripheral neuropathy. *Diabetes Care.* 1993;16(8):1103-1115.
30. Chad D, Ross D, Molitch M, *et al.* Treatment of painful diabetic neuropathy with topical capsaicin — a double-blind multicentre investigation. *Pain.* 1990;42:387-8.
31. Chad DA, Aronin N, Lundstrom R, *et al.* Does capsiacin relieve the pain of diabetic neuoropathy? *Pain.* 1990;42:387-8.
32. Watson CP, *et al.* Post-herpetic neuralgia and topical capsaicin. *Pain.* 1988;35:289-297.
33. Watson CP, Evans RJ, Wait VR, Birkett N. Post-herpetic neuralgia: 208 cases. *Pain.* 1988;35:289-297.
34. Bernstein JE, Korman NJ, Bickers DR, Dahl MV, Millikan LE. Topical capsaicin treatment of chronic postherpetic neuralgia. *Journal of the American Academy of Dermatology.* 1989;21(2, Pt.1):265-270.
35. Bernstein JE, Bickers DR, Dahl MV, Roshal JY. Treatment of chronic postherpetic neuralgia with topical capsaicin. A preliminary study. *Journal of the American Academy of Dermatology.* 1987;17(1):93-96.
36. Bernstein JE. Capsaicin in the treatment of dermatologic disease. *Cutis.* 1987;39:352-3.
37. Peikert A, Hentrich M, Ocas G. Topical 0.025% capsaicin in chronic post-herpetic neuralgia: Efficacy, predictors of response and long-term course. *Journal of Neurology.* 1991;238(8):452-456.
38. Bjerring P, Arendt-Nielsen L, Soderberg V. Argon laser induced cutaneous sensory and pain thresholds in post-herpetic neuraligia. Quantitative modulation by topical capsaicin. *Acta Dermato Venereologica* (Stockholm). 1990;70(2):121-125.

39. Hawk RJ, Millikan LE. Treatment of oral postherpetic neuralgia with topical capsaicin. *International Journal of Dermatology*. 1988;27(5):336.
40. Watson CPN, Evans RJ, Watt VR. The post-mastectomy pain syndrome and the effect of topical capsaicin. *Pain*. 1989;38:177-186.
41. Watson CP, Evans RJ. The postmastectomy pain syndrome and topical capsaicin: a randomized trial. *Pain*. 1992;51(3):375-379.
42. Deal CL, Schnitzer TJ, Lipstein E, *et al.* Treatment of arthritis with topical capsaicin: a double-blind trial. *Clinical Therapeutics*. 1991;13(3):383-395.
43. McCarthy G, McCarty D. Effect of topical capsaicin on asteoarthritis of the hands. *Journal of Rheumatology*. 1992;19:604-7.
44. Sicuteri F, Fusco BM, Marabini S, *et al.* Beneficial effect of capsaicin application to the nasal mucosa in cluster headache. *Clinical Journal of Pain*. 1989;5:49-53.
45. Marks DR, Rapoport A, Padla D, *et al.* A double-blind, placebo-controlled trial of intranasal capsaicin for cluster headache. *Cephalalgia*. 1993;13(2):114-116.
46. Chesire WP, Snyder CR. Treatment of reflex sympathetic dystrophy with topical capsaicin. *Pain*. 1990;42: 307-11.
47. Rayner HC, Atkins RC, Westerman RA. Relief of local stump pain by capsaicin cream [Letter]. *Lancet*. 1989;ii:1276-1277.
48. Fusco BM, Alessandri M. Analgesic effect of capsaicin in idiopathic trigeminal neuralgia. *Anesthesia and Analgesia*. 1992;74(3):375-377.
49. Heal the burn: Pepper and lasers in cancer pain therapy. *Journal of the National Cancer Institute*. 1994;86(18):1381.
50. Morgenlander JC, *et al.*, Capsaicin for the treatment of pain in the Guillain-Barrè syndrome [Letter]. *Annals of Neurology*. 1990;28(2):199.
51. Bernstein JE, *et al.* Effects of topically applied capsaicin on moderate and severe psoriasis vulgaris. *Journal of the American Academy of Dermatology*. 1986;15(3):504-507.
52. Locock RA. Capsicum. *Canadian Pharmaceutical Journal*. 1985;118:517-519.
53. Skofitsch G, Donnerer J, *et al.* Comparison of Nonivamide and Capsaicin with regard to their pharma cokinetics and effects on sensory neurons. *Arzneimittel Forschung*. 1984;34:154-6.
54. Szolesanyi J. Capsaicin, irritation, and desensitization. In: Green BG, Mason JR, Kare MR, eds. *Chemical Senses*. New York: Marcel Dekker; 1990.
55. Lynn B. Capsaicin: actions on nociceptive C-fibres and therapeutic potential [Review article]. *Pain*. 1990;41:61-69.
56. Nagy JI, Emson PC, Iversen IL. A re-evaluation of the neurochemical and antinociceptive effects of intrathecal capsaicin in the rat. *Brain Research*. 1981;211:497-502.
57. Fitzgerald M. Capsaicin and sensory neurones — A review. *Pain*. 1983;15:109-130.
58. Nagy JI. Capsaicin's action on the nervous system. *Trends in Neurosciences*. 1982;5:362-5.
59. Nagy JI. A chemical probe for sensory neuron mechanism. In: Iversen LL, Iverson SD, Snyder SH, eds. *Handbook of Psychopharmacology*. New York: Plenum; 1982:185.
60. Buck SH, Burks TF. Capsaicin: Hot new pharmacological tool. *Trends in Pharmacological Sciences*. 1983; 4:84-7.
61. Virus RM, Gebhart GF. Pharmacological action of capsaicin: Apparent involvement of substance P and serotonin. *Life Science*. 1979;25:1273-84.
62. Lembeck F, Gamse R, Juan H. Substance P and sensory nerve endings. In: von Euler US, Pernow B, eds. *Substance P.* New York: Raven Press; 1977:169.
63. Jancso G, Kiraly E, Such G, Joo F, Nagy A. Neurotoxic effect of capsaicin in mammals. *Acta Physiol Hung*. 1987;69:295-313.
64. Baranowski R, Lynn B, Pini A. The effects of locally applied capsaicin on conduction in cutaneous nerves in four mammalian species. *British Journal of Pharmacology*. 1986;80:267-76.
65. Gamse R, Petsche V, Lembeck F, Jansco G. Capsaicin applied to peripheral nerve inhibits axonal transport of substance P and somatostatin. *Brain Research*. 1982;239:447-62.
66. Kenins P. Responses of single nerve fibers to capsaicin applied to the skin. *Neuroscience Letters*. 1982;29:83-88.
67. Buck SH, Burks TF. The neuropharmacology of capsaicin: Review of some recent observations. *Pharmacological Reviews*. 1986;38:179-226.

68. Jessel TM, Iverson LL, Cuello AC. Capsaicin-induced depletion of substance P from primary sensory neurons. *Brain Research.* 1978;152:183-8.
69. Sambaiah K, Satyanarayana MN. Hypocholesterolemic effect of red pepper and capsaicin. *Indian Journal of Experimental* Biology. 1980;18:898-9.
70. Kawada T, *et al*. Effects of capsaicin on lipid metabolism in rats fed a high fat diet. *Journal of Nutrition*. 1986;116:1272-1278.
71. Futrell JM, Rietschel RL. Spice allergy evaluated by results of patch tests. *Cutis*. 1993;52:288-90.
72. Niinimaki A, Hannuksela M, Makinen-Kiljunen S. Skin prick tests and in vitro immunoassays with native spices and spice extracts. *Annals of Allergy, Asthma, & Immunology*. 1995;75:280-6.
73. Agrawal RC, Sarode AV, Lalitha VS, Bhide SV. Chili extract treatment and induction of eye lesions in hamsters. *Toxicology Letters*. 1985;28:1-7.
74. Visudhiphan S, Poolsuppasit S, Piboonnukarintr O, Tumliang S. The relationship between high fibrinolytic activity and daily capsicum ingestion in Thais. *The American Journal of Clinical Nutrition.* 1982;35:1452-8.
75. Smith JG, Crounse RG, Spence D. The effects of capsaicin on human skin, liver and epidermal lysomes. *Journal of Investigative Dermatology.* 1970;54:170-3.
76. Carpenter SE, Lynn B. Vascular and sensory responses of human skin to mild injury after topical treatment with capsaicin. *British Journal of Pharmacology*. 1981;73:755-58.
77. Tandan R, Lewis G, Fries T. Safety of topical capsaicin in diabetic neuropathy. *Neurology*. 1990;40 (Supplement):160.
78. McMahon SB, Lewin G, Bloom S. The consequences of long-term topical capsaicin application in the rat. *Pain.* 1991;44:301-10.
79. Desai HG, Venugoplan K, Antia FP. Effect of red chilli powder on DNA content of gastric aspirates. *Gut*. 1973;14:974-6.
80. Pimparker BND, Donde UM. Effects of commonly used spices on human gastric secretion. *Journal of the Association of Physicians of India*. 1972;20:910-910.
81. Dugani A, Glavin GB. Capsaicin effects on stress pathology and gastric acid secretion in rats. *Life Science.* 1986;39:1531-1518.
82. Wang JP, Hsu MF, Teng CM. Antiplatelet effect of capsaicin. *Thrombosis Research*. 1984;36:497-507.
83. Surh YJ, Lee SS. Capsaicin in hot chili pepper: Carcinogen, co-carciogen or anticarcinogen? *Food and Chemical Toxicology*. 1996; 34:313-316
84. Farnsworth NR, Biugel A, Cordell C, *et al*. Potential value of plants as sources of new antifertility agents I. [Review]. *Journal of Pharmaceutical Sciences*. 1975;64(4):535-598.

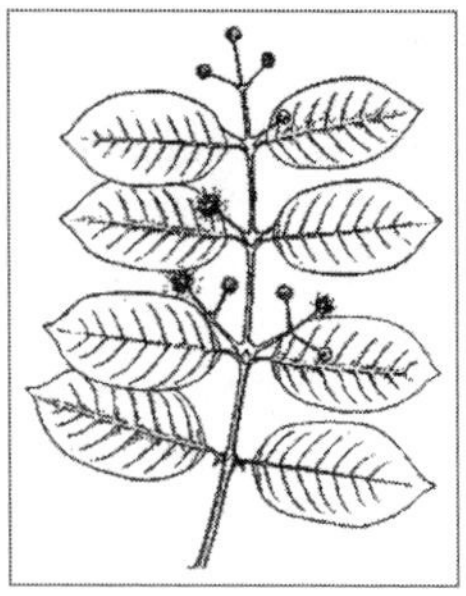

CAT'S CLAW

Uncaria tomentosa (Willd. Ex Roem.& Schult) DC. or *Uncaria guianensis* (Aubl.) J.F. Gmel.

THUMBNAIL SKETCH

Active Constituents
- Oxindole alkaloids, glycosides

Common Uses
- Gastrointestinal disorders, rheumatism, cancer, asthma, diabetes, menstrual irregularities.

Adverse Effects
- None noted.

Cautions/Contraindications
- Pregnancy, lactation, hemophiliacs undergoing certain treatments.

Drug Interactions
- None documented.
- Caution with various hormone or immunoglobulin based therapies.

Doses
- No established protocols were found.
- Standardization to alkaloid content is common.

INTRODUCTION

Family: Rubiaceae

Synonyms: Una de gato, Garabato, Paraguayo[1, 2]

Members of the genus *Uncaria* are found throughout Asia, Africa and South America.[3] The species found in South America are woody climbing vines growing up to 100 feet. The common name, cat's claw, comes from the curved thorns or 'hooks' used by the plant to fasten itself onto supporting plants.[2] While many South American plants are referred to as una de gato, the two species mentioned above are the ones primarily used medicinally.[4] These species are often considered to have identical therapeutic indications.[1, 2] They are also very similar in appearance with only slight differences in the presentation of the leaves and the hooks.[4]

The parts used medicinally are the dried inner stem bark or the root. It takes from three to eight years for plants to reach a suitable size to harvest. Cat's claw has long been used for various ailments by the indigenous peoples of South America and has recently gained popularity in both North America and Europe. Given this increase in demand, ecological concerns have been raised with regard to the sustainability of the crop.[3] Consequently, the Peruvian government has recently invested in an extensive planting campaign.[2, 4] Some consider that Una de gato may offer an alternative (and more suitable) crop to the illegal cultivation of 'coca'.[1] Since most cat's claw supplements available in North America appear to be made from *Uncaria tomentosa*, the following discussion will be limited to this species.

Constituents[2, 4-8]

- Oxindole alkaloids including: uncarine F, isopteropodine, pteropodine, isorhynchophylline, rhynchophylline and mitraphylline.
- Quinovic acid glycosides
- Triterpenes including: oleanolic acid
- Polyphenols including: catechins, rutin, quercetin
- Miscellaneous: tannins

The alkaloid content of plants seem to vary appreciably from one year to the next.[9]

THERAPEUTIC USES & RELEVANT PHARMACOLOGY

COMMON USES

Uncaria tomentosa has been used traditionally in the management of many conditions notably: rheumatism, peptic ulcers, intestinal disorders, certain cancers, asthma, inflammatory conditions and menstrual irregularities.[3, 4] North American practitioners and patients have noted relief in cases of diverticulitis, diabetes, gastritis, colic and 'leaky bowel syndrome'.[10, 11]

PHARMACOLOGY

Oxindole alkaloids extracted from the root were found to have immunomodulatory properties, increasing phagocytosis in both *in vitro* and *in vivo* experimental models.[12] It has been suggested that cat's claw may act as an immunostimulating agent, activating cell-mediated immune function as well as 'normalizing immunoglobulins'.[1]

Extracts made from the bark of *Uncaria tomentosa* have been shown *in vitro* to exert a protective antimutagenic effect against photomutagenesis induced by 8-methoxy-psoralen (8-MOP) plus UVA in *S. typhimurium* TA 102.[13] One *in vivo* study, demonstrated that the "mutagenic activity of the urine" of an adult male smoker was "dramatically" decreased when the volunteer consumed an aqueous decoction made from the bark of *Uncaria tomentosa.* This decrease in mutagenicity was maintained for eight days after the administration of the decoction ended. The authors of this study suggest that agents found in the extract have an antioxidant effect.[13] In addition, an oxindole alkaloid (uncarine F) has been shown to exert an antiproliferative effect against leukemic cell lines *in vitro.* The authors of the study suggest that this agent may prove useful in the management of certain acute leukemias.[5]

Extracts made from the bark of *Uncaria tomentosa* were shown to possess anti-inflammatory properties *in vivo*, using the carrageenan-induced edema test in rat paw. This anti-inflammatory action could be due to agents with 'intrinsic anti-inflammatory effect' or due to the existence of a synergy between multiple constituents.[14]

Glycosides extracted from the bark of *Uncaria tomentosa* have also been shown to possess antiviral properties (against vesicular stomatitis virus) *in vitro*.[6] In a review article, Jones describes a six-year trial of HIV positive patients (n=14) in which administration of a "standardized cat's claw root extract rich in alkaloids" increased T helper cell counts and delayed or prevented the onset of symptoms.[2] A number of review articles made reference to ongoing studies into the use of *Uncaria tomentosa* in the treatment of various conditions, notably HIV and cancer.[2, 3, 11]

ADVERSE EFFECTS

No adverse effects could be found. This herbal medicine is considered non-toxic by most authors;[1, 4] however, plants with high tannin content, such as cat's claw, may affect the kidneys and liver or irritate the gastrointestinal tract.[15]

CAUTIONS/CONTRAINDICATIONS

Many of the plants commonly referred to as una de gato are considered poisonous. Consequently, proper identification of plants used in the manufacture of this herbal supplement is of particular importance.[2]

The safety of cat's claw products in pregnancy or lactation has not yet been established.[4] In addition, a patent for an Austrian product suggests that hemophiliacs receiving fresh blood plasma or therapy with cryoprecipitates should avoid concurrent use of *Uncaria tomentosa.*[4]

DRUG INTERACTIONS

No cases of documented drug interactions could be found.

European manufacturers caution against concurrent use with: passive vaccines composed of animal sera, intravenous hyperimmunoglobulin therapy, insulin and "other hormone products." The rational behind these concerns could not be found.[4]

DOSAGE REGIMEN

Little information could be found with regard to the therapeutic dosage of *Uncaria tomentosa*. A hydroalcoholic tincture (50% water/alcohol) has been proposed as the most effective dosage form because of the increased alkaloid content.[4] Products commonly available on the Canadian market contain 200 to 300 mg of concentrated extract of *U. tomentosa* bark standardized to oxindole alkaloid and polyphenol content.

REFERENCES

1. Duke J. Una de Gato. *The Business of Herbs*. 1994;May/June:12-13.
2. Jones K. Cats Claw. *Herbs for Health*. 1996;Sep/Oct:42-46.
3. Foster S. Cat's Claw. *Health Foods Business*. 1995;June:24-25.
4. Jones K. *Cat's Claw: Healing Vine of Peru*. Seattle, WA: Sylvan Press; 1995:152.
5. Stuppner H, Sturm S, Geisen G, Zillian U, Konwalinka G. A differential sensitivity of oxindole alkaloids to normal and leukemic cell lines. *Planta Medica*. 1993;59(Supplement issue):A583.
6. Aquino R, De Simone F, Pizza C, *et al*. Plant metabolites, structure and in vitro antiviral activity of quinovic acid glycosides from *Uncaria tomentosa* and *Guettarda platypoda*. *Journal of Natural Products*. 1989;52(4):679-685.
7. Hemingway S, Phillipson J. Alkaloids from South American species of *Uncaria* (Rubiaceae). *Journal of Pharmacy and Pharmacology*. 1974;26(Supp.):113P.
8. de Matta S, Monache F, Ferrari F, Marini-Bettolo G. Alkaloids and procyanidins of an *Uncaria sp*. from Peru. *Farmaco*. 1976;31(7):527-35.
9. Laus G, Keplinger D. Separation of sterioisomeric oxindole alkaloids from *Uncaria tomentosa* by high performance liquid chromatography. *Journal of Chromatography*. 1994:243-249.
10. Steinberg P. *Uncaria Tomentosa* (Cats Claw). A wondrous herb from the Peruvian rain forest. *Townsend Letter for Doctors*. 1994;May:442-443.
11. Steinberg P. Cat's Claw Update (*Uncaria tomentosa*). That wondrous herb from the Peruvian rain forest. *Townsend Letter for Doctors*. 1995;Aug/Sep:70-71.
12. Wagner H, Kreutzkamp B, Jurcic K. The alkaloids of *Uncaria tomentosa* and their phagocytosis-stimulating action. *Planta Medica*. 1985;5:419-23.
13. Rizzi R, Re F, Bianchi A, et al. Mutagenic and antimutagenic activities of *Uncaria tomentosa* and its extracts. *Journal of Ethnopharmacology*. 1993;38(1):63-77.
14. Aquino R, De Feo V, De Simone F, *et al*. Plant metabolites: New compounds and anti-inflammatory activity of *Uncaria tomentosa*. *Journal of Natural Products*. 1991;54(2):453-459.
15. Marles RJ, Associate Professor, Department of Botany, Brandon University, Brandon, Manitoba. Review of Medicinal Plant Modules for CCNM; 1997.

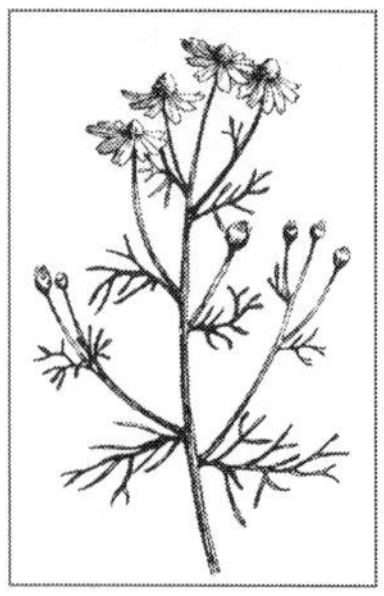

GERMAN CHAMOMILE

Matricaria recutita L.

THUMBNAIL SKETCH

Active Constituents
- Volatile oil (chamazulene, (-)α-bisabolol, spiroethers)
- Apigenin and other flavonoids

Common Uses

Internal
- Gastrointestinal discomfort, peptic ulcer, gastritis, indigestion and diarrhea
- Mild insomnia and anxiety
- Pediatric colic and teething

External
- Inflammatory skin conditions
- Canker sores and irritation of the gums and mouth

Adverse Effects
- Contact dermatitis
- Vomiting in very high doses

Cautions / Contraindications
- Individuals with a known allergy to members of the Sunflower (Compositae/Asteraceae) family

Drug Interactions
- None known

Doses
- 2-4 g of dried flowers (usually as an infusion/tea) three times daily

INTRODUCTION

Family: Asteraceae (also known as Compositae)

Synonyms: *Matricaria chamomilla* L., Single chamomile, Hungarian chamomile, PinHeads, Matricaria, Wild chamomile, Sweet false chamomile.[1-5]

German chamomile is one of two species of chamomile commonly used medicinally, the other being Roman or English Chamomile (*Chamaemelum nobile* (L.) All.). The primary indications of both are similar, even though the constituents are slightly different. Outside of the United Kingdom, German chamomile is the one which has been both evaluated most extensively and used therapeutically.[6]

German chamomile is a small (0.6m), fragrant, annual herb native to most of Europe and Western Asia and naturalized throughout North America.[4] As a commercially viable crop, more than 4000 tons of the chamomiles are produced annually,[5, 7] mainly in Eastern Europe, The Balkans and parts of South America.[4] The bulk of this is German Chamomile.[5] Most of the cultivated crop is destined for Europe, especially Germany,[5] rather than North America where the herb has been relegated by the public to the role of a beverage.[8] The flowers, preferably picked a few days before opening, are the parts used medicinally.[1]

The fact that the Germans often refer to German chamomile as 'alles zutraut', meaning capable of anything, gives some idea of the high regard in which this plant is held.[9, 10] Its panacea-like properties and numerous indications have led many people to refer to it rather confusingly as 'European ginseng'. Chamomile tea is used as a digestive, hypnotic and antispasmodic, finding particular favor in the treatment of children's ailments.[5] As Brown has noted, it should not be forgotten that it helped Peter Rabbit get over a particularly over-indulgent trip to Farmer McGregor's vegetable garden.[9] It takes a brave skeptic to argue with evidence like that.

Constituents[1, 3, 4, 7, 11]

The flowers contain:

- Terpenoids: azulene, chamazulene, α-bisabolol, α-bisabololoxide A, B, C, matricin, farnesol
- Flavonoids: apigenin, apiin, luteolin, quercetin, and rutin
- Coumarins: umbelliferone, herniarin
- Miscellaneous: capric acid, polysaccharides, spiroethers, and tannins

The yield of the medicinally important volatile oil fraction, rich in terpenoids and spiroethers, is dependent on both the age and locale of the plant.[7] Matricin is converted to chamazulene in the extraction process.[9] While standardization is not universal, German products are normally authenticated by measuring chamazulene and α- bisabolol content.[7, 9]

THERAPEUTIC USES & RELEVANT PHARMACOLOGY

PHARMACOLOGY

The medicinal properties of German chamomile may be attributed to several different components.[5, 7] While most attention is paid to the volatile oil fraction, it is now becoming increasingly apparent that other constituents have therapeutically useful properties.

Volatile Oil

The constituents of the volatile oil portion are known to have a variety of medicinal properties including anti-inflammatory[5, 7, 12] and spasmolytic actions.[5, 7, 13]

(-)-α-*bisabolol*

(-)-α-bisabolol is reported to be one of the most powerful anti-inflammatory products present in German chamomile oil.[5, 7, 11, 14] This activity is greater than that exerted by a synthetic racemic mixture, (+)α-bisabolol or various bisabololoxides present.[7, 11, 14] Results from *in vivo* studies suggest an antiulcerogenic action against various noxious substances and traumatic stimuli including indomethacin, stress and ethanol.[5, 7, 15] It has also been shown to have antibacterial and antifungal activity. [5, 7] An antispasmodic property has been demonstrated, which is greater than that of the total oil and equivalent to that of papaverine.[1]

Azulene Component

Azulene components have been shown to possess both antiallergenic[5, 7] and anti-inflammatory properties.[5, 7, 13] Following oral administration, matricin was shown to exert a more pronounced anti-inflammatory action in the rat paw carrageenin test than either chamazulene or guaiazulene. [5, 16] The anti-inflammatory action of chamazulene, but not its precursor matricin, appears to be partly due to inhibition of leukotriene synthesis.[17] In addition, chamazulene appears to have antioxidant properties.[17, 18] The hepatoregenerative action of the volatile oil seen in rats is also attributed to the azulene portion.[7]

Cis-spiroethers

Cis-spiroethers have been shown to possess anti-inflammatory[3, 7] and antispasmodic properties.[12, 19] They were shown to have a prolonged spasmolytic action in the digestive tract of mice following oral absorption; however, they were also absorbed into systemic circulation.[19]

Flavonoids

The flavonoid apigenin was shown to have an anti-inflammatory action *in vitro* superior (10x) to matricin, suggesting that the anti-inflammatory action of the whole plant is not solely dependent on the essential oil content.[13] The flavonoids have been shown to have antispasmodic activity with apigenin being more potent that papaverine.[12] In addition, recent animal studies have demonstrated that apigenin present in an aqueous extract of German chamomile flower has an affinity for central benzodiazepine receptors, competitively inhibiting the binding of flunitrazepam.[20] It has also been reported that the flavonoids found in German chamomile have antihistaminic properties.[21]

Polysaccharides

The high molecular weight polysaccharides appear to have immunostimulant properties.[22, 23]

Whole Extracts

While the individual agents responsible are as yet unknown, the volatile oil has been shown to decrease uric acid levels *in vivo*.[24] In addition, results from *in vivo* studies show that the essential oil of the herb increases bile secretion and biliary cholesterol concentration.[25] Ethanolic extracts of the German chamomile have also been shown to inhibit the growth of polio and herpes virus *in vitro*.[26]

COMMON USES

Digestive Upset

The most widely accepted use of chamomile is as a digestive aid and carminative. It is considered useful in the management of many gastrointestinal disorders such as: colic, indigestion, gastritis, diarrhea and peptic ulcer disease. This phytomedicine seems particularly suitable when there is an etiology of stress or tension.[9] A commercial product, Kamillosan®, was shown to exert a spasmolytic effect on the smooth musculature of the intestine in isolated guinea pig ileum.[12]

Mouth and Gum Irritation

The treatment of mouth and gum irritation with chamomile mouthwash is an approved indication according to guidelines established by Commission E, a federal German advisory body.[27] It is thought to be effective in the management of minor mucosal irritations.[5, 7] In an uncontrolled trial of patients (n=98), chamomile was found to decrease stomatitis resulting from chemotherapy.[28] Unfortunately, these findings were not supported by a later, more sophisticated, double blind, placebo controlled trial (n=164) where chamomile mouthwash was shown to be ineffective in decreasing 5-Fluorouracil (5FU) induced stomatitis.[29]

Skin Irritations

The use of chamomile-based products as a topical treatment of many skin conditions, such as insect bites, eczema and diaper rashes, is common place in Europe, especially Germany.[5, 9] External application of chamomile has been shown to be effective in decreasing inflammation[7, 30, 31] and promoting cellular regeneration.[5] Kamillosan®, a proprietary product containing chamomile, as been shown to aid in the treatment of dermatitis of the lower legs when added to conventional treatment protocols.[5] It has also been used as adjunctive therapy in the management of more serious conditions such as stasis ulcers. Several studies have demonstrated that topically applied extracts of fresh chamomile have greater anti-inflammatory action than those made from the dried flowers.[13, 30] The therapeutic action of chamomile may not be limited to the outer layers of skin since *in vivo* studies have shown that the flavonoids applied topically can penetrate to the deeper layers as well.[32]

Insomnia and Anxiety

Chamomile tea is often used to treat insomnia and nervous tension due to its reputed mild hypnotic effect.[5, 7, 23] A sedative action has been noted during cardiac catheterisation in humans following oral administration.[5] While a mechanism of action has yet to be determined, as mentioned above certain flavonoids are known to bind to central benzodiazepine receptors. Apigenin has also been reported to exert a distinct anxiolytic action in mice, with a sedative effect being noted at higher doses.[20] Some authors attribute this hypnotic effect to the possible presence of tryptophan in the flowers, a fact that has yet to be substantiated.[5]

ADVERSE EFFECTS

Cases of allergic reactions to chamomile preparations or the plant itself have been widely documented.[5, 7, 33-40] The vast majority of these are limited to contact skin irritation,[38, 40,] most commonly amongst people frequently in contact with the fresh plant (i.e., florists and gardeners).[34, 38] Two cases of immediate anaphylactic reactions following oral consumption have been noted.[37, 39] Even though allergic sensitivity is quite rare, given the possible outcomes it would be prudent to be cautious.[7, 33] The sesquiterpene lactones with exocyclic α-methylene rings are considered the constituents primarily responsible for this allergic potential which is also shown by other members of this family.[5, 7, 35, 41] Contact irritation appears to be more common with topical use of Roman chamomile than German chamomile.[42]

It is important to note that in most cases of allergic reaction to chamomile, including the incidents of anaphylactic reactions, no attempt was made to authenticate the product itself. This has led many to suggest that the vast majority of allergic reactions may be a result of adulteration with other unidentified plants. For example, German chamomile products containing Stinking Dog Fennel (*Anthemis cotula* L.), which has an established allergenic potential, have been sold erroneously under the name of chamomile.[7, 35]

Direct adverse reactions to chamomile appear to be very rare.[7] Consumption of large doses has been noted to cause emesis.[3, 7, 9]

LD_{50} of oral (-)α-bisabolol in rats is 14.85g/kg and in mice 11.35g/kg[7]
LD_{50} for orally administered chamazulene in rats is 10g/kg[7]
LD_{50} of oral German chamomile oil in mice is 2.5mL/Kg[25]
LD_{50} of oral German chamomile oil in rats exceeded 5g/Kg[43]

CAUTIONS/CONTRAINDICATIONS

Cross-sensitivity is known to exist between different members of the Asteraceae (also known as Compositae) family.[7, 33-35] Given this, individuals with a known allergy to other members of the Asteraceae/Compositae family (e.g., ragweed, asters, chrysanthemums) should be cautious in taking products containing German chamomile.[3, 5, 9] Individuals with existing asthma, urticaria or other allergic conditions should also use chamomile products with caution due to a chance of exacerbation of their symptoms.[3]

German chamomile and the constituent (-)α-bisabolol have been shown to have no teratogenic potential in animal studies.[36] Resorption of fetuses and reduction in birth weight were observed in rats given very high doses of German chamomile.[36] However, no specific contraindications or warnings for use in pregnancy or lactation were found in the literature.[9] In addition, no information was found regarding the potential for sensitization of infants when breast-fed by mothers drinking chamomile tea. However, Newall cautions against applying chamomile products to the gums of teething children.[3] While no reason was given, it is assumed that this warning relates to the potential induction of an allergenic response.

DOSE REGIMEN

Infusion:

The most popular dosage form of chamomile is an infusion. Instructions for the preparation of an infusion are given below:

Pour hot water (150mL) over a heaped tablespoonful of German chamomile flowers (approx. 3g), cover, and after 5-10 minutes, pass through a tea strainer. Unless otherwise prescribed for gastrointestinal complaints a cup of the freshly prepared tea is drunk three or four times a day between meals. For inflammation of the mucous membranes of the mouth and throat, use the freshly prepared tea as a wash or gargle.[27]

Since a large proportion of the medicinally active components are contained in the volatile oil, it is important to cover the container while making the infusion.[44]

Other Oral Dose Regimens

- 1-4mL liquid extract (1:1,45% ethanol) three times daily[1]
- 3-10mL tincture (1:5, 45% ethanol) three times daily[1]
- 2-4g of dried flower heads three times daily[1]

External:

- Topical preparations are usually 3-10% w/w of chamomile.[1, 9]

Since adulteration is common place, attempts should be made to authenticate the source of the plant contained in any product.[7] While not widely available in North America, European products such as Kamillosan® exist that are standardized and authenticated.[5, 35]

REFERENCES

1. Bradley P. *British Herbal Compendium*. Bournemouth: BHMA; 1992:239.
2. Wren R. Potter's *New Encyclopedia of Botanical Drugs and Preparations.* Saffron Walden: C.W. Daniel Company; 1988:362.
3. Newall C, Anderson L, David Phillipson J. *Herbal Medicines: A Guide for Health Care Professionals.* London: The Pharmaceutical Press; 1996:296.
4. Leung A, S F. *Encyclopedia of Common Natural Ingredient Used in Food, Drugs and Cosmetics.* 2nd ed. New York, NY: John Wiley and Sons; 1996:649.
5. Berry M. The Chamomiles. *The Pharmaceutical Journal.* 1995;254:191-193.
6. Tyler V. *The Honest Herbal.* 3rd ed. Binghampton, NY: Pharmaceutical Products Press; 1993:375.
7. Mann C, Staba EJ. *The Chemistry, Pharmacology, and Commercial Formulations of Chamomile. Herbs, Spices and Medicinal Plants.* 1984;1:235-280.
8. Brown D. Anxiolytic effects of chamomile modulated through central benzodiazepine receptors. *Quarterly Review of Natural Medicine.* 1996;4(2):87-88.
9. Brown D. *Herbal Prescriptions for Better Health.* Rocklin, CA: Prima Publishing; 1995:349.
10. Tyler V. *The Honest Herbal.* 3rd ed. Binghamton, NY: Pharmaceutical Products Press; 1993:375.
11. Isaac O. Pharmakologische Untersuchungen von Kamillen-Inhaltsstoffen.1.Zur Pharmakologie des (-)-alpha Bisabolols under der Bisabololoxide (Ubersicht)/Pharmacological investigations with Compounds of Chamomile 1. On the Pharmacology of (-)-α-Bisabolol and Bisabolol oxides (Review). *Planta Medica.* 1979;35:118-123.
12. Achterrath-Tuckermann U, Kunde R, Flaskamp E, *et al.* Pharmacological investigations with com pounds of Chamomile V. Investigations on the spasmolytic effect of compounds of chamomile and kamillosan on the isolated guinea gig ileum. *Planta Medica.* 1980;39:38-50.
13. Della Loggia R, Carle R, Sosa S, Tubaro A. Evaluation of the anti-inflammatory activity of chamomile preparations. *Planta Medica.* 1990;56:657-658.

14. Jakovlev V, Isaac O, Thiemer K, Kunde R. Pharmacological investigations with compounds of chamomile II. New investigations on the antiphlogistic effects of (-) - alpha bisabolol and bisabolol oxides. *Planta Medica.* 1979;35:125-140.
15. Szelenyi I, Isaac O, Thiemer K. Pharmacological experiments with compounds of chamomile III. Experimental studies of the ulceroprotective effect of chamomile. *Planta Medica.* 1979;35:218-227.
16. Jakovlev V, Isaac O, Flakamp E. Pharmacological investigations with compounds of chamomile VI. Investigations on the antiphlogistic effects of chamazulene and matricine. *Planta Medica.* 1983;49:67-73.
17. Safayhi H, Sabieraj J, Sailer E, Ammon H. Chamazulene: An antioxidant-type inhibitor of leukotriene B4 formation. *Planta Medica.* 1994;60(5):410-3.
18. Rekka E, Kourounakis A, Kourounakis P. Investigation of the effect of chamazulene on lipid peroxidation and free radical processes. *Research Communications in Molecular Pathology and Pharmacology.* 1996;92(3):361-4.
19. Holzl J, Ghassemi N, Hahn B. Preparation of 14C-spiro ethers by chamomile and their use by an investigation of absorption. Planta Medica. 1986;52:533.
20. Viola H, Wasowski C, Levi de Stein M, *et al.* Apigenin, a component of *Matricaria recutita* flowers, is a central benzodiazepine receptors-ligand with anxiolyic effects. *Planta Medica.* 1995;61:213-216.
21. Miller T, Wittstock U, Lindequist U, Teuscher E. Effects of some components of the essential oil of chamomile, Chamomila recutita on histamine release from rat mast cells. *Planta Medica.* 1996;62:60-61.
22. Wagner H. The immune stimulating polysaccharides and heteroglycans of higher plants. A preliminary communication. *Arzneimittelforschung.* 1984;34(6):659-661.
23. Mills S. *The Essential Book of Herbal Medicine.* 2nd ed. London: Penguin Publ; 1991:677.
24. Von Grochulski A, Borkowski B. Influence of chamomile oil on experimental glomerulonephritis in rabbits. *Planta Medica.* 1972;21:289-292.
25. Ikram M. Medicinal Plants as hypocholesterlemic agents. *Journal of the Pakistan Medical Association.* 1980;30:278-282.
26. Suganda A, Amoros M, Fauconnier B. Effets inhibiteurs de quelques extraits bruts et semi purifies de plantes indigenes Francaises sur la multiplication de l'herpes virus humain 1 et du poliovirus humain 2 en culture cellulaire. *Journal of Natural Products.* 1983;46(5):626-632.
27. Blumenthal M, Brusse WR, Goldberg A, *et al. The Complete German Commission E Monographs.* Austin, TX: American Botanical Council; 1998:685.
28. Carl W, Emrich L. Management of oral mucositis during local radiation and systemic chemotherapy:A study of 98 patients. *Journal of Prosthetic Dentistry.* 1991;66:361-9.
29. Fidler P, Loprinzi C, O'Fallon J, *et al.* Prospective evaluation of a chamomile mouthwash for prevention of 5 FU induced oral mucositis. *Cancer.* 1996;77(3):522-5.
30. Tubaro A, Zilli C, Redaelli C, Della Loggia R. Evaluation of anti-inflammatory activity of a chamomile extract after topical application. *Planta Medica.* 1984;51:359.
31. Korting H, Schafer-Korting M, Hart H, *et al.* Anti-inflammatory activity of hamamelis distillate applied topically to the skin. *European Journal of Clinical Pharmacology.* 1993;44:315-318.
32. Merfort I, Heilmann J, Hagedorn-Leweke U, Lippold B. *In vivo* skin penetration studies of chamomile flavones. *Pharmazie.* 1994;49:509-11.
33. Paulsen E, Andersen K, Hausen B. Compositae dermatitis in a Danish dermatology department in one year. *Contact Dermatitis.* 1993;29:6-10.
34. Hausen B. The sensitizing capacity of Compositae plants III. Test results and cross reactions in Compositae-sensitive patients. *Dermatologica.* 1979;159:1-11.
35. Hausen B, Busker E, Carle R. The sensitizing capacity of Compositae Ppants. VII. Experimental investigations with extracts of *Chamomila recutita* (L.) Rauschert and *Anthemis cotula* L. *Planta Medica.* 1984;50:229-234.
36. Habersing S, Leuschner F, Isaac O, Theimer K. Pharmacological studies with compounds of Chamomile IV. Studies on toxicity of (-) alpha bisabolol. *Planta Medica.* 1979;37:115-123.
37. Benner M, Lee H. Anaphylactic reaction to chamomile tea. *Journal of Allergy and Clinical Immunology.* 1973;52:307-308.
38. Van Ketel W. Allergy to *Matricaria chamomila. Contact Dermatitis.* 1987;16:50-51.
39. Casterline C. Allergy to chamomile tea. *Journal of the American Medical Association.* 1980;4:330-331.
40. Hausen B. A 6-year experience with Compositae mix. *American Journal of Contact Dermatitis.* 1996;7(2):94-9.
41. Mitchell J, Dupuis G. Allergic contact dermatitis from sesquiterpenoids of the Compositae family of plants. *British Journal of Dermatology.* 1971;84:139-150.

42. Harris B, Lewis R. Advances in aromatherapy — Chamomile Part 1. *International Journal of Alternative and Complementary Medicine*. 1994; September : 12.
43. Opdyke D. Chamomile oil — German. *Food and Cosmetics Toxicology*. 1974;12:851-852.
44. Grieves M. *A Modern Herbal.* London: Pen-Johnson; 1931:912.

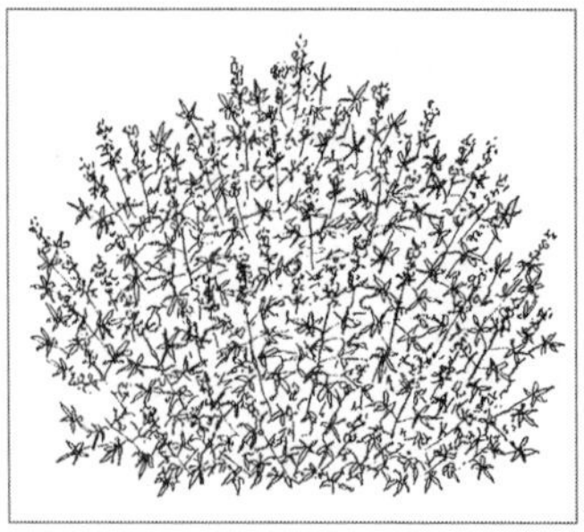

CHASTE TREE

Vitex agnus-castus L.

THUMBNAIL SKETCH

Active Constituents

The action of *Vitex agnus-castus* appears to be determined by a number of different constituents. The iridoid agnuside is often used as a marker molecule to confirm authenticity.

Common Uses

Symptoms of premenstrual syndrome, mastodynia, acne resulting from a hormonal imbalance, insufficient lactation, symptoms of menopause, situations associated with hyperprolactinemia, and menstrual cycle irregularities.

Adverse Effects

While rare, the following have been noted: nausea, headache, menstrual irregularities, diarrhea, dyspepsia, acne, and pruritus.

Cautions/Contraindications

- Avoid in pregnancy and children.

Drug Interactions

- Avoid with oral contraceptives and hormone replacement therapy.
- Theoretical interaction with dopamine antagonists such as haloperidol and metoclopramide

Doses

- 40 drops of an extract standardized to fruit content (9g/100mL) daily.
- Treatment should be continued for several months.

INTRODUCTION

Family: Verbenaceae

Synonyms: Chasteberry, Agnus-castus, Monk's pepper[1]

Chaste tree is a deciduous shrub native to Mediterranean Europe and central Asia. The distinctive purple peppercorn size berries are the parts used medicinally.[2] The plant has been used since the time of ancient Greece and Rome where it played a part in religious ceremonies and medicinal practice. It was reputed to decrease libido in women and was used to 'secure' chastity. It was included in monks' diets, was planted liberally in the grounds of many Catholic monasteries and worn in the clothing in order to promote celibacy.[2-4]

Chaste tree is considered of particular importance in women's health care. It is indicated for the unpleasant consequences of menses and menopause due to its amphoteric, or balancing quality.[5] *Vitex agnus-castus* is considered one of the major galactagues, increasing lactation in nursing mothers.[3, 4]

Constituents [1, 2, 6-11]

- Flavonoids: isovitexin, orientin, castican, chrysophanol D
- Iridoids: aucubin, agnuside, and eurostide
- Volatile oil: a mixture of monoterpenes and sesquiterpenes including cineol, limonene, and pinene
- Essential Fatty acids: linoleic acid
- Miscellaneous: vitamin C, carotenes, castine (a bitter principle)

It should be noted that the whole plant extract (rather than one constituent in particular) is considered medicinally active. The flavonoid agnuside is often used as a reference constituent as a measure of authenticity.[3]

Ketosteroids, with a structure similar to sex hormones, have been isolated from the leaves and flowers. The clinical relevance of this is unknown since these plant parts are rarely used medicinally. [4]

THERAPEUTIC USES & RELEVANT PHARMACOLOGY

WOMEN'S HEALTH CARE

Agnus-castus has been reported to be useful in the management of many 'female' conditions including: premenstrual syndrome, mastodynia, premenstrual acne, unpleasant consequences of menopause, insufficient lactation in nursing mothers, menopause and ailments resulting from corpus luteum insufficiency.

Premenstrual Syndrome

One study (n=36) of women diagnosed with pre-menstrual syndrome (PMS) found a generalized improvement in both the physical and psychological symptom picture at a dose of 40 drops of a proprietary brand of agnus-castus tincture (Agnolyt®) daily over three months. Normalization in the luteal phase was also noted.[12] This is supported by an uncontrolled, observational study conducted with women (n=1542, mean age=34.7 years) diagnosed with PMS in which Agnolyt® was shown to be useful. Results were based on patient and physician assessment. A majority of patients noted either complete relief (33%) or improvement (57%) in their symptoms. These favorable results were supported by the physician assessment (71%=very good; 21% = satisfactory). The dose given was 40 drops daily, with improvement being seen after 25 days.[13]

Other Menstrual Disorders

Loch *et al.* demonstrated in an uncontrolled observational study of 2447 women presenting with a variety of menstrual disorders (including menorrhagia, hypomenorrhea, hypermenorrhea, metrorrhagia and dysmenorrhea) that a *Vitex agnus-castus* tincture (42 drops daily, mean duration of treatment of 153 days) was therapeutically effective. Both patients and physicians noted an appreciable improvement in symptoms. Instances of multiple diagnoses and concurrent drug use were noted but not controlled for.[14] These favorable findings are supported by a multi-center trial in women (n=1571) presenting with menstrual disorders. At a dose of 40 drops of Agnolyt® daily, with a mean treatment time of 135 days, improvement was noted in 89.1% of cases.[15]

In a placebo controlled trial using another commercial product, Mastodynon®, Kubista *et al.* demonstrated a 74.5% improvement (as determined by the use of a 'pain scale') in women (n=55) suffering from severe mastopathy with cyclic mastodynia. There was no statistically significant change in prolactin or progesterone levels.[16]

Many studies have indicated that agnus-castus may prove useful in situations of abnormal menstrual cycle including: normalization of menstrual flow in women suffering from polymenorrhea;[17] decreased bleeding in cases of menorrhagia;[17] pregnancies in cases of both long-standing primary and secondary infertility;[17] increase in progesterone levels in women suffering from compromised corpus luteum function;[18] and secondary amenorrhea.[14]

Lactation

As mentioned above, one of the primary indications of agnus-castus is that of a galactagogue (i.e., increasing production of milk in nursing mothers). Two studies have supported this indication.[1, 19] In practice, the onset of action takes several weeks, but the increase in production is marked.[2, 3]

Hyperprolactinemia

In a randomized double blind, placebo controlled trial in women (n=52) suffering luteal phase defects due to latent hyperprolactinemia, a commercial brand of agnus-castus (Strotan®), given as 20mg daily, was shown to be beneficial. Latent hyperprolactinemia was evaluated by monitoring prolactin levels 15 minutes and 30 minutes after an IV injection of 200 micrograms of Thyroxin Releasing Hormone (TRH). After three months it was noted in the test group that prolactin levels were decreased, shortened luteal phases normalized and progesterone deficits eliminated when compared to the placebo group. With the exception of a luteal rise in 17 beta-estradiol in the test group, all other hormonal parameters were unchanged.[20]

Mechanism of Action

It has been suggested that the mechanism of action of agnus-castus is centrally mediated, rather than a direct hormone-like action.[21] Weiss hypothesized that by acting at the level of the pituitary, it promotes LH (luteinizing hormone) and inhibits FSH (follicle stimulating hormone) release.[22] This consequently results in an increase in progesterone levels at the expense of estrogen. Many practitioners have noted that chaste tree appears more progesteronal than estrogenic in nature.[4] However, a study demonstrated that agnus-castus did not influence FSH or LH, either basal levels or when stimulated by addition of luteinizing hormone releasing hormone (LHRH).[23]

Latent hyperprolactinemia has long been known to accompany many of the unpleasant symptoms of premenstrual syndrome, particularly mastodynia.[24-26] It has been hypothesized that the medicinal action of agnus-castus is primarily due to its action on prolactin levels.[21] *In vitro* and *in vivo* experiments have shown that components of agnus-castus inhibit secretion of prolactin, decreasing basal levels and when stimulated by administration of thyroxin releasing hormone (TRH).[27, 28] Further this action is antagonized with administration of a dopamine antagonist (haloperidol), suggesting that constituents present in agnus-castus bind directly to central dopamine receptors.[27, 28] It has also been noted that agnus-castus contains an agent or agents with affinity for both the D1 and D2 receptors.[23, 29] It appears that the action of agnus-castus on prolactin levels is not due to any cytotoxic effects.[29] While this goes some way to explaining the therapeutic properties of agnus-castus, a complete pharmacology is yet to be elucidated and it is unlikely that its medicinal action is solely due to its influence on the dopaminergic system.[21]

Other studies suggest that whether agnus-castus exerts an antagonistic or agonistic action on prolactin levels may be dependent on both basal levels and drug dose.[30] In a recent trial performed in healthy male subjects (n=20), it was demonstrated that at low doses an antagonistic quality was predominant, the reverse being seen at higher doses. It was also noted that there was a 'smoothing out' effect (decrease in the extent and frequency of prolactin concentration peaks and troughs) independent of the dose given. The authors make the assumption that this specific extract of agnus-castus contained both antagonistic and agonistic constituents acting possibly at different sites. It was also noted that the initial level of prolactin concentration also effected the action of the extract-tested. The unblinded nature of this study and the small number of participants should be noted. Male subjects were selected because they tend to have more stable prolactin levels than women.[30]

Miscellaneous

There were numerous instances of pregnancy reported in the trials discussed above, including in women with established infertility.[17, 18, 20, 31]

A number of uncontrolled studies have suggested that agnus-castus may prove useful in the management of acne vulgaris of a hormonal etiology.[32]

It has been reported that chaste tree, either alone or combined with other herbal medicines, may prove useful in the management of the unpleasant consequences of menopause, notably fluid retention, hot-flushing, anxiety and depression.[2]

ADVERSE EFFECTS

Adverse effects seem to be quite rare with agnus-castus. Situations of dry mouth, disturbed sleep, tachycardia, nausea, allergic skin reaction, vomiting, sensation of epigastric pressure, confusion, giddiness, acne, pruritus, alopecia, erythema and headache have been noted in some studies.[13, 14, 30]

Changes in menses including increased flow and changes in cycle have also been noted.[3] One instance of multiple follicular development was described in a patient undergoing unstimulated *in vitro* fertilization treatment upon introduction of a herbal medicine containing *Vitex agnus-castus*.[33] Although no similar situations are reported in the literature,[34, 35] the author of the original article suggests caution in this application.[36]

CAUTIONS/CONTRAINDICATIONS

Vitex agnus-castus should not be used in children or during pregnancy.[4] Although it is reputed to stimulate milk production,[1, 19] concerns have been raised regarding its use for this purpose given the lack of conclusive information.[1]

DRUG INTERACTIONS

It is advisable not to use agnus-castus with oral contraceptives or hormone replacement therapy.[4] *Vitex agnus-castus* should also be used with caution in individuals taking dopamine antagonists such as haloperidol and metoclopramide.[21]

DOSAGE REGIMENS

Many of the clinical trials mentioned above have been carried out using a commercial brand of alcohol based tincture standardized to fruit content (9g/100mL of tincture) called Agnolyt®. The suggested daily dose is 40 drops daily.[4]

OTHER REGIMENS

- Fruit: 0.5-1g three times daily[1]
- Tincture: 0.2-0.4mL (1:2) or 3 to 10mL (1:5) daily[4]

Many authors note that agnus-castus does not have an immediate action. Treatment should be uninterrupted and last for several months when used for most of the above indications. In certain situations, the duration of treatment should be appreciably longer (e.g., 5 to 7 months for anovulatory cycles and infertility and up to 18 months for secondary amenorrhea of longer than 2 years).[3]

REFERENCES

1. Newall C, Anderson L, David Phillipson J. *Herbal Medicines: A Guide for Health Care Professionals.* London: The Pharmaceutical Press; 1996:296.
2. Du Mee C. *Vitex agnus castus. Australian Journal of Medical Herbalism.* 1993;5(3):63-65.
3. Brown D. *Vitex agnus castus* Clinical Monograph. *Quarterly Review of Natural Medicine.* 1994;2(2):111-121.
4. Houghton P. Agnus castus. *The Pharmaceutical Journal.* 1994;253:720-721.
5. Mills S. *The Essential Book of Herbal Medicine.* 2nd ed. London: Penguin ; 1991:677.
6. Belic I, *et al.* Constituents of *Vitex agnus castus* seeds. Part 1. *Journal of the Chemical Society.* 1961:2523-2525.
7. Gomaa C, El-Moghazy M, Halim F, El-Sayyad A. Flavonoids and iridoids from *Vitex agnus castus. Planta Medica.* 1978;33:227.
8. Wollenweber E, Mann K. Flavonols from fruits of *Vitex agnus castus. Planta Medica.* 1983;48:126-127.
9. Rimpler H. Iridoids and Ecdysones from Vitex species. *Phytochemistry.* 1972;11:2653-2654.

10. Kustrak D, Kuftinec J, Blazevic N. The composition of the essential oil of *Vitex agnus castus*. *Planta Medica*. 1992;58(Supp.1):A681.
11. Zwavig J, Bos R. Composition of the essential fruit oil of *Vitex agnus castus*. *Pharmacy World and Science*. 1993;15(6): Supp H15.
12. Coeugniet E, Elek E, Kuhnast R. Premenstrual syndrome (PMS) and its treatment. *Arztezitchr Naturheilverf*. 1986;27(9):619-22.
13. Dittmar F, Bohnert K, Peeters M. Premenstrual syndrome: Treatment with a phytopharmaceutical. *Therapiewoche Gynakol*. 1992;5(1):60-8.
14. Loch E, Bohnert K, Peeters M. The treatment of menstrual disorders with *Vitex Agnus castus* tincture. *Der Frauenarzt*. 1991;32(8):867-70.
15. Marie-Snow J. *Vitex agnus-castus* L. *The Protocol Journal of Botanical Medicine*. 1996;1(4):20-23.
16. Kubista E, Muller G, Spona J. Treatment of mastopathy with cyclic mastodynia. Clinical results and hormone profiles. *Gynakologische Rundschav*. 1986;26:65-79.
17. Bleier W. Therapie von Zyklus und Blutungsstorungen und weiteren endokrin bedingten Erkrankungen der Frau mit pflanzlichen Wirkstoffen. *Zentralblatt Fur Gynakologie*. 1959;81(18):701-709.
18. Propping D, Katzorke T, Belkein I. Diagnosis and therapy of corpus luteum defiociency in general practice. *Therapiewoche*. 1988;38:2992-3001.
19. Bruckner C. In mitteleuropa genutze heilpflanzen mit milchsekretionsfordernder wirkung (galactagoga). *Gleditschia*. 1989;17:189-210.
20. Milewicz A, Gejdel E, Sworen H, *et al*. *Vitex agnus-castus* extract in the treatment of luteal phase defects due to latent hyperprolactinemia: Results of a randomised placebo-controlled double-blind study*Arzneimittelforschung* 1993;43(7):752-6.
21. Bohnert K. The Use of *Vitex agnus castus* for hyperprolactinemia. *Quarterly Review of Natural Medicine*. 1997;5(1):19-21.
22. Weiss R. *Herbal Medicine*. Beaconsfield: Beaconsfield Publishers; 1988:362.
23. Jarry H, Leonhardt S, Gorkow C, Wuttke W. *In vitro* prolactin but not LSH and FSH release is inhibited by com pounds in extracts of Agnus Castus: direct evidence for a dopaminergic principle by the dopamine receptor assay. *Experimental and Clinical Endocrinology*. 1994;102:448-454.
24. Muhlenstedt D, Bohnet H, Hanker J, Schneider H. Short luteal phase and prolactin. *International Journal of Fertility*. 1978;23(3):213-218.
25. Carroll B, Steiner M. The psychobiology of premenstrual dyphoria: The role of prolactin. *Psychoneuroendocrinology*. 1978;3:171-180.
26. Halbreich U, Assael M, Ben-David M, Bornstein R. Serum Prolactin in women with premenstrual syndrome. *Lancet*. 1976:654-656.
27. Sliutz G, Speiser P, Schultz A, Spona J, Zellinger R. *Agnus castus* extracts inhibit prolactin secretion of rat pituitary cells. *Hormone and Metabolic Research*. 1993;25:253-255.
28. Jarry H, Leonhardt S, Wuttke W. *Agnus castus* as dopaminergous effective principle in Mastodynon N. *Zeitschrift Phytother*. 1991;12:77-82.
29. Wuttke W. Dopaminergic Action of extracts of *Agnus castus*. [Abstract]. *Forschende Komplementarmedizen*. 1996;3(6):329-330.
30. Merz P, Gorkow C, Schroder A, *et al*. The effects of a special *Agnus castus* extract (BP1095e1) on prolactin secretion in healthy male subjects. *Endocrinology and Diabetes*. 1996;104:447-453.
31. Propping D, Katzorke T. Treatment of corpus luteum insufficiency. *Zeits Allgemeinmedizin*. 1987;63:932-3.
32. Amann W. *Akne vulgaris* und *agnus castus* (Agnolyt). *Zeits Allgemeinmedizin*. 1975;14:1645-1648.
33. Cahill D, Fox R, Wardle P, Harlow C. Multiple follicular development associated with herbal medicine. *Human Reproduction*. 1994;9(8)(Aug):1469-70.
34. Propping D. Multiple follicular development associated with a herbal medicine. *Human Reproduction*. 1995;10(8):2175.
35. Brown D. Vitex and multiple follicular development. *Quarterly Review of Natural Medicine*. 1995;3(2):105-106.
36. Cahill D. Comment. *Human Reproduction*. 1995;10(8):2175-6.

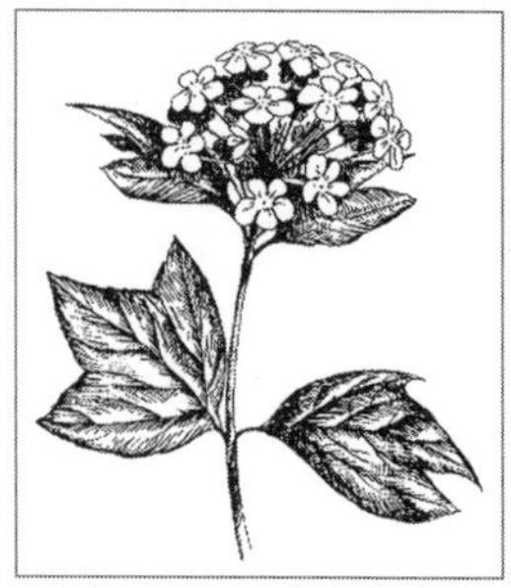

CRANBERRY

Vaccinium macrocarpon Ait.

THUMBNAIL SKETCH

Active Constituents

- Fructose
- An unidentified large molecular weight compound

Common Uses

- Prevention of urinary tract infections

Adverse Effects

- None known

Cautions/Contraindications

- None known

Drug Interactions

- None known

Doses

- 150 mL to 600 mL cranberry juice daily
- 300 to 400 mg concentrated cranberry juice capsules twice daily

INTRODUCTION

Family: Ericaceae

Synonyms: *Oxycoccus macrocarpus* (Ait.) Pursh[1]

Cranberry is native to the marshland of Northern Europe, Eastern Canada, and the Eastern United States. It is a leathery-leaved evergreen with characteristic shiny red berries and pale pink flowers.[2] Folk wisdom has long held that drinking cranberry juice will prevent urinary tract infections. Early clinical trials generally supported this claim; however, there were some negative findings and much controversy over the hypothesized mechanism of action. A recent large clinical trial aimed at ending the controversy found cranberry juice to be clinically effective in the prevention of urinary tract infections, but has generated controversy of its own.

Constituents[1, 2]

The berries contain:

- Proanthocyanidins
- Fructose
- Flavonol glycosides: leptosine
- Catechin
- Triterpenoids
- Organic Acids: citric acid, malic acid, benzoic acid, quinic acid
- Miscellaneous: vitamin C, unidentified large molecular weight molecule

THERAPEUTIC USES & RELEVANT PHARMACOLOGY

PREVENTION AND TREATMENT OF URINARY TRACT INFECTIONS

Many early trials of the effectiveness of cranberry for the prevention and/or treatment or urinary tract infections involved small numbers of participants and were not blinded or controlled.[3-6] Similar criticism may be made of relatively recent clinical trials that have suggested that cranberry juice may be useful for the prevention and/or treatment of urinary tract infections.[7, 8] One non-blinded, uncontrolled clinical trial involved 28 elderly patients in a long-term health care facility (a population at high risk for urinary tract infections) who drank 120 to 180 mL of Ocean Spray Cranberry Juice Cocktail® daily for 7 weeks. Mid-stream clean catch urines (or catheterized urines for 3 patients) were obtained biweekly for 7 weeks. The authors report that 19 of the 28 patients showed no evidence of urinary tract infection during the study period, while in the remaining 9 they found leukocytes and/or nitrates in the urine and significant presence of gram negative bacilli. The authors conclude that their study provides evidence that drinking cranberry juice product may prevent urinary tract infections.[7] In a similar study, 21 patients took 12 capsules containing 800 mg cranberry (Pharmacaps ®) daily. There was no incidence of urinary tract infections in 20 patients. The same cranberry product was tested in 6 patients with pre-existing urinary tract infections and no cures were reported.[9] Larger, randomized, double-blinded studies were definitely needed.

In an attempt to fill this void, a recent randomized, double-blind, placebo-controlled trial was conducted with 153 elderly women who ingested 300 mL of commercially available cranberry beverage or placebo daily for 6 months. The authors concluded that the frequency of bacteriuria with pyuria was significantly decreased (after 4 to 8 weeks) in the cranberry group in comparison with the placebo group. In addition, there was a decrease in the rate of antibiotics prescribed by physicians to treat urinary tract infections in the cranberry group, suggesting a clinically relevant effect of ingesting cranberry juice.[8] However, this study was criticized in several letters.[10-13] These criticisms, including the difficulties of obtaining "clean-voided specimens",[12] and that the two groups may not have had the same base-line frequency of urinary tract infections,[10, 13] are adequately addressed by the authors.[14] Another small, (n=17) randomized, controlled, cross-over trial confirms these findings.[15]

Mechanism of Action

The original hypothesis was that cranberry juice acted by increasing urine acidity;[5, 6, 16-18] however other studies have challenged this theory.[8, 19-21] The most popular theory currently is that cranberry possesses "anti-adherence" properties, which prevent bacteria from attaching to the lining of the urinary tract.[22-24] For example, two compounds have been found in cranberry that inhibit the adhesion of *Escherichia coli* to urinary tract cells. Fructose, found in all fruit juices, and another as yet unidentified compound (found in cranberry and blueberry juice only) have been shown to inhibit *Escherichia coli* fimbrial adhesions.[25]

MISCELLANEOUS

Anticancer Activity

In vitro screening tests have suggested that the proanthocyanidin fraction of cranberry has potential anticarcinogenic activity.[26]

ADVERSE EFFECTS

None reported.

CAUTIONS/CONTRAINDICATIONS

None reported.

DRUG INTERACTIONS

None reported.

DOSAGE REGIMENS

Prevention of urinary tract infections:

- 150 mL to 600 mL cranberry juice daily[7, 22]
- 300 to 400 mg concentrated cranberry juice capsules twice daily[27]

Note: Cranberry juice should not be used as a substitute for antibiotics in acute urinary tract infections.

REFERENCES

1. Marles RJ, Associate Professor, Department of Botany, Brandon University, Brandon, Manitoba. Review of Medicinal Plant Modules for CCNM; 1997.
2. Leung AY, Foster S. *Encyclopedia of Common Natural Ingredients Used in Food, Drugs, and Cosmetics.* 2nd ed. New York, NY: John Wiley and Sons Inc; 1996:649.
3. Papas PN, Brusch CA, Ceresia GC. Cranberry juice in the treatment of urinary tract infections. *Southwestern Medicine*. 1966; 47(1): 17-20.
4. Zinsser HH. Newer antibacterial drugs in urological infections. *Medical Clinics of North America.* 1964; 48: 293-304.
5. Bodel PT, Cotran R, Kass E. Cranberry juice and the antibacterial activity of hippuric acid. *Journal of Laboratory and Clinical Medicine.* 1959;64:881.
6. Kahn DH, Panariello V, Saeli J, *et al.* Effect of cranberry juice on urine. *Journal of the American Diet Association*. 1967; 51: 251.
7. Gibson L, Pike L, Kilbourn JP. Effectiveness of cranberry juice in preventing urinary tract infections in long-term care facility patients. *The Journal of Naturopathic Medicine*. 1991; 2(1): 45-7.
8. Avorn J, Manone M, Gurwitz JH, Glynn RJ, Choodnovskiy I, Lipsitz LA. Reduction of bacteriuria and pyuria after ingestion of cranberry juice. *Journal of the American Medical Association*. 1994; 271: 751-754.
9. Kilbourne JP. Cranberry juice appears to prevent urinary tract infections. *CCML Newsletter*. 1986;January.
10. Katz LM. Reduction of bacteriuria and pyuria using cranberry juice [Letter]. *Journal of the American Medical Association*. 1994; 272(8): 589.
11. Hamilton-Miller JMT. Reduction of bacteriuria and pyuria using cranberry juice [Letter]. *Journal of the American Medical Association*. 1994; 272(8): 588.
12. Goodfriend R. Reduction of bacteriuria and pyuria using cranberry juice [Letter]. *Journal of the American Medical Association*. 1994;272(8):588.
13. Hopkins W, J., Heisey D, M., Jonler M, Uehling DT. Reduction of bacteriuria and pyuria using cranberry juice (letter). *Journal of the American Medical Association*. 1994;272(8):588-9.
14. Avorn J, Maonone M, Gurwitz JH, Glynn RJ, Choodnosky I, Lipsitz LA. Reduction of bacteruria and pyuria using cranberry juice [Reply to letters]. *Journal of the American Medical Association.*1994;272(8):589.
15. Haverkorn MJ, Mandigers J. Reduction of bacteriuria and pyuria using cranberry juice. *Journal of the American Medical Association*. 1994;272(8):590.
16. Schultz AS. Efficacy of cranberry juice on urinary pH. *Journal of Community Health Nursing*. 1984;1:155-169.
17. Moen DV. Observations on the effectiveness of cranberry juice in urinary infections. *Wisconsin Medical Journal*. 1962; 61:282-283.
18. Kinney AB, Blount M. Effect of cranberry juice on urinary pH. *Nursing Research*. 1979;28:287-290.
19. Fellers CR, Redmon BC, Parrott EM. The effect of cranberries on urinary acidity and blood alkali reserve. *Journal of Nutrition*. 1933;6:455-463.
20. Nickey NE. Urine pH: effect of prescribed regimens of cranberry juice and ascorbic acid. *Archives of Physical Medicine and Rehabilitation.* 1975;55:556.
21. McLeod DC, Nahata MC. Methenamine therapy and urine acidification with ascorbic acid cranberry juice. *American Journal of Hospital Pharmacology*. 1978;35:654.
22. Sobota AE. Inhibition of bacterial adherence by cranberry juice: Potential use for the treatment of urinary tract infection. *Journal of Urology*. 1984;131:1013-1016.
23. Zafriri D, Ofek I, Adar R, *et al*. Inhibitory activity of cranberry juice on adherence of type I and type P fimbriated *Escherichia coli* to eukaryotic cells. *Antimicrobial Agents and Chemotherapy*. 1989;33(1):92-98.
24. Schmidt D, Sobota A. An examination of the anti-adherence activity of cranberry juice on urinary and nonurinary bacterial isolates. *Microbios*. 1988;55:173-181.
25. Ofek I, Goldhar J, Zafriri D, Lis H, *et al*. Anti-*Escherichia coli* adhesion activity of cranberry and blueberry juices [Letter]. *New England Journal of Medicine*. 1991;324:1599.
26. Bomser J, Madhavi DL, Singletary K, Smith MAL. In vitro anticancer activity of fruit extracts from *Vaccinium* species. *Planta Medica*. 1996;62:212-6.
27. Brown D. *Herbal Prescriptions for Better Health.* Rocklin, CA: Prima Publishing; 1996:349.

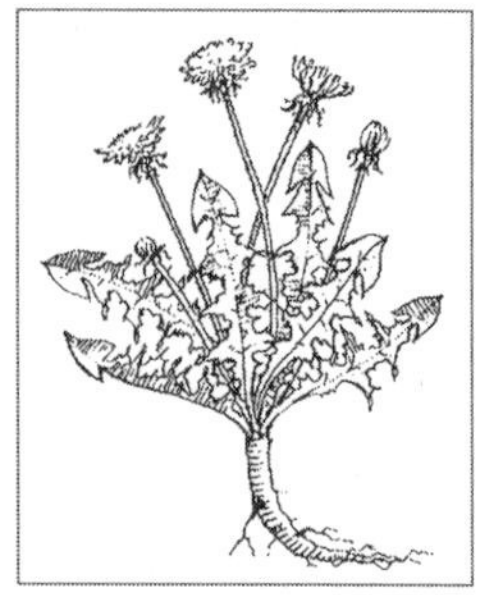

DANDELION

Taraxacum officinale G.H. Weber ex Wiggers

THUMBNAIL SKETCH

Active Constituents

- Terpenes/terpenoids
- Bitter principle
- Phytosterols
- Inulin
- Minerals (potassium)

Common Uses

- Root: Hepatobiliary disorders, dyspepsia, loss of appetite
- Leaves: Water retention.

Adverse Effects

- Possible contact dermatitis

Cautions/Contraindications

- Root: occlusion of the bile ducts, empyema, and paralytic ileus
- Leaves: occlusion of the bile ducts

Drug Interactions

- Leaf may potentiate the action of diuretics

Doses

- 4-10g of dried leaf three times daily
- 3-5g of dried root three times daily
- 4-10mL leaf liquid extract (1:1 in 25% alcohol) three times daily
- 5-10mL root tincture (1:5 in 45% extract) three times daily

INTRODUCTION

Family: Asteraceae (also known as Compositae)

Synonyms: Lion's tooth, Fairy clock, Wet-a-bed, Pissenlit, Dent-de-Lion, Irish daisy, Puffball, Swine's snout[1-3]

Taraxacum officinale is a perennial herb native to Europe but now found throughout North America.[4] Historically, members of the *Taraxacum* genus have been used by many cultures for their therapeutic properties. Dandelion is considered one of the primary herbs in the British herbal tradition, the roots being used for liver and digestive problems and the leaves for their 'diuretic' properties in cases of edema. This latter action is demonstrated eloquently by the French name, Pissenlit.[2, 3] Dandelion has also been used in conditions as varied as fevers, boils, diarrhea and hemorrhoids.[5] It has been used in China and the Indian subcontinent for various conditions including: snakebites, abscesses, appendicitis and for its nutritional value.[3]

Constituents[1, 2, 4, 6-8]

- Terpenoids including the triterpenoids: taraxerol, taraxacin, lactucin, and taraxasterol
- Acids: Chlorogenic acid, caffeic acid
- Carbohydrates: fructose, glucose, inulin, and sucrose. (During the summer the fructose in the root is converted into inulin, to be re-converted back in the winter.)
- Vitamins/Minerals: leaves are rich in potassium (297mg/100g), vitamin A (14 000 IU/100g), vitamin C, B complex, zinc, manganese, copper.
- Phytosterols: sitosterol, stigmasterol, taraxasterol, and campesterol. (The composition of the sterol portion found in the leaves undergoes extensive seasonal fluctuation.)
- Flavonoid glycosides: luteolin 7-glucoside, luteolin 7-diglucosides

Many references are made to the 'bitter principle' (also called taraxin) found primarily in dandelion root. This portion consists mainly of a mixture of sesquiterpene lactones and taraxacoside.[9]

THERAPEUTIC USES & RELEVANT PHARMACOLOGY

LIVER FUNCTION

Dandelion root plays a major part in modern herbal practice where it is considered to be a safe treatment used in the management of many liver related conditions.[2, 10] It is considered to be a both a choleretic (promoting production of bile) and a cholagogue (causing contraction of the bile duct initiating the flow of stored bile).[1, 3] These properties are firmly part of herbal tradition, and the limited clinical data available tend to support them. For example, studies have shown that administration of dandelion increased bile flow in dogs and rats and aided in the management of a variety of gall-bladder conditions.[3, 11] In addition, a product in which dandelion is one of nine ingredients has been used to treat hepatitis.[12]

Given the importance of the liver as an organ of elimination within the herbal tradition, dandelion root is thought to be a useful and protective adjunctive therapy to chemotherapy. [13]

DIURETIC ACTION

Racz-Kotilla *et al.* demonstrated (in rats and mice) that dandelion possessed diuretic properties when given in high doses. This study noted that an extract made from the leaves had a more pronounced diuretic action than the root. They found the 4% aqueous solution of dandelion leaf (15 mL/kg) had a diuretic effect comparable to furosemide at a dose of 80mg/kg.[14] This appears to confirm the distinction between leaf and root noted by herbalists.[2] Also noted was that a 4% aqueous leaf extract (8mL/kg) given for thirty days resulted in a marked weight loss.[14] In a more recent *in vivo* trial, no real diuretic effect was noted when an extract of *Taraxacum officinale* was administered to female wistar rats. Although no specifics were given regarding dose, the dandelion root was used in the preparation of the extract. Even though the diuretic action of dandelion has been shown in animal studies, the exact mechanism is as yet unknown. It appears that there may be numerous constituents playing a role in this function, including sesquiterpene lactones (found in the terpenoid portion), inulin and potassium.[15]

Since dandelion is rich in potassium, herbalists often advocate its use with herbs that have the potential for inducing hypokalemia.[2]

MISCELLANEOUS

Anti-microbial

Extracts made from dandelion pollen have been shown to exert an antimicrobial action against *Proteus, Escherichia* and *Salmonella in vitro*.[1]

Digestion

Dandelion root is described as a 'digestive bitter' and is often used in the treatment of dyspepsia and to stimulate the appetite.[2, 16, 17]

Hypoglycemia

A hypoglycemic action was noted in rabbits following esophageal administration. The fall in blood sugar was pronounced at high doses and it has been suggested that dandelion could be acting in a similar fashion to conventional sulphonylurea hypoglycemics.[18] Other trials have found contradictory results.[9]

Genitourinary

Investigators have hypothesized that the historical role of dandelion in the management of kidney stones could be due to the degradation of potential mucopolysaccharide foci by the saponins present in the plant.[19]

ADVERSE EFFECTS

Contact dermatitis has been noted after frequent exposure to the fresh herb.[20, 21] This is unlikely to be clinically important since most herbal products are made from the dried material.[15] Even when given as a large part of the diet (32%) for a prolonged period of time (209 days), dandelion root was not shown to have carcinogenic potential in rats.[22]

CAUTIONS/CONTRAINDICATIONS

- Leaf: Dandelion leaf should be used with caution in cases of occlusion of the bile ducts.[23]
- Root: Dandelion root should be used with caution in cases of: occlusion of the bile ducts and/or gall bladder, empyema and paralytic ileus.[23]
- Possible cross reactivity has been noted between different members of the Asteraceae/Compositae (Sunflower) family, including dandelion, in sensitive individuals.[24]
- Historical/anecdotal evidence suggests avoidance of excessive doses in pregnancy or lactation but no evidence has been published to support this claim.[6]

Since Dandelion is most often considered to be a weed by many gardeners, it is very often heavily sprayed with a variety of herbicides and pesticides. Thus, clients should be cautioned against collecting this herb from gardens, by roadsides or from crop fields.[3] It has also been noted that *Taraxacum officinale* growing in urban areas may contain enough heavy metals (lead, zinc and copper) to be potential harmful if taken orally.[25]

DRUG INTERACTIONS

No specific interactions between this plant and any pharmaceutical preparations could be found. Houghton suggests caution in using any herbal diuretic with conventional diuretics.[15]

DOSAGE REGIMEN

- 3-5g of dried root, by infusion or decoction, three times daily[23]
- 5-10mL of tincture from the root (1:5, 25% ethanol) three times daily[23]
- 4-10g of dried leaf, by infusion, three times daily[23]
- 4-10mL of leaf liquid extract (1:1 in 25% alcohol), three times daily[23]

It should be noted that the constituents of this plant, and arguably their medicinal action, change dramatically with the seasons. Generally speaking the roots are best collected between June and August when they are most bitter.[3]

REFERENCES

1. Cordatos E. *Taraxacum officinale. Textbook of Natural Medicine.* Seattle,WA: Bastyr University; 1992.
2. Mills S. *The Essential Book of Herbal Medicine*. 2nd ed. London: Penguin; 1991:677.
3. Blanchert K. Dandelion: Leaves are rich source of vitamins and minerals. *Alternative and Complementary Therapies*. 1995;1(2):115-117.
4. Leung A, Foster S *Encyclopedia of Common Natural Ingredients Used in Food, Drugs and Cosmetics*. 2nd ed. New York, NY: John Wiley and Sons; 1996:649.
5. Hobbs C. *Taraxacum officinale*: A monograph and literature review. *Eclectic Dispensatory*. Portland: Eclectic Medical Publication; 1989.
6. Newall C, Anderson L, David Phillipson J. *Herbal Medicines: A Guide for Health-care Professionals*. London: The Pharmaceutical Press; 1996:296.

7. Clifford M, Shutler S, Thomas G, Ohiokepehai O. The chlorogenic acids content of coffee substitutes. *Food Chem.* 1987;24:99-107.
8. Williams C, Goldstone F, Greenham J. Flavonoids, Cinnamic acids and coumarins from the different tissues and medicinal preparations of *Taraxacum officinale*. *Phytochemistry.* 1996;42(1):121-127.
9. Marles RJ, Associate Professor, Department of Botany, Brandon University, Brandon, Manitoba. Review of Medicinal Plant Modules for CCNM; 1997.
10. Stelling K. Restoring the Liver. *Canadian Journal of Herbalism*. 1991;12(11):7-10.
11. Faber K. The dandelion — *Taraxacum officinale* Weber. *Pharmazie*. 1958;13(7):423-435.
12. Sankaran J. Livr-Doks in viral hepatitis. *The Antiseptic*. 1977;74:621-626.
13. Stelling K, Salama, S, Salib M. Phytotherapy as an adjunct in cancer treatment. *Canadian Journal of Herbalism*. 1995(Winter):34-36.
14. Racz-Kotilla E, Racz G, Solomon A. The action of *Taraxacum officinale* extracts on the body weight and diuresis of laboratory animals. *Planta Medica*. 1974;26:212-217.
15. Houghton P. Bearberry, dandelion and celery. *The Pharmaceutical Journal*. 1995;255:272-273.
16. Hoffman D. *Holistic Herbal.* Rockport, MA: Element Books; 1996:256.
17. Chevallier A. *The Encyclopedia of Medicinal Plants.* London: Reader's Digest; 1996:336.
18. Akhtar MS, Khan Q, Khaliz T. Effects of *Portulaca oleracae* (kulfa) and *Taraxacum officinale* (dhudhal) in nor moglycaemic and alloxan-treated hyperglycaemic rabbits. *Journal of the Pakistan Medical Association*. 1985;35:207-210.
19. Grases F, Melero G, Costa-Bauza A, *et al*. Urolithiasis and phytotherapy. *International Urology and Nephrology*. 1994;26(5):507-11.
20. Lovell C, Rowan M. Dandelion dermatitis. *Contact Dermatitis*. 1991;25:185-188.
21. Dawe R, Green C, MacLeod T, Ferguson J. Daisy, dandelion and thistle contact allergy in the photosensitive dermatitis and actinic reticuloid syndrome. *Contact Dermatitis*. 1996;35:109-10.
22. Hirono I, Mori H, Kato K, Ushimaru Y. Safety examination of some edible plants. Part 2. *Journal of Environmental Pathology Toxicology and Oncology*. 1977;1:72-74.
23. Bradley P. *British Herbal Compendium*. Bournemouth: BHMA; 1992:239.
24. Fernandez C, Martin-Esteban M, Fiandor A, *et al.* Analysis of cross-reactivity between sunflower pollen and other pollens of the compositae family. *Journal of Allergy and Clinical Immunology*. 1993;92(5):660-7.
25. Cook C, Sgardelis S, Pantis J, Lanaras T. concentrations of Pb,Zn and Cu in Taraxacum spp. in relation to urban pollution. *Bulletin of Environmental Contamination and Toxicology.* 1994;53:204-210.

DEVIL'S CLAW

Harpagophytum procumbens DC.

THUMBNAIL SKETCH

Active Constituents

- Iridoid glycosides (harpaside, harpagoside)

Common Uses

- Inflammation of the joints including osteo-arthritis, rheumatoid arthritis and gout
- Indigestion and dyspepsia

Adverse Effects

- Mild digestive upset

Cautions/Contraindications

- Active peptic ulcer

Drug Interactions

- None

Doses

- 100-250 mg of dried tuber three times daily
- 1-2mL (1:1, 25% ethanol) liquid extract three times daily

INTRODUCTION

Family: Pedaliaceae

Synonyms: Harpagophytum, Grapple plant, Wood spider[1-3]

Devil's claw is a herbaceous plant native to Southern Africa, notably the Transvaal. It produces brilliant red/purple flowers and woody barbed fruit, which is responsible for its descriptive name. Decoctions of dried roots have long been taken as a tea by the indigenous peoples for a variety of digestive and rheumatic conditions.[2] It was introduced to Europe by Mehnert and became so popular that in 1976, it was estimated that 30 000 arthritic patients in the United Kingdom alone were using it.[4] The secondary tuber is the part principally used medicinally.[3]

Constituents[1, 3, 5-9]

- Iridoid glycosides: harpagide, harpagoside, and procumbide
- Phenolic Acids: chlorogenic acid, cinnamic acid
- Flavonoids: kaempferol, luteolin

Harpagoside, which appears to be the constituent of most interest, is primarily found in the secondary tubers.[3] The flowers, stem and ripe fruit appear to be devoid of this agent.[10]

THERAPEUTIC USES & RELEVANT PHARMACOLOGY

PHARMACOLOGY

Devil's claw has been reputed to have anti-inflammatory and anti-rheumatic properties.[2, 9, 11, 12] It is commonly used in the management of many inflammatory joint diseases such as osteo-arthritis, rheumatoid arthritis and gout.[9, 11, 12]

MUSCULOSKELETAL (ANTI-INFLAMMATORY)

Many authors have suggested that devil's claw can exert an anti-inflammatory action. Aqueous extracts of devil's claw were shown to possess anti-inflammatory activity in both rats and mice following intraperitoneal administration.[13, 14] The activity appeared greater in chronic rather than acute situations.[15] The anti-inflammatory properties were abolished after oral administration[13] or after an acid treatment.[14] Although harpagoside alone did not have appreciable anti-inflammatory properties, it did appear to exert a peripheral analgesic action.[14]

One study reported that an aqueous extract of devil's claw may possess an anti-inflammatory action comparable to phenylbutazone.[1] However, extracts of devil's claw were shown to possess no appreciable action in reducing rat hind paw edema induced by either carragennan or *Mycobacterium butyricum* when compared to standard NSAID agents.[16, 17] Even at doses far higher (100X) than the "standard recommended dose" of devil's claw, no inflammatory action was seen nor any inhibitory action on prostaglandin synthetase action noted.[16]

In an attempt to demonstrate a possible mechanism of anti-inflammatory action, Moussard *et al.* found that 500 mg of devil's claw (standardized to 3% total glucoiridoids per unit dose) had no influence on eicosanoid production. Human volunteers (aged 20-35 years) were divided into a control group (n=9) and treatment group (n=25). The volunteers took either the placebo or 4 caps of devil's claw daily for 21 days. The influence on both cyclooxygenase and lipoxygenase pathways were determined by using the spontaneously clotting whole human blood model performed on samples taken before and after the investigation. There was no statistically significant difference in blood clotting times between the two groups.[18]

Given the popularity of devil's claw as an herbal remedy, it is surprising to find only a few clinical trials. In one positive trial, 43 patients suffering from a range of degenerative arthritides were treated with 1.5 g daily of devils claw (Arkocaps®). Symptom improvement was noted after eight days, with marked improvement in pain (89%), range of motion (84%) and time needed for stiffness to wear off (86%).[19]

In contrast, several negative trials have been published. In an uncontrolled trial conducted in the United Kingdom, thirteen volunteers (34-71 years of age) suffering from various arthritic conditions (seropositive arthritis, seronegative rheumatoid arthritis, and psoriatic arthritis) were selected because they had failed to respond to conventional pharmaceutical care. Each was given 410 mg of aqueous extract three times daily for 6 weeks. While 4 patients showed some improvement in certain areas (more specific details were not published), there was no significant change in the symptoms of the group as a whole as determined by a variety of objective and subjective measures. It should be noted that the patients continued taking their conventional antirheumatic medications for the duration of this trial.[4] Another more recent randomized, placebo controlled, double blind four week study of 118 patients presenting with low back pain found that devils claw treatment was not significantly better than placebo treatment in two out of three outcome measures. The primary outcome measure was the amount of a specific opiod analgesic (Tramadol®) taken by patients in the last 3 weeks of the study. Secondary outcome measures included relief according to the Arhus low back pain index and the number of patients pain-free at the study's conclusion. While the number of patients pain free at the conclusion of the trial was significantly higher in the treatment group than in the placebo group, there was no significant difference between the groups with respect to the Arhus low back pain index or the amount of analgesic ingested.[20] This study has been criticized because the consumption of analgesic could not be equated with the subjective experience of pain.[21]

DIGESTIVE

Weiss classifies devil's claw as a 'bitter tonic' useful in the management of various gastrointestinal complaints including dyspepsia and digestive upsets due to poor gallbladder and/or pancreatic function.[2] An *in vitro* study has indicated that the iridoid components of devil's claw influence guinea pig ileum. Harpagoside was noted to decrease the contractile response caused by either acetylcholine or barium chloride. The authors infer that this could be a result of an action on the mechanism that controls influx of calcium into the cells.[22] Harpagide was also shown to exert a dose dependent action on the contractile response of guinea pig ileum, augmenting the response at low dose but inhibiting it at a higher one.[22]

MISCELLANEOUS

Cardiovascular

Crude methanolic extracts of *Harpagophytum procumbens* exert a dose dependent protective effect on experimental ventricular arrhythmias induced by various means in both rat and isolated rabbit heart.[23, 24] Some authors have suggested that this action is in part due to an inhibition of calcium influx into the myocardial cells since it was shown to be protective against arrhythmias induced by digitalis. This action appears to be the result of a synergistic interplay of constituents rather than solely the harpagoside.[24] Also noted was a positive inotropic effect at low doses and a negative inotropic effect at higher doses.[22, 24]

Antimicrobial

Extracts made from the secondary roots of devil's claw exerted weak anti-fungal action against various fungi.[25]

ADVERSE EFFECTS

A "slight digestive upset" was reported by two patients participating in one study.[19] One individual in another study reported morning frontal throbbing headache, tinnitus, severe anorexia and loss of appetite;[4] however, no attempt appears to have been made to determine whether these effects were due to the devil's claw product being investigated.

CAUTIONS/CONTRAINDICATIONS

Given the action of devil's claw as a classic bitter, theoretically it may increase gastric acid secretion. This fact has led to a caution of its use in cases of active peptic ulcer disease.[2, 9] Historically the use of devil's claw has been contraindicated in pregnancy due to its alleged 'abortifacient' action.[1] Although this situation could be due to a simple mistranslation, until more information is known, it is still a valid point of concern.[26]

DRUG INTERACTIONS

No interactions between this herb and any pharmaceutical preparations could be found. Given the influence in animal studies of *Harpagophytum procumbens* on cardiac muscle (mentioned above), its use in high doses may interact with cardiac and hypo/hypertensive therapy.[1]

DOSAGE REGIMENS

Many of the clinical trials described above used doses in the range of 400 to 500 mg dried herb three times daily.

Other doses often quoted include:[9]

For digestive indications:

- 500 mg of dried tuber in decoction three times daily
- 1mL of tincture (1:5; 25% ethanol) three times daily

For other indications:[9]

- 1.5-2.5g of dried tuber in decoction three times daily
- 1-2mL of liquid extract (1:1, 25% ethanol) three times daily
- 100 to 250 mg dried tuber three times daily

While many products are standardized to harpagoside content, it would be prudent to use whole plant extracts until the importance of this constituent is verified.

REFERENCES

1. Newall C, Anderson L, David Phillipson J. *Herbal Medicines: A Guide for Health Care Professionals.* London: The Pharmaceutical Press; 1996:296.
2. Weiss R. *Herbal Medicine.* Beaconsfield: Beaconsfield Press; 1988:362.
3. Leung A, Foster S. *Encyclopedia of Common Natural Ingredients Used in Food, Drugs and Cosmetics.* 2nd ed. New York, NY: John Wiley and Sons; 1996:649.
4. Grahame R, Robinson B. Devil's Claw (*Harpagophytum procumbens*): pharmacological and clinical studies. *Ann Rheum Dis*. 1981;40:632.
5. Wren R. *Potter's New Encyclopedia of Botanical Drugs and Preparations*. Saffron Walden: C.W. Daniel Company; 1988:362.
6. Ziller K, Franz G. Analysis of the water-soluble fraction from the roots of *Harpogophytum procumbens*. *Planta Medica*. 1979;37:340-348.
7. Kikuchi T, Matsuda S, Kubo Y, Namba T. New iridoid glucosides from *Harpagophytum procumbens* DC. *Chemical and Pharmaceutical Bulletin*. 1983;31:2296-2301.
8. Burger J, Vincent Brandt E, Ferreira D. Iridoid and phenolic glycosides from *Harpogophytum*. *Phytochemistry*. 1987;26: 1453-1457.
9. Bradley P. *British Herbal Compendium*. Bournemouth: BHMA; 1992:239.
10. Czygan F, Krueger A. Pharmaceutical biological studies of the genus harpagophytum. Part 3. Distribution of the iridoid glycoside harpagoside in the different organs of *Harpagophytum procumbens* and *Harpagophytum zeyheri*. *Planta Medica*. 1977;31:305-307.
11. Chevallier A. *The Encyclopedia of Medicinal Plants.* London: Reader's Digest; 1996:336.
12. Hoffman D. *Holistic Herbal.* Rockport, MA: Element Books; 1996:256.
13. Soulimani R, Younos C, Mortier F, Derrieu D. The role of stomachal digestion on the pharmacological activity of plant extracts, using as an example of *Harpagophytum procumbens*. *Canadian Journal of Physiology and Pharmacology*. 1994;72(12):1532-6.
14. Lanhers M, Fleurentin J, Mortier F, *et al*. Anti-inflammatory and analgesic effects of an aqueous extract of *Harpagophytum procumbens*. *Planta Medica*. 1992;58:117-123.
15. Erdos A, Fontaine R, Friehe H, *et al*. Beitrag zur pharmakologie und toxokologie verschieder extrakte, sowie des harpagoside aus Harpagophytum procumbens DC. *Planta Medica*. 1978;34:97-108.
16. Whitehouse L, Znamirowska M, Paul C. Devil's Claw (*Harpagophytum procumbens*):No evidence for anti-inflammatory activity in the treatment of arthritic disease. *Canadian Medical Association Journal*. 1983;129:249-251.
17. Mcleod D, Revell P, Robinson D. Investigations of *Harpagophytum procumbens* (Devil's Claw) in the treatment of experimental inflammation and arthritis in the rat. *British Journal of Pharmacology*. 1979;66:140-41.
18. Moussard C, Alber D, Toubin M, Thevenon N, Henry J. A drug used in traditional medicine, *Harpagophytum procumbens*: No Evidence for NSAID-like effect on whole blood eicosanoid production in humans. *Prostaglandins Leukotrienes and Essential Fatty Acids*. 1992;46:283-286.
19. Pinget M, Lecomte A. The effects of harpagophytum capsules (Arkocaps) in degenerative rheumatology. *Medecine Actuelle*. 1985;12:65-67.
20. Chrubasik S, Zimpfer C, Schutt U, Ziegler R. Effectiveness of *Harpagophytum procumbens* in treatment of acute back pain. *Phytomedicine*. 1996;3(1):1-10.
21. Barnes J. *Harpagophytum procumbens* extract for acute low back pain requires further investigation. *Focus on Alternative and Complementary Therapies*. 1996;1(1):6-7.

22. Occhiuto F, Circosta C, Ragusa S, *et al*. A drug used in traditional medicine: *Harpagophytum procumbens* DC.IV. Effects on some isolated muscle preparations. *Journal of Ethnopharmacology*. 1985;13:201-208.
23. Circosta C, Occhiuta F, Ragusa S, *et al.* A drug used in traditional medicine: *Harpagophytum procumbens* DCII.Cardiovascular activity. *Journal of Ethnopharmacology*. 1984;11:259-74.
24. Costa De Pasquale R, Busa G, Circosta C, *et al.* A drug used in traditional medicine: *Harpagohytum procumbens* DC III. Effects on hyperkinetic ventricular arrythmias by reperfusion. *Journal of Ethnopharmacology*. 1985;13:193-199.
25. Guerin J, Revelliere H. Activite antifongique d'extraits vegetaux a usage therapeutique. II. Etude de 40 extraits sur 9 souches fongiques. *Annales Pharmaceutiques Francaises*. 1985;43:77-81.
26. Tyler V. *The Honest Herbal.* 3rd ed. Binghamton, NY: Pharmaceutical Products Press; 1993:375.

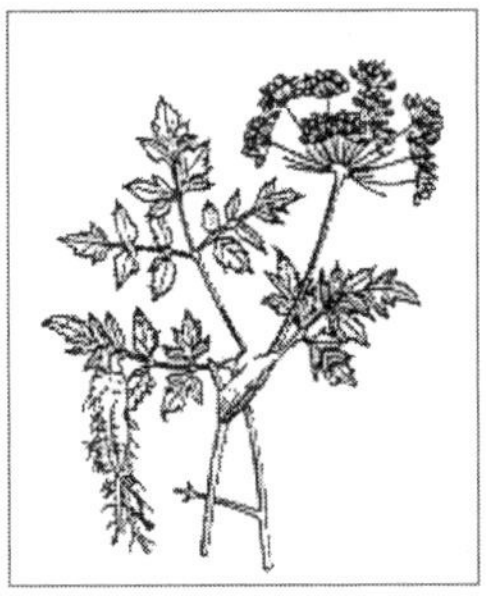

DONG QUAI

Angelica sinensis (Oliv.) Diels

THUMBNAIL SKETCH

Active Constituents

- Components of both the alcohol and aqueous soluble portions have been shown to possess therapeutic properties.

Common Uses

- Women's Health Care including the unpleasant consequences of menopause, dysmenorrhea, amenorrhea.
- Most classical indications are dependent on a suitable Traditional Chinese Medical (TCM) diagnosis.

Adverse Effects

- Rare, but include diarrhea and phototoxic skin reaction.

Cautions /Contraindications

- Dong quai should be avoided during pregnancy, hypermenorrhea, hemorrhagic disease and women with a history of spontaneous abortion.

Drug Interactions

- While no examples of drug interactions could be found, caution is recommended in cases of concomitant administration with oral anticoagulants.

Doses

- 3-10 g of raw herb (or equivalent) daily

INTRODUCTION

Family: Apiaceae (also known as Umbelliferae)

Synonyms: Tang kuei, Dang gui, Female ginseng, Female tonic, Woman's herb, Toki, Tangwi, *A. polymorpha* Maxim. Var. *sinensis* Oliv.[1-4]

Dong quai is a fragrant perennial plant that is arguably one of the oldest and most established therapeutic agents used within the Traditional Chinese Medicine model. It is classified as a tonic, an agent which can strengthen and invigorate the whole individual or specific organ groups. While dong quai exerts its tonifying action on many sites, it is classically considered to be one of the major 'blood' tonics often used to 'build the blood'. Even though it has numerous applications, it was considered to be of particular importance in the management of 'female' conditions such as menopause and dysmenorrhea.[5] It is in the realm of women's health care that most people will encounter the use of dong quai within the Western world.

Angelica sinensis is native to South-Western China. The root, with its distinctive aromatic odor and bitter-sweet/pungent taste, is the part used medicinally. The larger roots are more prized than the smaller ones. As a general rule, the larger the root, the sweeter the taste and the better the quality. It can be ingested in various ways. The fresh root may be either steamed or fried in vinegar, or the dried root can be taken as a soup.[1, 3]

Similar plants are often used in place of *Angelica sinensis*. These include: *Angelica acutiloba* (Siebold & Zucc.) Kitag (Korean or Japanese dong quai), *Ligusticum glaucescens* Franch (wild chin quai) and *Levisticum officinale* Koch (European dong quai). While these do possess therapeutically useful qualities, they are considered by most to be inferior to *Angelica sinensis*.[5]

Another member of the same genus, *Angelica archangelica* L. (Angelica), shares some of the same constituents and actions as its Chinese cousin, but it is used primarily as a digestive tonic, especially in cases of dyspepsia and flatulence.[6] In fact angelica is used extensively in the liquor industry where it is used as a flavoring in liqueurs such as benedictine and chartreuse.[2]

Constituents[1, 2, 5, 7, 8]

- Volatile Oil: ligustilide, n-butylidene phthalide, n-valerophernone-O-carboxylic acid.
- Furanocoumarins: psoralen, bergapten, archangelicin.
- Organic acids: ferulic acid, succinic acid, myristic acid.
- Miscellaneous: vitamin A, vitamin E, various members of the vitamin B group, polysaccharides including-AR-4E-2, angelica immunostimulating polysaccharide (AIP)

THERAPEUTIC USES & RELEVANT PHARMACOLOGY

CARDIOVASCULAR

Traditional Use

Within the Traditional Chinese Medicine (TCM) model dong quai is prescribed for conditions of 'blood deficiency', a situation that often presents with symptoms including: pale lips and tongue, dull/pale face with sallow complexion, depression and fatigue, poor memory, oligomenorrhea and amenorrhea.[9] While many of these symptoms may be equated with the Western concepts of anaemia and cardiovascular disease, it is important to realize that conditions diagnosed following a TCM tradition cannot be directly equated with a conventional medical diagnosis.

Cardiac Activity

Several experimental studies suggest that extracts of *Angelica sinensis* exert an inhibitory action on cardiac muscle contraction. Both aqueous and alcoholic extracts of *Angelica sinensis* have been shown to antagonize arrhythmias induced by a variety of agents (including epinephrine, strophanthin, digitalis, atropine, datura flower) in both *in vivo* and *in vitro* models.[5, 7, 10] A quinidine-like action (prolonged atrial refractory period, lowered cardiac excitability) was demonstrated in anesthetized dogs given an ether extract of *Angelica sinensis* root.[7, 10] In addition, a 2% fluid extract of *Angelica sinensis* has been shown to markedly increase coronary blood flow and decrease myocardial oxygen consumption in the isolated heart of guinea pigs.[7]

Vascular Action

It has been demonstrated that *Angelica sinensis* exerts a predominately hypotensive effect *in vivo*.[5, 7, 10, 11] This drop in blood pressure appears to be rapid and short lived.[10,5] It was thought that this action was in part due to a decreased cardiac out-put, but this has been shown not to be the case. It is more likely due to a vasodilatory action resulting from muscarinic and histaminic receptor stimulation.[7] Early investigations suggested that the hypotensive action was solely due to the non-volatile components, and the volatile constituents were thought to have a stimulating action. This has since been shown not to be the case.[7, 10]

Anti-thrombotic Action

In vitro experiments have demonstrated that aqueous extracts of *Angelica sinensis* could suppress platelet aggregation induced by ADP and collagen.[10,7] The agent thought to be predominantly responsible for this action is ferulic acid. It has been postulated that the decrease in platelet aggregation could be due to inhibition of cyclo-oxygenase and thromboxane A2 resulting in a subsequent decrease in the production of bio-active eicosonoids.[10] Osthole, extracted from a related species (*Angelica pubescens* Maxim.) has also been shown to decrease platelet aggregation by inhibiting thromboxane B_2.[12] It has also been postulated that the anti-thrombotic action could be due to a decrease in fibrinogen levels and blood viscosity.[10] This influence on the blood coagulating system is far from certain with some suggesting that an effect cannot be demonstrated.[11]

Miscellaneous

Angelica sinensis root when added to the feed (5% w/w) of albino rats and rabbits with experimental hyperlipidemia exerted a demonstrable antilipidemic effect. While the exact mechanism is unknown, it does not appear to be due to an effect on cholesterol absorption.[7]

WOMEN'S HEALTH

Traditional Use

Dong quai is considered to be useful in the management of a variety of conditions including: abnormal/suppressed/difficult menstruation;[2, 5, 7, 8] dysmenorrhea;[1, 2, 5, 7-9] dysfunctional uterine bleeding[2, 5, 8] (see contraindications); premenstrual syndrome;[5] preparation for conception;[1, 8, 9]

aiding recovery after birthing;[1, 9] and the unpleasant consequences of menopause.[13, 14] As mentioned above, many of these conditions are diagnosed and treated using models outside of the conventional medical model.

Menstrual Problems

A common Chinese patent formula which contains *Angelica sinensis* root (Xiao Yao Powder) was seen to decrease symptoms of premenstrual syndrome (PMS) in 10 women.[7] In addition, dong quai root has been shown to have an action on uterine tissue using various animal models. It appears that this effect is dependent on the extract used.[7, 10] The volatile oil fraction causes direct muscular relaxation, completely abolishing contractions in a dose dependent fashion.[5, 7, 10] The active constituent appears to be ligustilide.[10] The volatile oil antagonizes excitation caused by either histamine or epinephrine, while the non-volatile fractions have an opposite action resulting in strong uterine contractions.[5, 7, 10] The alcoholic extract has a more pronounced effect than the aqueous one.[7] When administered parenterally, there is no difference between the fractions; they all cause excitation.[7]

Intrauterine pressure was shown to influence the action of dong quai on rabbit uterine fistula. When the existing pressure was elevated, contraction became slower and more rhythmic.[7] It has been suggested that this action is responsible for dong quai's effectiveness in the treatment of dysmenorrhea.[5, 9]

Menopause

A product containing *Angelica sinensis* (Angelica-Paeonia Powder) was shown to alleviate symptoms commonly seen with menopause in 43 cases (specific details of this trial were not available at the time of preparation of this monograph).[7] In addition, a recent trial of a botanical formula containing *Angelica sinensis* (and *Arctium lappa* L., Asteraceae; *Glycyrrhiza glabra* L., Fabaceae; *Leonurus cardiaca* L.; Lamiaceae and *Dioscorea villosa* L.; Dioscoreaceae) conducted at the National College of Naturopathic Medicine found that symptoms of menopause where decreased when compared to a placebo group. As was correctly noted by the authors, given the small sample number (n=13) no definite conclusions can be made.[14] No conclusions can be drawn for *Angelica sinensis* in particular from this investigation since the other herbal ingredients in the botanical formula have demonstrable therapeutic actions in their own rights.

The many positive actions of dong quai on the female reproductive system have long been considered to result from 'phytoestrogenic' properties. This assumption is now being questioned because many of the actions of this herb are probably not estrogen dependent.[9, 15] Studies in mice have found dong quai to be devoid of estrogenic action.[5, 7] Conversely, both aqueous and petroleum ether extracts, when given intraperitoneally and subcutaneously, respectively, are reported to have an estrogen-like action.[11]

The evidence supporting the therapeutic usefulness of *Angelica sinensis* comes predominantly from the Asian medical model. Unfortunately, there is a distinct lack of quality clinical information. It should also be noted that what little evidence there is from a western conventional standpoint normally involves products in which dong quai is only one of many ingredients. More research is required before the traditional uses of dong quai can be supported using evidence from a biomedical paradigm.

MISCELLANEOUS

Antimicrobial

An aqueous decoction of dong quai has been shown to exert a weak antimicrobial action against a variety of bacteria including: *E coli, Salmonella typhi, Shigella dysenteriae*.[7]

Metabolic

When added to the feed of rats (5-6% of diet), *Angelica sinensis* was shown to reduce or prevent testicular disease resulting from vitamin E deficiency.[7]

Central Nervous System

Parenteral administration of tang kuei essential oil from Japan has been shown to exert tranquilizing, hypnotic and anesthetic actions in a variety of animal models.[11]

Analgesic Action

Dong quai is used within TCM for various conditions associated with pain primarily due to a TCM diagnosis of "blood stagnation."[9] This analgesic action appears dependent on the quality and origin of the pain.

ADVERSE EFFECTS

Even though tang kuei extract from Japan accelerated the death of mice that had been given carbon tetrachloride, in practice adverse effects caused by *Angelica sinensis* appear to be very rare.[11] The LD_{50} of dong quai administered intravenously to mice was 100.6g/kg.[10]

Diarrhea is possible because of dong quai's relaxant action on the smooth muscle of the digestive tract.[2, 16] This appears more likely if the individual has a "weak" digestive system already.[5] Concerns have been raised regarding the presence of furancoumarins (psoralen and bergapten) in *Angelica sinensis* and the subsequent increased possibility of a photosensitization resulting in a dermatitis like skin reaction.[15, 16] Examples of phototoxic reactions have been noted when high doses of psoralens from other plants (e.g. celery) have been administered in conjunction with UV light.[16]

It has been noted that parenteral administration of the volatile oil results in severe pain, nausea, hot flushes and chills. These reactions are usually self –limiting.[7] In addition it has been reported that the intravenous injection of the volatile components of the plant may cause renal failure.[10] A case of anaphylactic shock resulting from the injection of a product containing Angelica has also been noted.[7]

CAUTIONS / CONTRAINDICATIONS

Given its action on uterine smooth muscle, dong quai should not be used during the first trimester of pregnancy or in individuals with a history of spontaneous abortion.[5] Given the lack of information, many suggest that consumption of dong quai should be avoided at any stage of pregnancy except when used by an appropriately trained health-care provider.[2]

Practitioners of Traditional Chinese Medicine advise that 'tonic' herbs, such as dong quai, should not be used during acute illness (i.e., the flu and colds.)[3, 5] In addition, dong quai should be avoided in cases of hemorrhagic disease and hypermenorrhea.[5]

DRUG INTERACTIONS

- Plant medicines rich in coumarins may interfere with concomitant anticoagulant therapy.[17]

DOSAGE REGIMEN

- 3-10 g of raw herb (or equivalent) daily[18]

REFERENCES

1. Noe J. *Angelica Sinensis*: A Monograph. *Journal of Naturopathic Medicine*. 1997;7(1):66-72.
2. Foster S, Chongxi Y. *Herbal Emissaries: Bringing Chinese Herbs to the West.* Rochester, VT: Healing Arts Press; 1992:356.
3. Bensky D, Gamble A. *Chinese Herbal Materia Medica.* Seattle,WA: Eastland Press; 1986:556.
4. Marles RJ, Associate Professor, Department of Botany, Brandon University, Brandon, Manitoba. Review of Medicinal Plant Modules for CCNM; 1997.
5. Zhu D. Dong Quai. *American Journal of Chinese Medicine*. 1987;15:117-125.
6. Mills S. *The Essential Book of Herbal Medicine*. 2nd ed. London: Penguin; 1991:677.
7. Chang H-M, But P. *Pharmacology and Applications of Chinese Materia Medica.* Singapore: World Scientific Press; 1986.
8. Chevallier A. *The Encyclopedia of Medicinal Plants.* London: Reader's Digest; 1996:336.
9. Belford-Courtney R. Comparison of Chinese and Western uses of *Angelica sinensis*. *Australian Journal of Medical Herbalism*. 1993;5(4):87-91.
10. Mei Q, Yi T-J, Cui B. Advances in the pharmacological studies of radix *Angelica Sinensis* (Oliv) Diels (Chinese Danggui). *Chinese Medical Journal*. 1991;104(9):776-781.
11. Yoshiro K. The physiological action of Tang Kuei and Cnidium. *Bulletin Oriental Healing Arts Institute of U.S.A*. 1985;10(7):269-78.
12. Ko F, Wu T, Liou M, Huang T, *et al.* Inhibition of platelet thromboxane formation and phosphoinostides break down by osthole from *Angelica pubescens. Thrombosis and Haemostasis*. 1989;62(3):996-9.
13. Hudson T. Balancing the Female Hormonal System. *Gaia Symposium Proceedings*. Ashland, MA: Gaia Herbal Research Institute; 1993:119.
14. Hudson T, Standish L, Breed C, *et al.* Clinical and endocrinological effects of a menopausal botanical formula. *Journal of Naturopathic Medicine*. 1997;7(1):73-82.
15. Reichert R. Phyto-estrogens. *Quarterly Review of Natural Medicine*. 1994;2(1):27-33.
16. Tyler V. *The Honest Herbal*. 3rd ed. Binghamton, NY: Pharmaceutical Products Press; 1993:375.
17. Newall C, Anderson L, David Phillipson J. *Herbal Medicines: A Guide for Health Care Professionals.* London: The Pharmaceutical Press; 1996:296.
18. Teegarden R. *Chinese Tonic Herbs.* New York, NY: Japan Publishing Inc; 1985:197.

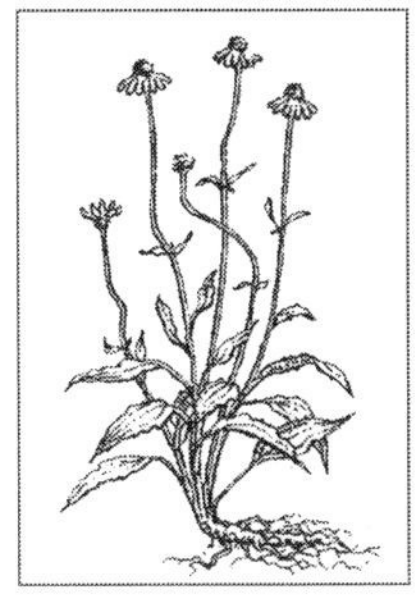

ECHINACEA

E. angustifolia DC., *E. purpurea* (L.) Moench, *E. pallida* (Nutt.) Nutt.

THUMBNAIL SKETCH

Active Constituents
- Polysaccharides
- Glycoproteins
- Alkamides
- Caffeic acid derivatives such as echinacoside, cichoric acid and cynarin

Common Uses
- *Internal:* supportive treatment of colds, flus, infections of the upper respiratory tract and lower urinary tract
- *External:* skin abrasions and ulcerations

Adverse Effects
- None known

Cautions/Contraindication
- *Internal:* Progressive systemic diseases (e.g., tuberculosis, multiple sclerosis); auto-immune conditions (e.g., diabetes mellitus, lupus, rheumatoid arthritis); use controversial in HIV/AIDS
- *External:* none known

Drug Interactions
- Theoretically opposes the effects of immunosuppressants

Doses

Internal:
- Dried herb: 1g three times daily
- Hydroalcoholic tincture (1:5; 45% ethanol): 2 to 5 mL three times daily
- Liquid Extract (1:1; 45% ethanol): 0.5 to 1 mL three times daily
- Expressed Juice (E. purpurea): 6-9 mL daily in divided doses

External
- Semi-solid preparations should contain at least 15% expressed juice (*E. purpurea*)

INTRODUCTION

Family: Asteraceae (also known as Compositae or Sunflower family)

Synonyms: Purple coneflower, Purple Kansas coneflower, Black simpson, Red sunflower, Comb flower, Cock up hat, Missouri snakeroot, Kansas snakeroot and Indian head[1, 2]

Echinacea species, indigenous to the North American mid-west (from Saskatchewan to Texas)[3, 4] were used extensively as medicinal herbs by native North American tribes[5] reportedly to treat a variety of ailments, including mouth sores, toothaches, colds, sore throats, burns and snake bites.[1, 6-8] Its use for snake bites gave rise to several common names (Missouri and Kansas Snake-root). *Echinacea angustifolia* (narrow-leaved purple cone flower) is the smallest of these plants (growing to only 0.5 m) with flowers approximately 2.5 cm long. Although commercial cultivation has been initiated, much of the medicinal supply is still wild-harvested. *Echinacea pallida* (pale purple cone flower) is larger, growing to approximately 1 m in height and producing a characteristic large, purple flower. *Echinacea purpurea* (common purple cone flower) can be distinguished by its oval leaves. The entire medicinal supply of this third species is cultivated.[3, 4] The roots are primarily used medicinally; however, there is evidence that the aerial parts of *E. purpurea* also have some medicinal action.[4, 9]

HFC Meyer, a German physician working, in Nebraska, is credited with introducing echinacea to the medical profession when he began selling a patent formula containing a root extract of *E. angustifolia* in the 1870s. In 1887 Meyer brought echinacea to the attention of John King, a well-known eclectic physician, and John Uri Lloyd, a prominent pharmacist and manufacturer, who undertook a number of trials of the product and then began marketing echinacea products as anti-infective agents.[1, 2] By 1915, echinacea products were available from many other pharmaceutical companies, including Merck, Wyeth and Parke Davis.[2] Although the eclectics embraced the use of echinacea, it was widely criticized by the 'regular' medical establishment of the time who argued that there was no scientific evidence to support its use.[10] However, from 1916 to 1950 *E. angustifolia* and *E. pallida* roots were listed as official drugs in the National Formulary of the United States.

To meet the growing European demand for echinacea, a German company (Madaus AHG) attempted to import *E. angustifolia* seeds from the United States. However, the species imported was subsequently demonstrated to be *E. purpurea*. The majority of European research on echinacea in the last 50 years was conducted using the Madaus product Echinacin®, which is made from the expressed juices of the aerial parts of *E. purpurea* combined with 22% ethanol (as a preservative).[1, 11]

Several hundred articles and three major books[12-14] have been written about echinacea. In addition, Bauer and Wagner provide an excellent review.[8] A large proportion of the literature was originally published in German. Key studies will be summarized in the following sections.

Constituents[8, 15-22]

Although the three species are often considered interchangeable clinically, their chemical constituents differ. One study found no characteristic chemical differences between the aerial parts of the three species; however, the alkylamides in the roots did differ significantly.[22] *E. angustifolia* may be distinguished from *E. purpurea* because the former contains isobutylamides, echinacoside and cynarin, and the latter contains distinctive polyacetylenes and polyenes.[19] Echinacoside (the chemical to which many echinacea products are standardized) has been found in both *E. angustifolia* and *E. pallida* (but not *E. purpurea*); however, cynarine, a quinic acid derivative has only been detected in *E. angustifolia* and may be useful for discriminating between it and the other two species.[8] In addition, echinacein, the isobutylamide generally thought to cause the 'tingling of the tongue' associated with echinacea products, has only been identified as a constituent of *E. angustifolia.*

E. angustifolia

- Carbohydrates: sucrose, pentosans, fructose
- Polysaccharides: inulin storage (fructans), hetero-polysaccharides (structural)
- Phenolic compounds: caffeic acid derivatives, echinacoside, 3-malonylglucoside cynarin (roots only), chlorogenic, isochlorogenic acid (leaves and stems)
- Flavonoids: a variety including luteolin, kaempferol and quercetin derivatives, rutoside
- Fatty Acids: linoleic, oleic, cerotic and palmitic acids
- Polyacetylenes: a variety of polyynes and polyenes
- Alkylamides: echinacein and a variety of others including pyrrolidides, piperidides, isobutylamides (pattern of alkylamides differs from *E. purpurea*)
- Alkaloids: tussilagine, isotussilagine (pyrrolizidines that do not contain 1,2-unsaturated necine ring system necessary to confer liver toxicity)
- Miscellaneous: betaine hydrochloride, phytosterols, n-triacontanol, behenic acid ethyl ester

E. purpurea

- Carbohydrates: fructose
- Polysaccharides: a variety of hetero-polysaccharides (structural) including arabinogalactan, xyloglucans
- Phenolic compounds: caffeic acid derivatives, chicoric acid, caftaric acid & derivatives (mainly aerial parts)
- Flavonoids: several including a variety of kaempferol, quercetin and rutin derivatives, rutoside
- Fatty Acids: linoleic, oleic, cerotic and palmitic acids
- Polyacetylenes: a varitey of polyynes and polyenes
- Alkylamides: echinacein and a variety of isobutylamides (pattern of alkylamides differs from *E. angustifolia*)
- Alkaloids: tussilagine, isotussilagine (pyrrolizidines that do not contain 1, 2-unsaturated necine ring system necessary to confer liver toxicity)
- Miscellaneous: glycine betaine, cyanidins, glycoproteins

E. pallida

(The polyacetylenes of *E. pallida* are very susceptible to oxidation, thus the chemical composition of the roots depends on storage conditions.)[19]

- Carbohydrates: sucrose, petosans
- Polysaccharides: inulin storage (fructans), hetero-polysaccharides (structural)
- Phenolic compounds: caffeic acid derivatives, echinacoside, des-rhamnosyl-verascoside, 6-0-caffcoyl-echinacoside (roots only), caftaric acid & derivatives (mainly aerial parts), chlorogenic, isochlorogenic acid (leaves and stems)

- Flavonoids: a variety including luteolin, kaempferol and quercetin derivatives, rutoside
- Fatty Acids: linoleic, oleic, cerotic and palmitic acids
- Polyacetylenes: a variety of polyynes and polyenes; ketoalkynes and ketoalkenes
- Alkylamides: traces
- Miscellaneous: betaine hydrochloride, cyanidins

THERAPEUTIC USES & RELEVANT PHARMACOLOGY

IMMUNOLOGICAL ACTIVITY

The immunostimulatory action of echinacea appears to depend on the synergistic action of several constituents; although several different compounds have been shown to possess immunological activity, echinacea's effects on the immune system cannot be attributed to any single compound.[8] Most of the scientific research has been conducted with isolated fractions of *E. purpurea* (often a polysaccharide extract) and *E. angustifolia*. Very little research has reported on *E. pallida*.

In vitro and In vivo Studies

Research teams have demonstrated that extracts of *E. purpurea*: increase phagocytosis significantly *in vitro*[23-29] and *in vivo;*[22-24, 28, 30] increase proliferation of phagocytes in spleen and bone marrow;[24] stimulate migration of granulocytes to the peripheral blood;[24, 26] stimulate macrophages to excrete tumor necrosis factor (TNF);[16, 17, 23, 24] stimulate macrophages to secrete interleukin-1 (IL-1)[16, 24] and interleukin-6 (IL-6);[24] stimulate monocytes to produce IL-1, IL-6, and tumor necrosis factor;[25] stimulate macrophages to produce interferon-B_2 ;[16] independently and directly activate macrophages to cytotoxicity;[16, 17, 30, 31] increase properdin levels;[32] increase the number of PMN and activate the adherence of PMN to the endothelial cells.[25] In addition, studies revealed that *E. purpurea* extracts appear to have no action on T lymphocytes;[31] no induction of lymphokine (MAF) production;[31] no significant stimulation of B cell proliferation;[16,31] and no enhancement of specific immune responses (antibody production).[24]

Studies with *E. angustifolia* extracts have demonstrated a statistically significant increase in the phagocytic activity of peritoneal macrophages in mice.[33]

Given that the majority of studies discussed above were completed with defined-composition extracts, it is difficult to extrapolate the results of these studies to consumption of the varied commercially available preparations of echinacea species in clinical settings.

Human Trials

Roesler *et al.* demonstrated that many of the effects of *E. purpurea* extracts previously noted *in vitro* or in animal models were also found when an extract was given i.v. to human test subjects.[25] Effects demonstrated in humans include: adherence to endothelial cells;[25] phagocytosis;[23, 32, 34, 35] migration from bone marrow into the peripheral blood,[25] and production of IL-6.[36] However, direct conclusions about the efficacy of marketed echinacea products are not possible from these findings.

Most clinical trials have been conducted with i.v or i.m. injections of 0.1 to 0.7 mL Echinacin® and small sample sizes (n<20) are the norm. Melchart *et al.* provide an excellent review of 26 clinical trials published to date. Of these, they report that 18 were randomized and 11 double-blinded; 6 were trials of echinacea alone and 20 tested preparations containing echinacea in combination with other products. Due to the poor quality (only 8 trials scored more than half the maximum quality score), and heterogeneity of the study conditions, a formal meta-analysis was not possible. However, the authors of the review concluded that there was some evidence of benefit due to the administration of echinacea in 22 of 36 treatment groups (in contrast with the 30 test groups felt to have positive results by the authors of the individual studies). The reviewers call for further, high quality clinical trials to provide definitive evidence as to the efficacy of echinacea.[37]

In one study 24 healthy males were administered either an alcoholic extract of *E. purpurea* or placebo orally (30 drops three times daily for 5 days). For those on the active treatment, stimulation of granulocyte phagocytosis reached a maximum (120% above base line) on day 5 and slowly decreased within 3 days to the normal range.[35] In another study, the effect of Echinacin® as an adjuvant in the treatment of recurrent vaginal candida infection (n=203) was tested. Individual infections were treated with econazol nitrate over 6 days and participants were also given either Echinacin® or placebo for 10 weeks. The recurrence rate in the control group was 60.5% and only 5%-16% in the active treatment group (depending on route of administration: oral or parenteral).[38]

Another recent placebo-controlled, double-blind, clinical trial of a liquid extract of *E. pallida* (90 drops = 900 mg) involved 160 consecutive patients at a family practice centre diagnosed with an upper-respiratory tract infection (URTI). The duration of treatment was 8 to 10 days with symptoms scored at 3-4 days and 8-10 days after entering the study. Patients taking *E. pallida* had significantly shorter duration of illness (reduced from 13 to 9.8 days in bacterial infection and to 9.1 days in viral infection) as compared to placebo. The specific clinical symptoms assessed (chills, weakness, muscle pain, headache) all disappeared more quickly in the active treatment group as compared with placebo.[39] These results are similar to those of an earlier study with *E. purpurea* (though not blinded or placebo-controlled).[40] Two other double-blind, placebo-controlled clinical trials of *E. purpurea* tested its efficacy in the treatment/prevention of the common cold and treatment of influenza. In one (n=108), ingestion of the expressed juice was able to decrease the frequency of infections of the common cold in highly susceptible people over an 8-week period, and decrease the severity of infections which did occur in the treatment group.[41] In the other (n=180), a dose of 450 mg of *E. purpurea* root daily was found no better than placebo; however, at a dose of 900 mg daily it significantly reduced flu symptoms, including weakness, chills, sore throat, muscle aches and headache.[42] A Canadian study found no difference between *E. angustifolia* (250 mg three times daily) and placebo for altering the duration, severity or symptoms of the common cold (n=190) in a double-blind, prospective trial.[43] However, this study can be criticized due to the low dose of *E. angustifolia* (750 mg daily) used in the trial. Most authors recommend 900 to 1000 mg daily.

OTHER RELATED ACTIVITY

Local Activity in Tissues

Historically echinacea species were used for the treatment of snake bites and were reported to reduce the spread of venom. Scientific investigation of this phenomenon occurred primarily in the 1950s and centered on the effect of echinacea on hyaluronidase. All these studies were conducted with the German product Echinacin®, which is made from the expressed juices of the aerial parts of *E. purpurea* combined with 22% ethanol (as a preservative).[1, 11] Echinacin® has been shown to inhibit hyaluronidase production *in vitro* and *in vivo*.[8, 44, 45] One study suggested that 0.04 mL of Echinacin® was equivalent to 1 mg of cortisone using a modified spreading test in rats.[46] It has been hypothesized that in addition to a direct effect on hyaluronidase production, Echinacin® may also stimulate changes in fibroblasts resulting in an indirect effect on the hyaluronic acid-hyaluronidase system.[47, 48]

Anti-Inflammatory Activity

Investigations of the anti-inflammatory properties of echinacea have primarily been limited to *Echinacea angustifolia*. In 1956, Keller isolated two active fractions from echinacea species and showed that Fraction A had some cortisone-like activity.[49] Later Bonadeo *et al.* isolated a polysaccharide fraction (which may be identical to Keller's Fraction A) and suggested that its anti-inflammatory mechanism of action may be the formation of a hyaluronic acid-polysaccharide complex which indirectly inhibits hyaluronidase.[50, 51] More recently, two research teams have confirmed the anti-inflammatory activity of *Echinacea angustifolia*. A raw extract applied topically inhibited edema (initiated by croton oil) in the ears of rats in a dose-dependent manner[52, 53] and was found to be more potent than benzidamine (a topical NSAID)[52] and approximately half as potent as topical indomethacin.[53] Given iv 1 hour prior to injection with carrageenan, the same extract inhibited edema in the paws of rats.[52] More recently, several alkylamides isolated from *E. angustifolia* were shown to inhibit both cyclooxygenase and 5-lipoxygenase *in vitro*.[18] Inhibition of 5-lipoxygenase *in vitro* has also been reported in an alkylamide fraction isolated from *Echinacea purpurea* roots.[54]

In a clinical study patients with chronic inflammation (9 due to viral infections; 14 due to bacterial infections) were administered Echinacin® (1 ampoule i.m. once daily for 7 days). There was an increase in the total lymphocyte count, with a decreased percentage of T4 cells.[55] Similar results were obtained in another study of patients suffering from contact eczema (n=4), neurodermatitis (n=6), herpes simplex (n=8) and Candida infection (n=10). Echinacin® was applied topically daily for 7 days. After 7 days, the proportion of T-helper cells was decreased, but an overall lymphocytosis was observed.[56]

Anti-bacterial and Anti-viral Activity

Echinacea has been shown to have only very weak activity as an anti-viral, anti-bacterial or anti-fungal agent. Several extracts of *E. angustifolia* (echinacoside and an alcoholic extract) have shown limited inhibitory activity against *Staphylococcus aureus*,[57] *Escherichia coli*,[58] *Pseudomonas aeruginosa*[58] and *Trichomonas vaginalis*[59] *in vitro*. Several compounds isolated from *E. purpurea* were also shown to have weak activity against *Escherichia coli* and *Pseudomonas aeruginosa*.[58] Echinacea does not appear to be clinically useful as an antibiotic.

Several teams of researchers have noted the anti-viral activity of echinacea. The brand Echinacin® (*E. purpurea*) was reported to have some activity (in mice) against encephalomyocarditis virus (EMC virus) and vesicular-stomatitis virus (VSV).[60] In addition, extracts of *E. purpurea* were found to have some activity against influenza, herpes, VSV, and poliovirus *in vitro*.[61, 62] Extracts of *E. pallida* have also been reported to exhibit some inhibition of VSV.[63] Given that the anti-viral activity observed requires the presence of 0-2-diethylamino ethyl dextran (DEAE) (*in vivo*)[60] and did not develop in the presence of hyaluronidase (*in vitro*),[61] an "interferon-like" mechanism of action without the induction of interferon has been hypothesized.

MISCELLANEOUS

Anti-cancer

Echinacin® (*E. purpurea*) 60 mg/m^2 (i.m. daily days 3-10 and then twice weekly) was given as part of an immunotherapy protocol was given to 15 outpatients with metastasizing, far-advanced colorectal cancers that included cyclophosphamide (LDCY) 300 mg/m2 every 28 days and thymostimulin 30 mg/m2 days 3-10 and then twice weekly. Stimulation of the phagocytic activity of peripheral blood leukocytes was noted 14 days after the low-dose cyclophosphamide and attributed to the effect of the Echinacin®. Mean survival time was 4 months and 2 patients survived more than 8 months.[64] Given the advanced stage of the disease in these patients, comparison of these survival times with others reported in the literature was not possible. A randomized, placebo-controlled trial is needed to assess the effects of this protocol on survival. A second study has suggested that components of echinacea may have the potential to promote anti-cancer activity.[65]

Protection Against Radiation

One study in irradiated rats suggests that *Echinacea purpurea* promoted the effective functioning of the vitamin E redox system by mobilizing the body's stores of liposoluble vitamin A, carotene, and vitamin E.[66]

Prevention and/or Treatment of Skin Photodamage

One study suggests that echinacea species has a dose-dependent protective effect on the free radical-induced degradation of Type III collagen. The authors suggest that echinacea products may be useful in the prevention and/or treatment of photodamage of the skin.[67]

WHICH ECHINACEA IS BEST?

Echinacea angustifolia is the favored species in North America and is often the only species listed in North American reference texts. It has been argued that it is largely the favorite simply because of familiarity – it is native to North America and knowledge about this species has been handed down through generations of herbalists and Native healers. However, *E. angustifolia* is largely still harvested from wild sources, which raises concerns about both the sustainability and quality of the supply. Limited efforts are currently underway to cultivate *E. angustifolia* for medicinal purposes.

In contrast, *Echinacea purpurea* is the only species which is currently commercially cultivated. In addition, the vast majority of both pharmacological and clinical studies have been conducted with *E. purpurea* – primarily with the commercial product Echinacin®, which is the expressed juice of the aerial parts of the plant, with alcohol added as a preservative. Echinacin® was used in the creation of the Commission E monograph in Germany.

One study found that the ethanolic root extracts of all three species caused a 20-30% increase in phagocytosis *in vitro* and *in vivo*,[28] with *E. purpurea* appearing slightly (non-significantly) more active than the other two species. Another trial found that *E. purpurea* was significantly more active *in vitro* than the other species;[68] however, Bergner criticizes this trial because the researchers used only 30% alcohol to make the extracts of each of the species and he notes that tinctures of *E. angustifolia* used clinically are usually made with 80% alcohol. The different alcohol concentrations would likely result in the extraction of different compounds from the plant material. He also argues that the sources of the three species were not reported.[69]

ADVERSE EFFECTS

Of all the studies reviewed for this monograph, only one reported any acute toxicity (mild "influenza-like" symptoms after i.v. administration of 5 mg of polysaccharide extract of *E. purpurea*)[25] and there were no reports of chronic toxicity of echinacea. Many reviews, including the German Commission E, indicate that there are no known toxic effects, although a temperature increase of 0.5 - 1°C is common with i.v, i.m., or s.c. injections of Echinacin®.[3, 8, 70] Using the Lorke method on mice, LD_{50} values of >2500 and >5000 mg/kg have been found for a polysaccharide mixture from the aerial parts of *E. purpurea* and from a cell culture of *E. purpurea* respectively.[71] The animals died not from the echinacea, but from the hyperosmolar solution injected in such large amounts. *E. purpurea* cell cultures have also been tested for possible gene toxicity in human lymphocyte cultures and found to have no significant toxic effects in short or long term experiments.[72] No hepatotoxic effects have been found (or are expected) with the pyrrolizidine alkaloides in echinacea species because they do not contain the 1,2-unsaturated necine ring system.[73, 74] Finally, some concern has been raised given the reported *in vitro* stimulation of the secretion of TNF and the potential roles of TNF in cachexia and endotoxic shock;[75] however, Bergner argues that an increase in the secretion of TNF has only been demonstrated by using purified polysaccharides derived from *E. purpurea* cells cultured *in vitro* and that these polysaccharides are not present in most commercial products.[76]

In the past, *Echinacea purpurea roots* have been adulterated with *Parthenium integrifolium* L., Asteraceae (Missouri snakeroot), which may have caused other adverse effects.[4]

Individuals with allergies to the sunflower family (Asteraceae or Compositae) may experience mild allergic symptoms when ingesting echinacea.[70, 77]

CAUTIONS/CONTRAINDICATIONS

❖*Internal:* Echinacea should be used with caution by patients with progressive systemic diseases (e.g., tuberculosis, leucoses, multiple sclerosis);[70] or auto-immune conditions (e.g., diabetes mellitus, lupus, rheumatoid arthritis). Use of echinacea is also controversial in HIV/AIDS.

However, Bergner argues that these cautions are not necessary. He argues that no clinical evidence exists to support these claims and cites historical evidence that echinacea has actually been used to treat tuberculosis[78, 79] and leukemia.[80]

❖*External:* None known.[8, 70]

DRUG INTERACTIONS

None reported by the German Commission E;[70] however, its effects oppose the action of immunosuppressants.

DOSAGE REGIMENS

Echinacea has widely been reported to lose its ability to stimulate the immune system if taken continuously for extended periods of time; however, there appears to be little scientific evidence to clearly support or confirm this claim.[81] Bergner argues that oral doses of echinacea have never been shown to lose their effectiveness, citing recent clinical trials which demonstrated continued effects from echinacea at 8 weeks or more.[76] This opinion is supported by Kerry Bone.[82] However, Hobbs reviews the literature and incorporates his extensive clinical experience to recommend that echinacea products be taken cyclically: 10 to 14 days on with a 3 day rest period.[7] The German Commission E monograph suggests that echinacea should not be taken continuously (internally or externally) for more than 8 weeks.[70]

Internal:

- Dried herb: 1g three times daily[83]
- Hydroalcoholic tincture (1:5; 45% ethanol): 2-5 mL three times daily[83]
- Liquid Extract (1:1; 45% ethanol): 0.5-1 mL three times daily[83]
- Expressed Juice (*E. purpurea*): 6-9 mL daily in divided doses[70]

External:

- Semi-solid preparations should contain at least 15% expressed juice (*E. purpurea*)[70]
- Many products are standardized to echinacoside content (approximately 4%). This is a method of demonstrating authenticity (for *E. angustifolia*) rather than a measure of therapeutic potency.

REFERENCES

1. Awang DVC, Kindack DG. Echinacea. *Canadian Pharmaceutical Journal*. 1991;124(512-516).
2. Hobbs C. Echinacea — a literature review. *Herbalgram*. 1994;30:33-47.
3. Murray MT. *The Healing Power of Herbs*. Rocklin, CA: Prima Publishing; 1992:246.
4. Foster S. Echinacea: The cold and flu remedy. *Alternative and Complementary Therapies*. 1995;1(4):254-7.
5. Shemluck M. Medicinal and other uses of the Compositae by Indians in the United States and Canada. *Journal of Ethnopharmacology*. 1982;5:303-58.
6. Vogel V. *American Indian Medicine*. Norman: University of Oklahoma Press; 1970.
7. Hobbs C. Echinacea: diminished immune stimulation over time? *Medical Herbalism*. 1994;6(2):3-5.
8. Bauer R, Wagner H. Echinacea species as potential immunostimulatory drugs. *Economic and Medical Plant Research*. 1991;5:253-321.
9. Bauer R. Echinacea drugs — effects and active ingredients [German]. *Zeitschrift fur Arztliche Fortbildung*. 1996;90(2):111-5.
10. Editorial. Echinacea. *Journal of the American Medical Association*. 1909;53:1836.
11. Brown DJ. Echinacea: Phytotherapy review and commentary. *Townsend Letter for Doctors*. 1995;January:134-5.
12. Hobbs C. The Echinacea Handbook. In: Miovich M, ed. Portland, OR: Eclectic Medical Publications; 1989.
13. Bauer R, Wagner H. Ein Handbuch für Ärtze, Apotheker und andere Naturwissenschaftler. Stuttgart: Wissenschaftliche Verlagsgesellschaft; 1990:182.
14. Foster S. Echinacea: *Nature's Immune Enhancer*. Rochester, VT: Healing Arts Press; 1991.
15. Hobbs C. The chemistry and pharmacology of Echinacea species. *Herbal Gram* (Supplement). 1994;30:1-7.
16. Luettig B, Steinmüller C, Gifford GE, *et al*. Macrophage activation by the polysaccharide arabinogalactan isolated from plant cell cultures of *Echinacea purpurea*. *Journal of the National Cancer Institute*. 1989;81(9):669-675.
17. Steinmuller C, Roesler J, Grottrup E, Franklin G, Wagner H, Lohmann-Mattes M-L. Polysaccharides isolated from plant cell cultures of *Echinacea purpurea* enhance the resistance of immunosuppressed mice against systemic infections with *Candida albicans* and *Listeria monocytogenes*. *International Journal of Immunopharmacology*. 1993;15(5):605-614.
18. Muller-Jakic B, Breu W, Probstle A, *et al*. *In vitro* inhibition of cyclooxygenase and 5-lipoxygenase by alkamides from Echinacea and Achillea species. *Planta Medica*. 1994;60:37-40.
19. Bauer R, Khan AI, Wagner H. TLC and HPLC Analysis of *Echinacea pallida* and *E. angustifolia* roots. *Planta Medica*. 1988;54:426-430.
20. Bauer R, *et al*. Alkamides from the roots of *Echinacea angustifolia*. *Phytochemistry*. 1989;28:505-508.
21. Bohlman F, Hoffmann M. Further amides from *Echinacea purpurea*. *Phytochemistry*. 1983;22:1173-1175.
22. Proksch A, Wagner H. Structural analysis of 4-0-methyl-glucuronoarabinoxylan with immuno-stimulating activity from *Echinacea purpurea* .*Phytochemistry*. 1987;26(7):1989-93.
23. Wagner H, *et al*. Immunologically active polysaccharides of *Echinacea purpurea* cell cultures. *Phytochemistry*. 1988;27:119-126.
24. Roesler J, Steinmuller C, Kiderlen A, *et al*. Application of purified polysaccharides from cell cultures of the plant *Echinacea purpurea* to mice mediates protection against systemic infections with *Listeria monocytogenes* and *Candida albicans*. *International Journal of Immunopharmacology*. 1991;13(1):27-37.
25. Roesler J, Emmendorffer A, Steinmuller C, *et al*. Application of purified polysaccharides from cell cultures of the

plant *Echinacea purpurea* to test subjects mediates activation of the phagocyte system. *International Journal of Immunopharmacology.* 1991;13(7):931-41.

26. Wildfeur A, Mayerhofer D. The effects of plant preparations on cellular functions in body defense [German]. *Arzneimittelforschung.* 1994;44(3):361-6.
27. Vömel T. Der einfluss einen pflanzelische immunostimulans auf die phagozytose von erythozyten durch das retikulohistozytäre system der isoliert perfundierten rattenleber. *Arzneimittelforschung.* 1985;35:1437-1439.
28. Bauer VR, Jurcuc K, Puhlmann J, Wagner H. Immunological *in vivo* and *in vitro* examinations of Echinacea extracts. *Arzneimittelforschung.* 1988;38:276-281.
29. Stotzem CD, Hungerland U, Mengs U. Influence of *Echinacea purpurea* on the phagocytosis of human granulocytes. *Medical Science Research.* 1992;20:717-20.
30. Bukovsky M, Kostalova D, Magnusova R, Vaverkova S. Testing for immunomodulating effects of ethanol-water extracts of the above-ground parts of the plants Echinaceae (Moench) and Rudbeckia L.J. [Slovak]. *Ceskoslovenska Farmacie.* 1993;42(5):228-31.
31. Stimpel M, Proksch A, Wagner H, *et al.* Macrophage activation and induction of macrophage cytotoxicity by purified polysaccharide fractions from the plant *Echinacea purpurea. Infection and Immunity.* 1984;46(3):845-849.
32. Mose JR. Effect of echinacin on phagocytosis and natural killer cells. *Medizinische Welt.* 1983;34:1463-1467.
33. Bukovsky M, Vaverkova S, Kostalova D. Immunomodulating activity of Echinacea gloriosa L., *Echinacea angustifolia* DC. and Rudbeckia speciosa Wenderoth ethanol-water extracts. *Polish Journal of Pharmacology.* 1995;47:175-77.
34. Wagner H, Proksch A. Immunomodulatory drugs of fungi and higher plants. In: Farnsworth N, Hikino H, H. W, eds. *Economic and Medicinal Plant Research.* Orlando, FL: Academic Press; 1985:113-155.
35. Jurcic K, Melchart D, Holzmann M, *et al.* Two proband studies for the stimulation of granulocyte phagocitosis by Echinacea-containing preparations. *Zeitschrift fur Phytotherapie.* 1989;10:67-70.
36. Fong Y, Moldawer LL, Marano M, *et al.* Endotoxemia elicits increased circulating B2-IFN/IL-^ in man. *Journal of Immunology.*1989;142:2321-2340.
37. Melchart D, Linde K, Worku F, *et al.* Immunomodulation with echinacea - a systemic review of controlled clinical trials. *Phytomedicine.* 1994;1:245-254.
38. Coeugniet EG, Kuhnast R. Recurrent candidiasis: adjuvant immunotherapy with different formulations of Echinacin®. *Therapiewoche.* 1986;36:3352-3358.
39. Dorn M, Knick E, Lewith G. placebo-controlled, double-blind study of *Echinacea pallidae radix* in upper respiratory tract infections. *Complementary Therapies in Medicine.* 1997;5:40-42.
40. Braunig B, Dorn M, Knick E. *Echinacea purpurea* radix: zur starkung der korpereigenen abwehr bei grippalen infekten. *Zeitschrift fur Phytotherapie.* 1992;13:7-13.
41. Schoneberger D. The influence of immune-stimulating effects of pressed juice from *Echinacea purpuraea* on the course and severity of colds. Results of a recent double-blind study (in German). *Forum Immunologie.* 1992;8:2-12.
42. Braunig B, Dorn M, Limburg E, Knick E. *Echinacea purpurea* radix for strengthening the immune system in flu-like infections [in German]. *Zeitschrift fur Phytotherapie.* 1992;13:7-13.
43. Galea S, Thacker K. Double-blind, Prospective Trial Investigating the Effectiveness of a Commonly Prescribed Herbal Remedy in Altering Duration, Severity and Symptoms of the Common Cold. Family Medicine, Health Sciences North,Thunder Bay, unpublished. 1996.
44. Busing KH. Inhibition of hyaluronidase by Echinacin [German] *Arzneimittelforschung.* 1952;2:467-472.
45. Korting GW, Born W. Beeinflussung des trypanociden salvarson-effekts durch hyaluronidase und einen hyaluronidase-inhibitor (Echinacin). *Arzneimittelforschung.* 1954;4:424-6.
46. Koch FE, Haase H. Eine modifikation des spreading-testes im tierversuch, gleichzeitig ein beitrag zum wirkungsmechanismus von Echinacin. *Arzneimittelforschung.* 1953;2:464-7.
47. Koch FE, Uebel H. Experimentelle untersuchungen uber den einfu von *Echinacea purpurea* auf das hypophysen-nebennierenrinden-system. *Arzneimittelforschung.* 1953;3:133-7.
48. Tunnerhoff FK, Schwabe HK. Studies in human beings and animals on the influence of Echinacea extracts on the formation of connective tissue following the implantation of fibrin (in German). *Arzneimittelforschung.* 1956;6:330-334.
49. Keller H. German Patent 950 674 (11 October 1956). *Chemical Abstracts.* 1959;53:8550i.
50. Bonadero I, *et al.* Echinacin B: Active polysaccharide from Echinace. [Italian]. *Rivista Italiana Essenze Profumi Piante officinali, Aromi, Saponi, Cosmetici, Aerosol.* 1971;53:281-295.
51. Bonadero I, Lavazza M. Echinacina B: suo azione sui fibroblasti. [Italian]. *Rivista Italiana Essenze Profumi Piante officinali, Aromi, Saponi, Cosmetici, Aerosol.* 1972;54:195.
52. Tragni E, Tubaro A, Melis S, Galli CL. Evidence from two classical irritation tests for an anti-inflammatory action of

a natural extract, echinacea B. *Food and Chemical Toxicology*. 1985;23:317-319.
53. Tubaro A, Tragni E, Del Negro P, *et al.* Anti-inflammatory activity of a polsaccharide fraction of *Echinacea angustifolia*. *Journal of Pharmacy and Pharmacology.* 1987;39:567-569.
54. Wagner H, Breu W, Willer F, *et al*. *In vitro* inhibition of curadiridouate metabolism by some alkamides and prenylated phenols. *Planta Medica*. 1989;55:566-7.
55. Gaisbauer M, Zimmer290man W, Schleich T. Natura. Med. 1986;1:6-10.
56. Coeugniet EG, Elek E. Immunomodulation with viscum album and *Echinacea purpurea* extracts. *Onkologie*. 1987;10(3 (Supplement)):27-33.
57. Stoll A, Renz J, Brack A. Isolierung und konstitution des echinacosids, eines glykosids aus den wurzeln von *Echinacea angustifolia* D.C. *Helvetica Chimica Acta*. 1950;33:1877-93.
58. Schulte KE, Rucker G, Perlick J. Das vorkommen von polyacetylen-verbindungen in *Echinacea purpurea* Mnch. und Echinacea angustifolia DC. *Arzneimittelforschung*. 1967;17:825-829.
59. Samochowiec E, Urbanska L, Manka W, Stolarska E. Evaluation of the effect of Calendula officinalis and *Echinacea angustifolia* extracts on *Trichamonas vaginalis in vitro.* [Polish]. *Wiadomosci Parazytologiozne*. 1979;25(1):77-81.
60. Orinda D, Diedrich J, Wacker A. Antiviral activity of constituents of the compositae purpurea. [German]. *Arzneimittelforschung*. 1973;23:1119-1120.
61. Wacker A, Hilbig W. Virus inhibition by *Echinacea purpurea*. *Planta Medica*. 1978;33:89-102.
62. May G, Willuhn G. Antiviral effect of aqueous plant extracts in tissue culture. [German]. *Arzneimittelforschung*. 1978;28(1-4):1-7.
63. Cheminat A, Zawatzky R, Becker H, *et al*. Caffeoyl conjugates from *Echinacea* spp: Structures and biological functions. *Phytochemistry*. 1988;27:2787-94.
64. Lersch C, Zeuner M, Bauer A, *et al*. Nonspecific immunostimulation with low doses of cyclophosphamide (LDCY), thymostimulin, and *Echinacea purpurea* extracts (echinacin) in patients with far advanced colorectal cancers: preliminary results. *Cancer Investigation*. 1992;10(5):343-348.
65. Voaden DJ, Jacobson M. Tumor inhibitors. 3. Identification and synthesis of an oncolytic hydrocarbon from American coneflower roots. *Journal of Medicinal Chemistry*. 1972;15:619-623.
66. Paranich AV, Pocherniava VF, Dubinskaia GM, *et al.* Effect of supposed radioprotectors on oxidation-reduction of vitamin E in the tissues of irradiated rats. [Russian]. *Radiatsionnaia Biologiia, Radioecologiia*. 1993;33(5):653-7.
67. Facino RM, Carini M, Aldini G, Saibene L, Pietta P, Mauri P. Echinoside and caffeoyl conjugates protect collagen from free-radical-induced degradation: A potential use of Echinacea extracts in the prevention of skin photodamage. *Planta Medica*. 1995;61:510-514.
68. Beuscher N, Bodinet C, Willigmann I, Satzgitter DE. Immonomudulierende eigenschaften von wurzelextrakten verschiedener Echinacea-arten. *Zeitschrift fur Phytotherapie*. 1995;16:157-66.
69. Bergner P. Echinacea Species. *Medical Herbalism*. 1995;7(3):16.
70. Blumenthal M, Brusse WR, Goldberg A, *et al.* *The Complete German Commission E Monographs*. Austin, TX: American Botanical Council; 1998:685.
71. Lenk M. Acute toxicity of various polysaccarides from *Echinacea purpurea* in the mouse. *Zeitschrift fur Phytotherapie*. 1989;10:49-52.
72. Schimmer O, Abel G, Behninger C. Investigations on the genotoxic potency of a neutral polysaccharide from Echinacea cell cultures in cultured human lymphoclytes. *Zeitschrift fur Phytotherapie* 1989;10:39-42.
73. Mattocks AR. *Chemistry and Toxicology of Pyrrolizidine Alkaloids.* London: Academic Press; 1986.
74. Newall CA, Anderson LA, Phillipson JD. *Herbal Medicines: A Guide for Health Care Professionals.* London: The Pharmaceutical Press; 1996:296.
75. Reynolds JE. Martindale. *The Extra Pharmacopoeia*. 29th ed. London: The Pharmaceutical Press; 1989.
76. Bergner P. Contraindications for echinacea? *Medical Herbalism*. 1997;9(1):1,11-4.
77. Tyler VE. *Herbs of Choice. The Therapeutic Use of Phytomedicinals.* Binghamton, NY: Pharmaceutical Products Press; 1994:209.
78. von Unruh V. *Echinacea angustifolia* and *Inula helenium* in the treatment of tuberculosis. *Nat Eclect Med Assoc Quart*.1915;7:63.
79. Heesen W, Schroeder C. Die bedeutung des Echiancin in der tuberculose-therapie. *Med Monatsschr.* 1960;14:251-6c
80. McLeod D. Case history of chronic lymphatic leukaemia. Ajoene inhibition of platelet aggregation: Possible mediation by a hemoprotein. *The Modern Phytotherapist*. 1996;2(3):10.
81. Bergner P. Echinacea myth: Phagocytosis not diminished after ten days. *Medical Herbalism*. 1994;6(1):1.
82. Bone K. Long term use of echinacea. *Medical Herbalism* 1995;7(1-2):23.
83. Bradley P. *British Herbal Compendium.* Bournemouth, UK: The British Herbal Medical Association; 1992:239.

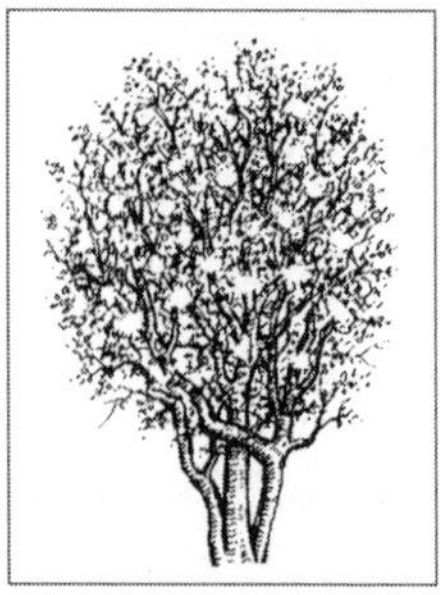

ELDER

Sambucus nigra L.

THUMBNAIL SKETCH

Active Constituents

- Flavonoids
- Triterpenes
- Essential oils
- Sterols
- Phenolic acids

Common Uses

Internal

- Ailments of the respiratory tract, especially with fever and phlegm: colds, flu, sinusitis, hay fever and bronchitis.

External

- Eczema, boils, dermatitis

Adverse Effects

- None noted with berries or flowers of American or European elder

Cautions/Contraindications

- Pregnancy and lactation
- Prolonged use is not recommended due to hypokalemic potential
- Intake should be limited to products made from the ripe berries or flowers only

Drug Interactions

- None noted.

Doses

- 3-5g dried flowers three times daily
- 3-5mL liquid extract (1:1, 25% ethanol) three times daily
- 10-25mL tincture (1:5; 25% ethanol) three times daily

INTRODUCTION

Family: Caprifoliaceae

Synonyms: Sambucus, Black elder, Common elder, Pipe tree, Bore tree, Bour tree, Hylder, Hylantree, Eldrum, Hollunder, Sureau, Sweet elder (canadensis), Rob elder (canadensis), Elderberry (canadensis); *S. nigra* L. ssp. *canadensis* (L.) R. Bolli[1-4]

Both *Sambucus nigra* L. (European elder) and *S. nigra* L. ssp. *canadensis* (L.) R. Bolli (American elder) are used medicinally. They share similar indications and appearance, except that the former is slightly larger, growing up to 10m in height as compared to 4 m for its North American cousin.[1, 5] *S. nigra* L. ssp. *canadensis* (L.) R. Bolli is native to Eastern United States and Canada with *Sambucus nigra* L. being common place throughout the hedgerows of the United Kingdom and Europe.[1, 5] Both species can now be found throughout North America. While the flowers are the part most commonly used medicinally, most parts, notably the leaves and berries, are considered to have therapeutic properties.[1, 3]

Although known for its healing properties, elder also has folkloric importance. It was considered a good charm, used to drive away robbers and kill snakes.[6] In rural England it was considered a grave offence to damage any part of the tree since it was thought to be intrinsically linked to 'Mother Earth'.[7]

Constituents

The below are limited to the investigational work on European elder.

Flowers:[1, 2, 5, 8-12]

- Flavonoids: quercetin, kaempferol, isoquercetin, rutin, astragalin.
- Triterpenes: ursolic acid, and amyrin, 30 hydroxyursolic acid
- Essential oil: fatty acids and alkanes
- Phenolic acids: chlorogenic acid, p-coumaric acid and caffeic acid
- Miscellaneous: Mucilage, tannins, potassium, pectin, proteins (plastocynin)

Leaf:

- Similar to above with cyanogenic glucosides (sambunigrin) also present.[5, 9, 13]

Berries:

- Fruit acids, tannins, anthocyanin pigments, pectin, traces of essential oil.[1]

Bark:

- Phytohemagglutins[14], lectin, triterpenoids[2] and cyanogenic glucosides.[4]

THERAPEUTIC USES & RELEVANT PHARMACOLOGY

Preparations made from various parts of the plant are suggested to be useful in the management of many conditions. Different parts are used for different indications.

FLOWERS

Elder flowers are used, alone or in combination with other herbal remedies such as peppermint, in the treatment of many respiratory conditions where there is fever and/or phlegm including: colds,[1, 7, 8, 15, 16] flu,[1, 7, 8, 15, 16] hayfever,[1, 7, 15] sinusitis,[1, 7, 15] recurrent ear infections,[1, 7] bronchitis,[1, 7] and croup.[1] Gargles made from the flower are used to ease sore and irritated throats.[1] Preparations of elder flower are particularly popular in pediatric cases.[16]

The flowers have also been used for many conditions of the genitourinary tract such as: cystitis,[1] and renal stones.[1] Generally, elder may be indicated in situations where diuresis is required.[7, 8, 15]

In addition, ointments, lotions and salves made from elder flowers are used to treat various skin conditions including: eczema, dermatitis, urticaria and generally irritated skin.[1]

BERRIES

The berries are considered to be useful as an antirheumatic and laxative.[1, 7, 15] Liquid extracts made from the berries are now commonly used in monodiets, juice fasts and detoxification protocols.

RELATED SPECIES

It should be noted that red elderberry (*Sambucus racemosa*) has long been used by the Haida, Saanich and Cowichan peoples of British Columbia in the treatment of many conditions ranging from women's health to those similar to the ones mentioned above.[17]

PHARMACOLOGY

Pharmacological findings provide preliminary explanations for some of elder's indications. Extracts of *Sambucus nigra* L. have been shown to exert a diuretic effect in rats, primarily as a result of the flavonoid and potassium content.[8,18] This may explain its use in disorders of the genitourinary tract. As well, a methanolic extract of the branch tips of red elderberry has been shown to exhibit activity against bovine respiratory syncytial virus.[17] Red elderberry has also been shown to have some antibacterial[19] and antifungal activity.[20] While the extracts of various species of Sambucus have been used as diagnostic tools (e.g., as an indication of immunocompetence), no human clinical trials could be found to substantiate the above indications.[2]

Other miscellaneous actions of elder have also been reported. For example, oral administration of an elder extract has been shown to have mild anti-inflammatory properties in rats [21] and lectins extracted from European elder have been shown to possess antispasmodic properties *in vitro*.[22]

ADVERSE EFFECTS

The flowers and ripe seeds appear to be free from adverse effects and are considered in the USA as being GRAS (generally regarded as safe).[2] Substances found in other parts of the plant, notably the cyanogenic glycosides, have the potential to cause gastrointestinal distress, including nausea, diarrhoea and vomiting.[2] Weiss cautions that the seeds of *Sambucus racemosa* may cause irritation to the mucous membranes.[23] Although the lectins have been shown to have teratogenic potential in pregnant mice, the doses administered were far above those possible in normal practice.[2]

CAUTIONS/CONTRAINDICATIONS

Newall cautions against both use in pregnancy and lactation and against long-term use due to the potential of hypokalemia resulting from prolonged diuresis.[2] No supporting evidence for this concern could be found from empirical sources.

DRUG INTERACTIONS

None recorded.

DOSAGE REGIMEN

Even though parts from the whole plant have been used historically, medicinal use should be limited to the flowers and ripe berries (which are usually boiled).[2, 4]

Internal

- 3-5g of dried flowers taken as a hot infusion three times daily[8]
- 3-5mL of liquid extract of dried flower (1:1, 25% ethanol) three times daily[8]
- 10-25mL of tincture of dried flower (1:5, 25% ethanol) three times daily[8]

External

- Elder Flowers can also be used externally in the form of poultices, ointments and salves.

Elder Flowers are also taken often in the form of cordials and for nutritious rather than medicinal reasons.[1, 23]

REFERENCES

1. Stelling K. Sambucus/Elder. *Canadian Journal of Herbalism*. 1991;12:15-18.
2. Newall C, Anderson L, David Phillipson J. *Herbal Medicines: A Guide for Health Care Professionals*. London: The Pharmaceutical Press; 1996:296.
3. Hutchens A. *Indian Herbology of North America*. Boston: Shambhala; 1991:382.
4. Marles RJ, Associate Professor, Department of Botany, Brandon University, Brandon, Manitoba. Review of Medicinal Plant Modules for CCNM ;1997.
5. Leung A, Foster S. *Encyclopedia of Common Natural Ingredients in Food, Drugs and Cosmetics*. 2nd ed. New York, NY: John Wiley and Sons; 1996:649.
6. Stelling K. Restoring the liver. *Canadian Journal of Herbalism*. 1991;12:7-10.
7. Chevallier A. *The Encyclopedia of Medicinal Plants*. London: Reader's Digest; 1996:336.
8. Bradley P. *British Herbal Compendium*. Bournemouth: BHMA; 1992:239.

9. Evans W. *Trease and Evans' Pharmacology.* 13th ed. London: Bailliere-Tindall; 1989:832.
10. Davidek J. Isolation of chromatographically pure rutin from flowers of elder. *Nature*. 1961;189:487-488.
11. Willuhn G, Richter W. On the constituents of *Sambucus nigra* II.The lipophillic components of the flowers. *Planta Medica*. 1977;31:328-343.
12. Toulemonde B, Richard H. Volatile constituents of dry elder (*Sambucus nigra.*L) flowers. *Journal of Agriculture and Food Chemistry*. 1983;31:365-70.
13. Jensen S, Nielsen B. Cyanogenic glucosides in *Sambucus nigra* L. *Acta Chemica Scandinavica*. 1973;27:2661-85.
14. Wren R. *Potter's New Encyclopedia of Botanical Drugs and Preparations*. Saffron Walden: C.W. Daniel Company; 1988:362.
15. Hoffman D. *Holistic Herbal.* Rockport, MA: Element Books; 1996:256.
16. Mills S. *The Essential Book of Herbal Medicine.* 2nd ed. London: Penguin Publ; 1991:677.
17. McCutcheon A, Roberts T, Gibbons E, *et al.* Antiviral screening of British Columbian medicinal plants. *Journal of Ethnopharmacology*. 1995;49:101-110.
18. Rebuelta M, *et al.* Etude de l'effet diuretique de differentes preparations des fleurs du sambucus nigra L. *Plantes Medicinales et Phytotherapie.* 1983;17:173-81.
19. McCutcheon A, Ellis S, Hancock R, Towers G. Antibiotic screening of medicinal plants of the British Columbian native peoples. *Journal of Ethnopharmacology*. 1993;37:213-223.
20. McCutcheon A, Ellis S, Hancock R, Towers G. Antifungal screening of medicinal plants of the British Columbian native peoples. *Journal of Ethnopharmacology*. 1994;44:157-169.
21. Mascolo N, *et al.* Biological screening of Italian medicinal plants for anti-inflammatory activity. *Phytotherapy Research*. 1987;1:28-31.
22. Richter A. Changes in the motor activity if smooth muscles of the rat uterus *in vitro* as the effect of phytohaemag glutins from *Sambucus nigra*. *Folia Biol*. 1973;21:33-48.
23. Weiss R. *Herbal Medicine*. Beaconsfield: Beaconsfield Publishers; 1988:362.

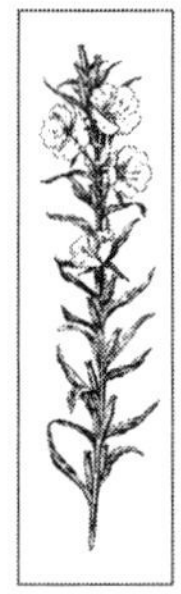

EVENING PRIMROSE

Oenothera biennis L.

THUMBNAIL SKETCH

Active Constituents

- Fixed oil containing gamma linolenic acid and linoleic acid

Common Uses

- Atopic eczema
- Diabetic neuropathy
- Women's Health Care including: premenstrual syndrome, mastalgia and endometriosis
- Rheumatoid arthritis
- Multiple sclerosis
- Sjögren's syndrome
- Psychiatric conditions: schizophrenia, hyperactivity in children, dementia
- Alcoholism
- Obesity

Cautions/Contraindications

- Mania and epilepsy

Drug Interactions

- None documented but concerns have been raised regarding use with: phenothiazines, non-steroidal anti-inflammatory drugs, corticosteroids, anticoagulants, and beta-adrenergic antagonists

Doses

- Adults: 2-8 grams daily in divided doses with food
- Children: 2-6 grams daily in divided doses with food

INTRODUCTION

Family: Onagraceae

Synonyms: Tree Primrose, Sundrop, King's cureall[1, 2]

Evening primrose is a biennial standing 1 to 3 meters in height.[3] The stem rises from a fibrous taproot with a flat basal rosette of leaves. The plant blooms in early summer, producing large yellow flowers. The capsular pods that form after the individual blooms die contain brown seeds rich in fixed oil.[4] Evening primrose is actually not a primrose (Family Primulaceae) at all, but a member of the fuchsia (Onagraceae) family. Its name arises from the fact that the flowers open in the evening in order to allow pollination by insects (especially moths). While *Oenothera biennis* L. is native to North America, it is now naturalized throughout Western Europe, brought there accidentally as sea trade increased between the two continents.[4]

Evening primrose has been used for both medical and culinary purposes in the past. The root was used as a vegetable because of its pungent flavor[4] and the whole plant was indicated in the management of many conditions including: gastrointestinal disorders, asthmatic coughs, neuralgia and whooping cough.[4, 5] These numerous indications gave rise to the plant being commonly referred to as King's cureall.[4]

The fixed oil from the seeds is now the primary form used therapeutically.[4] Evening primrose oil was one the first nutritional/botanical supplements to gain popularity in the renaissance of 'alternative medicine'. The popularity of evening primrose oil supplements is such that in 1993 a survey of complementary medicine use in Australia showed that over 12% of all women supplemented with this product.[6]

Constituents [2-4]

Given that the fixed oil of evening primrose oil is the part used medicinally, a discussion of the plant's constituents will be limited to the seeds.

Seeds: Approximately 14% fixed oil comprising approximately 70% cis-linoleic acid, 9% cis-gamma linolenic acid (GLA), oleic acid, palmitic acid and stearic acid.

THERAPEUTIC USES & RELEVANT PHARMACOLOGY

GENERAL PHARMACOLOGY

In understanding the suggested pharmacology of evening primrose oil, it is necessary to review some basic points regarding essential fatty acid (EFA) biochemistry and nomenclature. By definition, an essential fatty acid is one which the body cannot make. There are two basic types, omega 3 (derived from α-linolenic acid) and omega 6 (derived from linoleic acid). These essential fatty acids are polyunsaturated (containing more than one double bond). The naming of a particular fatty acid is made by determining the position of the first double bond from the methyl end of the carbon-carbon backbone of the molecule. For example, an omega 3 fatty acid contains a double bond between the third and fourth carbon atom. The essential fatty acids have a cis rather than a trans configuration and the omega 3 and omega 6 series are not interchangeable.[7, 8]

Both alpha-linolenic and linoleic acid can be modified via desaturation or elongation reactions. While neither alpha-linolenic acid nor linoleic acid have any direct biological effect, their metabolites have pronounced physiological properties. The enzymatic mechanism by which these changes occur is very similar, if not identical, in both the omega 3 and omega 6 series.[8] The physiological action of EFAs occurs in one of two primary ways. EFAs play a role in the physical properties of cell membranes, influencing their flexibility and fluidity and thus they impact membrane based receptors and systems. EFAs also act as precursors of biologically active eicasonoids such as prostaglandins and leukotrienes.[8]

In the omega 6 series, cis-linoleic acid (LA) is converted to gamma-linolenic acid (GLA) which in turn is converted to dihomogamma-linolenic acid (DGLA). The rate-limiting step for this process is the desaturation of LA to GLA by the enzyme delta-6 desaturase. The DGLA can then be metabolized further to form arachadonic acid (AA) by delta-5 desaturase. DGLA can also be acted upon by cyclo-oxygenase to form prostaglandin E_1 (PGE_1). PGE_1 is generally regarded as being beneficial, inhibiting inflammation and platelet aggregation, decreasing blood pressure and regulating the immune system. Conversely, arachidonic acid gives rise to harmful pro-inflammatory mediators.[7, 8] While it may be assumed that any increase in GLA would lead to a subsequent increase in both the anti-inflammatory and inflammatory moieties, this appears not to be the case. Administration of large amounts of GLA increases DGLA levels but not AA. It is thought that the beneficial metabolites of DGLA (including PGE_1) play a role in limiting the release of arachidonic acid from its phospholipid stores. Also while the conversion of GLA to DGLA is rapid, the activity of delta-5 desaturase is quite slow.[7, 8]

Since the body can manufacture GLA, it should not theoretically be considered an essential fatty acid. In practice this may not be the case due to the inefficiency of the rate limiting enzyme mentioned above, delta-6 desaturase. This enzyme system appears to be compromised in many situations including: aging,[4, 8, 9] diabetes,[8, 10, 11] excessive consumption of alcohol,[7, 8, 12, 13] viral infections,[7, 8, 14, 15] and atopic eczema.[7, 8] A deficiency in certain nutritional cofactors (e.g., zinc,[8, 16, 17] pyridoxine,[4, 8, 18] and magnesium[4, 8]) can also lead to a decreased activity of this enzyme system. The existence of a decreased rate of delta-6 desaturation in atopic individuals is not universally accepted.[19]

The therapeutic rationale for the use of evening primrose oil is that since it is rich in GLA it bypasses the rate limiting delta-6 desaturase stage.[4, 8, 20]

DERMATOLOGICAL CONDITIONS

Atopic eczema/dermatitis

The fact that delta-6 desaturation may be slower in atopic individuals has led to the suggestion that oral administration of evening primrose oil could be beneficial in the management of atopic eczema.[8] A number of clinical studies support this claim, showing that evening primrose oil significantly improved symptoms including itching, inflammation and dryness.[21-28] The evidence is not universally positive with a number of studies showing that evening primrose was not superior to placebo in the management of this condition.[29-33] Consequently, the use of evening primrose oil orally in the management of atopic eczema in North America remains controversial.[34-36] In contrast, evening primrose oil is considered suitable in the management of atopic eczema in many countries, including the United Kingdom, Germany, Australia and New Zealand.[20]

Several explanations for the failure of evening primrose oil in some studies have been suggested. Firstly, omega 3 EFAs (deep-sea fish oil) may be as important as omega 6, implying that combination products containing both may be more beneficial. Also, in some cases of atopy other desaturation steps apart from the delta-6 stage could be involved. Finally, not all cases of atopic eczema are due to disorders of fatty acid metabolism.[8]

Topical application of a cream containing 12.5% evening primrose oil to volunteers (n=20) with dry skin, significantly increased sebum content without changing transepidermal water loss. It should be noted that while the volunteers had an atopic disposition, they did not present with frank atopic dermatitis.[37] Evening primrose oil, when applied topically, did not prevent steroid induced epidermal atrophy caused by the twice daily application of 0.1% betamethasone valerate.[38]

Psoriasis

The supplementation of evening primrose oil and marine oil (i.e., omega 6 and omega 3) have proved unsuccessful in the management of psoriasis.[39]

Asthma

Oral administration of evening primrose oil appears not to be effective in the management of various forms of asthma.[19, 32, 40, 41]

Diabetic Neuropathy

As has already been noted, the ratio of linoleic acid and linolenic acid to their respective metabolites has been found to be elevated in diabetes.[8, 42, 43] In diabetic patients both delta-6 and delta-5 desaturase enzymes may be impaired.[8, 9] This impairment of normal fatty acid metabolism and subsequent production of physiological moieties may play an important role in the development of diabetic neuropathy.[43] By administering pre-formed gamma-linolenic acid (as in evening primrose oil), this imbalance may be corrected. The discovery that evening primrose oil may correct deficient nitric oxide in the nerve ischemia seen in diabetes implies that evening primrose's action may be more complex than was originally proposed.[44, 45] Also, recently the role played by cyclo-oxygenase activity in the neuroactivity of evening primrose oil appears to be an important factor to consider.[46, 47] A latency period noted in a recent animal study has led to the suggestion that the action of evening primrose oil may be mediated by metabolically generated compounds rather than one existing in the oil itself.[48]

A beneficial role for the use of evening primrose oil in the correction of the neurovascular disorders seen in diabetics has been demonstrated in a number of animal studies.[8, 48-52] Administration of 4 g of evening primrose oil (360 mg gamma-linolenic acid) daily for 6 months to diabetic patients (n=22) suffering from diabetic neuropathy caused an improvement (objective and subjective) when compared to placebo. Glycosylated hemoglobin levels were not influenced by evening primrose oil supplementation.[53] These positive findings were confirmed in a later double-blinded multicenter trial with patients (n=111) suffering from 'mild diabetic neuropathy'. The dose of evening primrose oil was higher than in the previous study (6 grams daily equivalent to 480 mg of gamma-linolenic acid) and the trial was carried out over a year. The response to evening primrose oil appeared more pronounced in those with lower starting glycosylated hemoglobin levels, suggesting satisfactory blood sugar control.[54] It appears that the gamma-linolenic acid content of a supplement does not determine its efficacy in managing diabetic neuropathy. In a recent animal study, evening primrose oil supplementation was shown to out-perform a number of other products rich in GLA (borage oil, blackcurrant oil and 'fungal' oil).[55]

WOMEN'S HEALTH CARE

Premenstrual syndrome

A number of studies have indicated that evening primrose oil may be of use in the management of premenstrual syndrome (PMS).[8, 56-60] The benefits are seen only following prolonged administration of four to six months.[8, 20] A proposed mechanism of action is that the PGE_1 generated could influence the actions of prolactin which is thought to play a role in the presentation of this syndrome.[8, 61] Women with premenstrual syndrome may also have difficulty in converting linoleic acid into gamma-linolenic acid.[62] However, on reviewing the available literature, Budeiri *et al.* concluded that evening primrose oil offered no benefit. They argued that most of the information comes from easily discounted, open studies and that the well-controlled studies were "small and modest" in design.[63] The above comments regarding the necessity of prolonged administration could play a part in these negative findings.

Mastalgia

Information from both placebo-controlled trials and open trials has shown that evening primrose oil is beneficial in the management of both cyclical and non-cyclical mastalgia.[64-68] The advantage of evening primrose oil over other more conventional therapies appears to be the lack of adverse effects.[65, 69] While one study suggested it was as effective as bromocriptine,[67] another suggested its effect to be only slightly greater than placebo.[66] The suggested mechanism of action is via prolactin modulation.[8] As with the case of PMS, benefits are only noted after prolonged administration, usually four to six months.[20]

Endometriosis

A combination product containing both gamma-linolenic acid and the omega 3 fatty acid eicosapentaenoic acid (Scotia HGA®) was shown in a placebo-controlled trial to decrease the symptoms of endometriosis in 90% of cases.[8]

Menopause

While evening primrose oil is often used in the management of menopause, it appears to offer no benefit over placebo in treating associated flushing and sweating.[70]

INFLAMMATORY AND AUTOIMMUNE CONDITIONS

Rheumatoid Arthritis

Various *in vitro* and *in vivo* trials have demonstrated that PGE_1 has anti-inflammatory properties. Since it has been suggested that evening primrose oil may increase the levels of this moiety, it may be therapeutically useful in the management of this condition.[8, 71] In a review of the relevant clinical trials, Joe and Hart conclude that the studies conducted varied in both design and quality and that the evidence supporting its use in the management of this condition is not conclusive. Any benefits noted appeared to be subjective rather than objective.[72] Short-term administration appears to provide no clinical benefits with relief being noted after six months in some studies.[71, 73, 74] Since two of the clinical trials were of limited duration[75, 76] this has been given as a possible explanation for their lack of positive results.[72]

In a double blind placebo controlled trial of patients (n=38, duration of 9 months) suffering from psoriatic arthritis, a combination product containing evening primrose oil and fish oil (Efamol Marine®) was seen to offer no therapeutic benefits.[77]

Multiple Sclerosis

An association between multiple sclerosis and levels of linoleic acid has been seen.[71, 73, 78, 79] There is some evidence to suggest that evening primrose oil may be beneficial in reducing the severity, duration of relapses of the disease and progression of the disease.[73, 80] The patients most likely to respond appear to be those with a recent diagnosis and less severe symptoms.[73, 81] The mode of action proposed is that the linoleic acid may be modifying an immune response and that the most benefit may be obtained by combining the therapy with a low animal fat/high polyunsaturated fat diet.[80] The need to use the more expensive evening primrose oil rather than linoleic acid has been questioned.[73]

Sjögren's Syndrome

Abnormalities in fatty acid metabolism have been noted in Sjögren's syndrome.[8] Supplementation with evening primrose oil has been shown to stimulate lachrymation and ease the lethargy often present with this condition.[8, 82, 83]

Cardiovascular Conditions

Essential fatty acids are known to play an important role in maintaining good cardiovascular health. Problems with essential fatty acid metabolism or inadequate consumption are known to increase cholesterol, increase platelet aggregation and increase blood pressure.[2] Combination products of omega 3 and omega 6 oils may be useful in the management of various cardiovascular conditions.[71, 84] Both human and animal studies suggest that evening primrose oil can decrease blood pressure and inhibit platelet aggregation.[8, 85]

In a double blind study, evening primrose oil supplementation was shown to result in symptomatic relief of patients suffering from Raynaud's phenomenon but no change in the objective measures were noted.[86]

PSYCHIATRIC CONDITIONS

Schizophrenia

While the exact pathophysiology of schizophrenia has yet to be determined, it has been suggested that abnormal essential fatty acid metabolism may be implicated. Decreased levels of linoleic acid in plasma phospholipids have been noted in schizophrenics. It has been suggested that they may have difficulty in producing PGE_1,[87] which may play a role in decreasing excessive central dopaminergic function (which is thought to play a role in the pathogenesis of the disease).[8, 88] Clinical research to date (placebo-controlled trials, open observational trials and reported case histories) has produced contradictory results.[8, 87-89] In a group of psychiatric patients suffering from tardive dyskinesia induced by neuroleptics, evening primrose oil was reported to cause a "marginally significant" improvement.[88] When four cofactors needed in essential fatty acid metabolism (zinc, pyridoxine, niacin and vitamin C) were added to the protocol, this improvement was increased, and included enhancement of memory and alleviation of schizophrenic symptoms.[8]

Hyperactivity

Abnormalities in essential fatty acid metabolism have been noted in cases of children with hyperactivity disorder, behavioral problems and learning difficulties.[90-94] It is interesting to note that both essential fatty acid requirements and the incidence of hyperactivity are higher in boys than girls.[92] A review of case studies suggests that supplementation with evening primrose oil may prove beneficial in treating hyperactivity.[95] However, in a placebo controlled, double blind study in hyperkinetic children (n=90, age 5 to 15), evening primrose oil supplementation did not improve behavioral patterns or change blood fatty acid composition compared to placebo.[73] It is important to note that the placebo used in this case was safflower oil, a substance rich in essential fatty acids.

Dementia

Supplementation with evening primrose oil may prove beneficial in the management of various kinds of dementia, including Alzheimer's disease and that caused by aging.[2, 8]

MISCELLANEOUS

Gastrointestinal Disorders

Evening primrose oil has been shown to "significantly improve stool consistency" when compared to both a fish oil supplement and placebo in ulcerative colitis. No difference in the other symptoms (stool frequency, rectal bleeding, disease relapse, sigmoidoscopic appearance or rectal histology) was seen.[96] In addition, relief was noted in a double-blind, placebo controlled crossover trial in women suffering from irritable bowel syndrome exacerbated premenstrually with supplementation of evening primrose oil.[8]

Post-Viral Fatigue Syndrome

Supplements containing evening primrose have been demonstrated to be effective in the management of "post-viral syndrome" (a.k.a. chronic fatigue syndrome, myalgic encephalomyelitis) in both placebo controlled trials and in clinical practice.[15, 97, 98] In a double-blind, placebo controlled trial of 63 adults with clear cases of "post-viral syndrome" taking a combination product of evening primrose oil and fish oil (Efamol Marine®), a pronounced improvement in symptoms (fatigue, myalgia, dizziness, poor concentration and memory) was noted.[15] This study was carried out on volunteers with a clear viral etiology to their condition.[15]

Alcoholism

Alcohol is known to have multiple effects on the metabolism of essential fatty acids; causing depletion of linoleic acid stores,[71] inhibiting the conversion of linoleic acid to gamma-linolenic acid,[12, 71] and stimulating the conversion of dihomogamma-linolenic acid to arachidonic acid.[71] While alcohol initially increases PGE_1 synthesis, long-term consumption causes a marked drop.[71] Abrupt cessation of alcohol consumption also causes a rapid fall in PGE_1 levels.[71] It has been hypothesized that administration of pre-formed gamma-linolenic acid may play a role in preventing alcohol toxicity and the development of alcohol addiction.[99] Human trials have shown that the administration of evening primrose oil decreases the need for tranquilizer use during the withdrawal phase and promotes the normalization of elevated liver enzymes.[71, 73] While long-term administration does not decrease relapse rate, it does appear to appreciably improve recovery of memory and visual-motor coordination.[71] Animal studies have demonstrated that administration of evening primrose oil may decrease the damaging effect on the brain and the teratogenic potential of alcoholism.[71, 100]

Renal Disease

Diets enriched with evening primrose oil have been shown to decrease the nephrotoxic effect of cyclosporine in rats.[101, 102] Evidence from *in vivo* trials also suggests that evening primrose oil supplementation may prove beneficial in the treatment of urolithiasis.[103-105]

Cancer

In vitro studies have shown that gamma-linolenic acid has anti-neoplastic properties.[71] The clinical relevance of this has yet to be determined.

Obesity

Evening primrose oil has been suggested useful in the management of obesity.[81] Clinical studies on humans have reported mixed results.[81, 106-108]

It is important to note that some authors suggest that insufficient vigorous clinical trials exist to justify many of the uses suggested for evening primrose oil.[2, 109]

ADVERSE EFFECTS

Evening primrose oil appears to be exceedingly safe.[71, 73, 110] Adverse effects in humans are very rare and limited to headache, nausea and diarrhea.[4, 8] Evening primrose oil has been shown in animal studies to have no carcinogenic properties.[111] At normal therapeutic doses (less than 4 grams daily), it is unlikely that evening primrose oil would be harmful if taken in pregnancy;[112] however, the composition of breast-milk can be manipulated by supplementing the maternal diet with evening primrose oil.[113]

CAUTIONS/CONTRAINDICATIONS

Evening primrose oil should not be used in mania due to a theoretical possibility of exacerbating the symptoms.[81] Evening primrose oil should be used with caution with patients suffering from epilepsy (see drug interactions).[2, 73, 81]

DRUG INTERACTIONS

No reports of interactions between evening primrose oil and conventional medication could be found. A possible increase in epileptic attacks has been postulated in schizophrenics on phenothiazines treated with evening primrose oil.[89] The clinical likelihood of this occurring in practice has been questioned.[8, 114] A theoretical interaction between gamma-linolenic acid and both non-steroidal anti-inflammatory drugs and corticosteroids has been suggested.[115] Whether this interaction would be synergistic or antagonistic is dependent upon whether the GLA is acting as a precursor of PGE_1 formation or if it modifies membrane composition.[8]

The therapeutic action of a product containing GLA, such as evening primrose oil, may be decreased with patients taking beta-blockers. This is due to the fact that cyclic AMP concentrations is in part mediated by beta adrenergic receptors as well as the action of PGE_1.[8] Evening primrose oil should be used with caution in patients taking conventional anticoagulant therapy.[81] Linoleic acid (in the form of safflower oil) has been shown to decrease neurotoxicity caused by lithium carbonate.[116]

DOSAGE REGIMENS

Most evening primrose oil supplements contain 8% gamma-linolenic acid.

- 2-8 grams daily in adults [2,20]

- 2-6 grams daily in children suffering from atopic eczema[2, 20]

Evening primrose oil is usually taken in divided doses. The incidence of nausea is more common when the supplement is taken on an empty stomach.[8] The therapeutic action of evening primrose oil may be limited if certain nutritional deficiencies such as zinc, vitamin C and pyridoxine exist.[8]

Other nutritional supplements exist which may contain more gamma-linolenic acid, such as borage oil (*Borago officinalis* L., Boraginaceae), blackcurrant oil (*Ribes nigrum* L., Grossulariaceae) and algal sources. These sources of GLA are generally considered less biologically active than that from evening primrose oil.[8] The vast majority of clinical evidence exists for evening primrose oil supplements.

It is important to remember that both omega 3 and omega 6 essential fatty acids are therapeutically important. Consequently, supplements combining both are becoming increasingly popular in practice.

REFERENCES

1. Wren R. *Potter's New Encyclopaedia of Botanical Drugs and Preparations.* Saffron Walden: C.W Daniel Company; 1988:362.
2. Newall C, Anderson L, Philipson JD. *Herbal Medicines: A Guide for Health-care Professionals.* London: The Pharmaceutical Press; 1996:296.
3. Leung A, Foster S. *Encylcopedia of Common Natural Ingredients Used in Food, Drugs and Cosmetics.* 2nd ed. New York, NY: John Wiley and Sons; 1996:649.
4. Briggs CJ. Evening primrose. *Canadian Pharmaceutical Journal.* 1986;119(5):249-54.
5. Hutchens A. *Indian Herbology of North America.* Boston, MA: Shambhala Press; 1991:382.
6. MacLennan A, Wilson D, Taylor A. Prevalence and cost of alternative medicine in Australia. *Lancet.* 1996;347:569-73.
7. Horrobin DF, Manku MS. Clinical biochemistry of essential fatty acids. *Omega-6 Essential Fatty Acids: Pathophysiology and Roles in Clinical Medicine* New York: Alan R. Liss; 1990:21-54.
8. Horrobin DF. Gammalinolenic acid: an intermediate in essential fatty acid metabolism with potential as an ethical pharmaceutical and as a food. *Reviews of Contemporary Pharmacotherapy.* 1990;1:1-45.
9. Horrobin D. Loss of delta-6-desaturase activity as a key factor in aging. *Medical Hypotheses.* 1981;7:1211-1220.
10. Jones D, Carter R, Haitas B, Mann J. Low phospholipid arachidonic acid values in diabetic platelets. *British Medical Journal.* 1983;286:173-175.
11. Tuna N, Frankhausen S, Goetz F. Total serum fatty acids in diabetes: relative and absolute concentrations of individual fatty acids. *American Journal of Medical Science.* 1968;255:120-130.
12. Brenner R, Peluffo R, Nervi A. Effect of ethanol administration on fatty acid desaturation. *Lipids.* 1980;15:263-268.
13. Horrobin DF. Essential fatty acids, prostaglandins and alcoholism: an overview. *Alcoholism, Clinical and Experimental Research.* 1987;11:2-9.
14. Behan P, Behan W. Essential fatty acids in the treatment of postviral fatigue syndrome. *Pathophysiology and Roles in Clinical Medicine.* 1990:275-282.
15. Behan P, Behan W, Horrobin D. Effect of high doses of essential fatty acids on the postviral fatigue syndrome. *Acta Neurologica Scandinavica.* 1990;82(3):209-16.
16. Bettger W, Reeves P, Moscatelli E, O'Dell B. Interaction of zinc and essential fatty acids in the rat. *Journal of Nutrition.* 1979;109:480-490.
17. Huang Y, Cunnane S, Horrobin D, Davignon J. Most biological effects of zinc deficiency corrected by gamma-linoleic acid but not linoleic acid. *Atherosclerosis.* 1982;41:193-207.
18. Cunnane S, Manku M, Horrobin D. Accumulation of linoleic and gamma-linolenic acids in tissue lipids of pyridoxine-deficient rats. *Journal of Nutrition.* 1984;114:1754-1761.
19. Leichsenring M, Kochsiek U, Paul K. (n-6)-Fatty acids in plasma lipids of children with atopic bronchial asthma. *Pediatric Allergy and Immunology.* 1995;6(4):209-12.
20. Brown D. *Herbal Prescriptions for Better Health.* Rocklin, CA: Prima Publishing; 1995:349.
21. Lovell CR, Burotn, JL, Horrobin DF, *et al.* Treatment of atopic eczema with evening primrose oil. *Lancet.* 1981(1):278.
22. Wright S, Burton JL. Oral evening primrose seed oil improves atopic eczema. *Lancet.* 1982(ii):1120-2.

23. Morse PF, Horrobin DF, Manku MS, *et al.* Meta-analysis of placebo-controlled studies of the efficacy of Epogam in the treatment of atopic eczema. Relationship between plasma essential fatty acid changes and clinical response. *British Journal of Dermatology*. 1989;121(75-90).
24. Bordoni A, Biagi PL, Masi M, *et al.* Evening primrose oil (Efamol) in the treatment of children with atopic eczema. *Drugs Under Experimental and Clinical Research*. 1987;14:291-7.
25. Stewart JCM, *et al.* Treatment of severe and moderately severe atopic dermatitis with evening primrose oil (Epogam); a multi centre study. *Journal of Nutritional Medicine*. 1991;2:9-15.
26. Schalin-Karrila M, Mattila L, Jansen CT, Votka P. Evening primrose oil in the treatment of atopic eczema: effect on clinical status, plasma phospholipid fatty acids and circulating blood prostaglandins. *British Journal of Dermatology*. 1987;117:11-19.
27. Anonymous. Oral medication treats symptoms and underlying cause of atopic eczema. *Hospital Medicine*. 1991;13(4):1-2.
28. Biagi PL, Bordoni A, Hrelia S, *et al.* The effect of gamma-linolenic acid on clinical status, red cell fatty acid composition and membrane microviscosity in infants with atopic dermatitis. *Drugs under Experimental and Clinical Research*. 1994;20(2):77-84.
29. Berth-Jones J, Graham-Brown RA. Placebo-controlled trial of essential fatty acid supplementation in atopic dermatitis [published erratum appears in Lancet 1993 Aug 28;342(8870):564] [see comments]. *Lancet*. 1993;341(8860):1557-60.
30. Bamford JTM, Gibson RW, Renier CM. Atopic eczema unresponsive to evening primrose oil (linolenic and gamma-linolenic acids). *Journal of the American Academy of Dermatology*. 1985;13:959-65.
31. Whitaker DK, Cilliers J, de Beer C. Evening primrose oil (Epogam) in the treatment of chronic hand dermatitis: disappointing therapeutic results. *Dermatology*. 1996;193(2):115-20.
32. Hederos CA, Berg A. Epogam evening primrose oil treatment in atopic dermatitis and asthma. *Archives of Disease in Childhood*. 1996;75(6):494-7.
33. Berg A. Epogam evening primrose oil treatment in atopic dermatitis and asthma. *Archives of Disease in Childhood.* 1996;75(6):494-7.
34. McHenry PM, Williams H, Bingham E. Management of atopic eczema. *British Medical Journal*. 1995;310:843-7.
35. Berth-Jones J, Graham-Brown RA. Evening primrose oil. Does not show promise in atopic dermatitis [letter; comment]. *British Medical Journal*. 1994;309(6966):1437.
36. Anon. No therapeutic effect for evening primrose oil in eczema. *Pharmaceutical Journal*. 1993;250:864.
37. Janosy I, Raguz J, *et al.* Effects of a cream containing 12.5% evening primrose oil on atopic disposition. *H & G Journal*. 1995;70:498-502.
38. Oliwiecki S, Armstrong J, Burton JL, Bradfield J. The effect of essential fatty acids on epidermal atrophy due to topical steroids. *Clinical and Experimental Dermatology.* 1993;18(4):326-8.
39. Oliwiecki S, Burton JL. Evening primrose oil and marine oil in the treatment of psoriasis. *Clinical and Experimental Dermatology*. 1994;19(2):127-9.
40. Stenius-Aarniala B, Aro A, Hakulinen A, *et al.* Evening primrose oil and fish oil are ineffective as supplementary treatment of bronchial asthma. *Annals of Allergy*. 1989;62:534-537.
41. Ebden P, Bevan C, Banks J, *et al.* A study of evening primrose seed oil in atopic asthma. *Prostaglandins, Leukotrienes and Essential Fatty Acids*. 1989;35:69-72.
42. Julu P. Gammalinolenic acid: A novel remedy for diabetic neuropathy in experimental animals. *Omega 6 Essential Fatty Acids: Pathophysiology and Roles in Clinical Medicine.* New York: Alan R Liss Inc; 1990:465-476.
43. Reichert RG. Evening primrose oil and diabetic neuropathy. *Quarterly Review of Natural Medicine*. 1995(Summer):141-5.
44. Omawari N, Dewhurst M, Vo P, Mahmood S, Stevens E, Tomlinson DR. Deficient nitric oxide responsible for reduced nerve blood flow in diabetic rats: effects of L-NAME, L-arginine, sodium nitroprusside and evening primrose oil. *British Journal of Pharmacology*. 1996;118(1):186-90.
45. Cameron NE, Cotter MA, Hohman TC. Interactions between essential fatty acid, prostanoid, polyol pathway and nitric oxide mechanisms in the neurovascular deficit of diabetic rats. *Diabetologia*. 1996;39(2):172-82.
46. Julu PO, Gow JW, Jamal GA. Endogenous cyclo-oxygenase substrates mediate the neuroactivity of evening primrose oil in rats. *Journal of Lipid Mediators and Cell Signalling.* 1996;13(2):115-25.
47. Fang C, Jiang Z, Tomlinson DR. Expression of constitutive cyclo-oxygenase (COX-1) in rats with streptozotocin-induced diabetes; effects of treatment with evening primrose oil or an aldose reductase inhibitor on COX-1 mRNA levels. *Prostaglandins, Leukotrienes and Essential Fatty Acids*. 1997;56(2):157-63.
48. Julu PO. Latency of neuroactivity and optimum period of treatment with evening primrose oil in diabetic rats. . *Journal of Lipid Mediators and Cell Signalling*. 1996;13(2):99-113.
49. Cameron NE, Cotter MA. Comparison of the effects of ascorbyl gamma-linolenic acid and gamma-linolenic acid in the correction of neurovascular deficits in diabetic rats. *Diabetologia*. 1996;39(9):1047-54.
50. Dines CD, Cotter MA, Cameron NE. Nerve function in galactosaemic rats: effects of evening primrose oil and doxazosin. *European Journal of Pharmacology.* 1995;281(3):303-9.

51. Cameron NE, Cotter MA, Dines KC, *et al*. The effects of evening primrose oil on nerve function and capillarization in streptozotocin-diabetic rats: modulation by the cyclo-oxygenase inhibitor flurbiprofen. *British Journal of Pharmacology.* 1993;109(4):972-9.
52. Stevens EJ, Lockett MJ, Carrington AL, Tomlinson DR. Essential fatty acid treatment prevents nerve ischaemia and associated conduction anomalies in rats with experimental diabetes mellitus [see comments]. *Diabetologia*. 1993;36(5):397-401.
53. Jamal GA, Charmichael H. The effect of gamma-linolenic acid on human diabetic peripheral neuropathy: a double-blind placebo-controlled trial. *Diabetic Medicine*. 1990;7:319-23.
54. Keen H, Payan J, Allawi J, *et al.* Treatment of diabetic neuropathy with gamma-linolenic acid. *Diabetes Care*. 1993;16:8-15.
55. Dines KC, Cotter MA, Cameron NE. Effectiveness of natural oils as sources of gamma-linolenic acid to correct peripheral nerve conduction velocity abnormalities in diabetic rats: modulation by thromboxane A2 inhibition. *Prostaglandins, Leukotrienes and Essential Fatty Acids*. 1996;55(3):159-65.
56. Puolakka J, Makarainen L, Viinikka L, Ylikorkala O. Biochemical and clinical effects of treating the premenstrual syndrome with prostaglandin synthesis precursors. *Journal of Reproductive Medicine*. 1985;30:149-153.
57. Horrobin D. The role of essential fatty acids and prostaglandins in premenstrual syndrome. *Journal of Reproductive Medicine*. 1983;28:465-8.
58. Brush MG. Efamol (evening primrose oil) in the treatment of premenstrual syndrome. In: Horrobin DF, ed *Clinical uses for essential fatty acids.* Buffalo, New York: Eden Press; 1982:p.155.
59. Collins A, Cerin A, *et al.* Essential fatty acids in the treatment of premenstrual syndrome. *Obstetrics and Gynecology*. 1993;81:93-8.
60. Steinberg S. The treatment of late luteal phase dysphoric disorder. *Life Sciences*. 1991;49(11):767-802.
61. Lurie S, Borenstein R. The Premenstrual Syndrome. *Obstetrical and Gynecological Survey*. 1990;45(4):220-228.
62. Brush MG, Watson SJ, *et al.* Abnormal essential fatty levels in plasma of women with premenstrual syndrome. *American Journal of Obstetrical Gynecology*. 1984;150:363-6.
63. Budeiri D, Li Wan Po A, Dornan JC. Is evening primrose oil of value in the treatment of premenstrual syndrome? *Controlled Clinical Trials.* 1996;17(1):60-8.
64. Pye JK, Mansel RE, Hughes LE. Clinical experience of drug treatments for masatalgia. *Lancet*. 1985(ii):373-7.
65. Mansel R, Pye J, Hughes L. Effects of essential fatty acids on cyclical mastalgia and non-cyclical breast disorders. *Omega-6 Essential fatty acids: pathophysiology and roles in clinical medicine.* New York: Alan R Liss; 1990:557-566.
66. Wetzig NR. Mastalgia: a 3 year Australian study. *Australian and New Zealand Journal of Surgery.* 1994;64(5):329-31.
67. Gateley CA, Miers M, Mansel R, Hughes L. Drug treatments for mastalgia: 17-year experience in the Cardiff mastalgia clinic. *Journal of the Royal Society of Medicine*. 1992;85:12-15.
68. Genolet P, Delaloye J, De Grandi P. Diagnosis and treatment of mastodynia (French). *Revue Medicales de la Suisse Romande*. 1995;115(5):385-90.
69. Anon. Cyclical breast pain- what works and what doesn't. *Drugs and Therapeutics Bulletin*. 1992;30(1):1-3.
70. Chenoy R, Hussain S, Tayob Y, *et al*. Effect of oral gammalinolenic acid from evening primrose oil on menopausal flushing. *British Medical Journal*. 1994;38:501-3.
71. Horrobin DF. Nutritional and medical importance of gamma-linolenic acid. *Progress in Lipid Research*. 1992;31:163-94.
72. Joe LA, Hart LL. Evening primrose oil in rheumatoid arthritis. *Ann Pharmacother*. 1993;27(12):1475-7.
73. Li Wan Po A. Evening primrose oil. *Pharmacy Journal*. 1991;246:670-6.
74. Belch JJ, Ansell D, Madhok R, *et al*. Effects of altering dietary essential fatty acids on requirements for non-steroidal anti-inflammatory drugs in patients with rheumatoid arthritis: a double blind placebo controlled study. *Annal of the Rheumatic Diseases.* 1988;47(2):96-104.
75. Hansen T, Lerche A, Kassis V, *et al*. Treatment of rheumatoid arthritis with prostaglandin E1 precursors cis-linoleic acid and gamma-linolenic acid. *Scandinavian Journal of Rheumatology.* 1983;12:85-8.
76. Jantti J, Seppala E, Vapaatalo H, Isomaki H. Evening primrose oil and olive oil in the treatment of rheumatoid arthritis. *Clinical Rheumatology* 1989;8:238-44.
77. Veale DJ, Torley HI, Richards IM, *et al.* A double-blind placebo controlled trial of Efamol Marine on skin and joint symptoms of psoriatic arthritis. *British Journal of Rheumatology.* 1994;33(10):954-8.
78. Horrobin D. Multiple sclerosis: the rational basis for treatment with colchicine and evening primrose oil. *Medical Hypotheses*. 1979;5(3):365-78.
79. Mertin H, Meade C. Relevance of fatty acids in Multiple Sclerosis. *British Medical Bulletin.* 1977;33:67-71.
80. Dworkin R, *et al.* Linoleic acid and multiple sclerosis: A reanalysis of three double-blind trials. *Neurology*. 1984;34:1441-5.
81. Barber HJ. Evening primrose oil: a panacea? *Pharmacy Journal*. 1988;240:723-5.
82. Horrobin D. Essential fatty acid and prostaglandin metabolism in Sjogren's syndrome, systemic sclerosis and rheumatoid

arthritis. *Scandinavian Journal of Rheumatology Supplement*. 1986;61:242-5.
83. Oxholm P, Manthorpe R, Prause J, Horrobin D. Patients with primary Sjogrens syndrome treated for two months with evening primrose oil. *Scandinavian Journal of Rheumatology*. 1986;15(2):103-8.
84. Werbach M. *Nutritional Influences on Illness*. 2nd ed. Tarzana: Third line press; 1993:700.
85. Mtabaji JP, Manku MS, Horrobin DF. Abnormalities in dihomo-gamma-linolenic acid release in the pathogenesis of hypertension. *American Journal of Hypertension*. 1993;6(6 Pt 1):458-62.
86. Belch J, Shaw B, O'Dowd A, *et al.* Evening primrose oil (Efamol) in the treatment of Raynauld's phenomenon: a double blind study. *Thrombosis and Haemostasis*. 1985;54(2):490-4.
87. Vaddadi K. The use of gamma-linolenic acid and linoleic acid to differentiate between temporal lobe epilepsy and schizophrenia. *Prostaglandins and Medicine*. 1981;6:375-379.
88. Vaddadi K, Courtney P, Gilleard C, *et al.* A double-blind trial of essential fatty acid supplementation in patients with tardive dyskinesia. *Psychiatry Research*. 1989;27:313-323.
89. Holman C, Bell A. A trial of evening primrose oil in the treatment of chronic schizophrenia. *Journal of Orthomolecular Psychiatry*. 1983;12:302-304.
90. Stevens L, Zentall S, Abate M, *et al.* Omega-3 fatty acids in boys with behaviour, learning and health problems. *Physiology and Behavior.* 1996;59(4/5):915-920.
91. Stevens L, Zentall S, Deck J, *et al.* Essential fatty acid metabolism in boys with attention-deficit hyperactivity disorder. *American Journal of Clinical Nutrition*. 1995;62(4):761-8.
92. Shreeve C. A state of perpetual motion. *World Medicine*. 1982;5(1):87-93.
93. Manku M, Morse-Fischer N, Horrobin D. Changes in human plasma essential fatty acid levels as a result of administration of linoleic acid and gamma-linolenic acid. *European Journal of Clinical Nutrition*. 1988;42:55-60.
94. Mitchell E, Aman M, Turbott S, Manku M. Clinical characteristics and serum essential fatty acid levels in hyperactive children. *Clinical Pediatrics*. 1987:406-11.
95. Blackburn M. Use of Efamol (Oil of Evening Primrose) for depression and hyperactivity in children. *Pathophysiology and Roles in Clinical Medicine*: Alan R Liss, INc; 1990:345-349.
96. Greenfield SM, Green AT, Teare JP, *et al.* A randomized controlled study of evening primrose oil and fish oil in ulcerative colitis. *Aliment Pharmacol Ther*. 1993;7(2):159-66.
97. Chilton SA. Cognitive behaviour therapy for the chronic fatigue syndrome. Evening primrose oil and magnesium have been shown to be effective [letter; comment]. *British Medical Journal*. 1996;312(7038):1098.
98. Lewith G. Chronic fatigue syndrome. *Update*. 1995(50):765.
99. Horrobin D. A biochemical basis for alcoholism and alcohol-induced damage including the fetal alcohol syndrome and cirrhosis; Interference with essential fatty acid and prostaglandin metabolism. *Medical Hypotheses*. 1980;6:929-42.
100. Varma P, Persaud T. Protection against ethanol-induced embryonic damage by administering gamma-linolenic acid and linoleic acids. *Prostaglandins, Leukotrienes and Medicine*. 1982;8(6):641-5.
101. Morphake P, Bariety J, Darlametsos I, *et al.* Alteration of cyclosporine (CsA)-induced nephrotoxicity by gamma linolenic acid (GLA) and eicosapentaenoic acid (EPA) in Wistar rats. *Prostaglandins, Leukotrienes and Essential Fatty Acids*. 1994;50(1):29-35.
102. Mills DE, de Antueno R, Scholey J. Interaction of dietary fatty acids and cyclosporine A in the borderline hypertensive rat: tissue fatty acids. *Lipids*. 1994;29(1):27-32.
103. Burgess NA, Reynolds TM, Williams N, *et al.* Evaluation of four animal models of intrarenal calcium deposition and assessment of the influence of dietary supplementation with essential fatty acids on calcification. *Urological Research*. 1995;23(4):239-42.
104. Tulloch I, Smellie WS, Buck AC. Evening primrose oil reduces urinary calcium excretion in both normal and hypercalciuric rats. *Urological Research*. 1994;22(4):227-30.
105. du Toit PJ, van Aswegen CH, Nel JD, *et al.* Pyelonephritis: renal urokinase activity in rats on essential fatty acid diets. *Urological Research*. 1994;22(3):127-30.
106. Haslett C, Douglas J, Chalmers S, *et al.* A double-blind evaluation of evening primrose oil as an antiobesity agent. *International Journal of Obesity*. 1983;7(6):549-53.
107. Garcia C, *et al.* Gamma linolenic acid causes weight loss and lower blood pressure in overweight patients with family history of obesity. *Swed J Biol Med*. 1986;4:8-11.
108. Vaddadi K, Horrobin D. Weight loss produced by evening primrose oil administration in normal and schizophrenic individuals. *IRCS J Med Sci*. 1979;7:52.
109. Kleijnen J. Evening primrose oil [editorial] [see comments]. *British Medical Journal*. 1994;309(6958):824-5.
110. Everett D, Greenough R, Perry C, *et al.* Chronic toxicities studies of Efamol evening primrose oil in rats and dogs. *Med. Sci. Res.* 1988;16:863-864.

111. Everett D, Perry C, Bayliss P. Carcinogenicity studies of Efamol evening primrose oil in rats and mice. *Med. Sci. Res.* 1988;16:865-866.
112. Lepik K. Safety of Herbal Medications in Pregnancy. *Canadian Pharmaceutical Journal*. 1997;130(3):29-33.
113. Cant A, Shay J, Horrobin DF. The effect of maternal supplementation with linolenic and gamma-linolenic acids on the fat com position and content of human milk. *Journal of Nutritional Science and Vitaminology*. 1991;37:573-9.
114. Stockley I. *Drug Interactions: A source book of adverse interactions, their mechanisms, clinical importance and management.* 3rd ed. London: Blackwell; 1994:932.
115. Brenner RR. Nutritional and hormonal factors influencing desaturation of essential fatty acids. *Progress in Lipid Research*. 1982;20:41-8.
116. Lieb J. Linoleic acid in the treatment of lithium toxicity and familial tremor. *Prostaglandin and Medicine*. 1980;4:275-279.

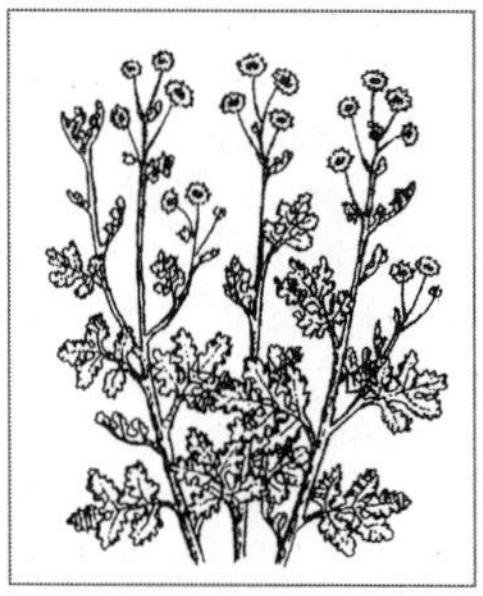

FEVERFEW

Tanacetum parthenium (L.) Schultz-Bip.

THUMBNAIL SKETCH

Active Constituents

- Sesquiterpene lactones notably parthenolide

Common Uses

- Prophylactic treatment of migraines
- Inflammatory joint disease

Adverse Effects

- Mouth ulceration and gastrointestinal upset
- Post-Feverfew Syndrome (including nervousness, tension, fatigue and joint ache) has been noted.

Cautions/Contraindications

- Contraindicated in pregnancy, lactation and children under 2 years of age.

Drug Interactions

- Theoretically interaction with anticoagulant therapy such as warfarin.

Doses

- A daily dosage of 125mg of a dried feverfew leaf preparation from authenticated *Tanacetum parthenium* containing at least 0.2% parthenolide for the prophylactic treatment of migraines.

INTRODUCTION

Family: Asteraceae (also known as Compositae)

Synonyms: Featherfew, Featherfoil, Motherherb, Flirtwort, Midsummer daisy, Pyrethrum, Febrifuge plant, Altamisa, *Chrysanthemum parthenium* (L.) Bernh., *Leucanthemum parthenium* (L.) Gren & Godron, *Pyrethrum parthenium* (L.)[1-4]

Feverfew is a herbaceous perennial native to most of Europe, especially the Balkans, but now naturalized throughout the Americas, Europe and the rest of the world.[5-7] It stands 15 to 60cm in height with several flowers existing on a common stalk. The flowers may be as large as 2cm with a yellow central disc and a single layer of outer white florets.[5, 6] The flowers have a strong odor and the bitter tasting leaves have a 'feather-like' appearance.[5, 8] The parts used medicinally are the aerial parts, especially the leaves.

Feverfew has been used medicinally for a variety of indications dating back to the days of Ancient Greece. Its use has been documented in many of the materia medica written in the Middle Ages. It was particularly popular in the management of fever (hence its name), headache, migraine, women's health care (threatened miscarriage, labor difficulties, menstrual irregularities), toothache, gastric upset and insect bites.[4, 8] The bitter dried powder could be taken orally either mixed with honey or wine or used topically by adding the herb to baths.[4] In a landmark decision, the Health Protection Branch of the Canadian federal government approved the use of a product standardized to parthenolide content for the prophylactic treatment of migraines.[9]

There have been numerous incidents in the past of other members of the Asteraceae family, such as German chamomile and tansy, being sold erroneously as Feverfew.[5, 6, 8] Confusion has also occurred because numerous Latin binomials have been applied to the plant.[5]

Constituents[3-8, 10]

- *Sesquiterpene lactones*: germacranolides (including parthenolide, artemorin and chrysanthemonin), eudesmanolides (including santamarin, reynosin and magnolialide) and guaianolides (including chrysartemin A, partholide and chrysanthemolide)
- *Others*: volatile oils (mainly monoterpene and sesquiterpene derivatives), pyrethrin and various flavonoids

Qualitative and quantitative differences exist between different chemical races of feverfew. For example, specimens rich in santamarin and reynosin have no parthenolide, and specimens rich in parthenolide have little or no reynosin or santamarin.[11]

THERAPEUTIC USES & RELEVANT PHARMACOLOGY

PHARMACOLOGY

Extracts of feverfew appear to influence production of physiologically active eicasonoids. While feverfew suppresses prostaglandin production,[12, 13] it neither inhibits cyclo-oxygenase[12, 13] nor thromboxane A_2 synthesis.[13, 14] Unlike classic non-steroidal anti-inflammatory drugs, constituents found in feverfew appear to inhibit cellular phospholipases, hence preventing the release of arachidonic acid and subsequent formation of inflammatory mediators.[15, 16] An additional action could be an inhibition of the activating factors of protein kinase C.[17] Compounds present in feverfew may also exert an inhibitory action directly on the prostaglandin synthetase enzyme system preventing the production of prostaglandins from arachidonic acid.[18] It has been suggested that non-sesquiterpene lactones may also play a part in this inhibition of eicasonoid synthesis.[16]

Extracts of feverfew have been shown to exert an antisecretory and anti-aggregatory effect on blood platelets and polymorphonuclear leucocytes.[4, 14, 15, 19] With respect to human platelet activity, there appears little difference between a crude chloroform feverfew extract and parthenolide.[17] Feverfew extract has been shown to decrease deposition of platelets on collagen substrates, leading some to suggest its use as an anti-thrombotic drug.[20] The antisecretory action seems to be dependent on the presence of compounds containing alpha-methylene butyrolactone units (e.g., parthenolide, 3-beta-hydroxyparthenolide, canin and artecanin).[21] This inhibition of secretory and aggregatory activity appears to be due to an action on cellular sulphydryl groups.[22, 23] Feverfew extracts have been shown to impede the production of HETE (12-hydroxyeicosateraenoac acid) for which a sulphydryl containing substance (glutathione) is a cofactor.[23] The proposed inhibitory action of phospholipase A_2 activity could also be due to a blockade of important sulphydryl containing components.[4] In addition, feverfew has been reported to inhibit release of serotonin by platelets and vitamin B12 binding protein from polymorphonuclear leucocytes.[19] Feverfew extract has also been shown to protect rabbit aortas against perfusion injury.[24]

Feverfew extracts also appear to inhibit the release of enzymes from polymorphonuclear leucocytes. This action appears more pronounced than that seen with conventional non-steroidal anti-inflammatory drugs such as indomethacin. This action could be responsible for feverfew's reputed effectiveness in the management of various arthritides and certain skin conditions such as psoriasis.[5, 6] In addition, an extract of feverfew has been shown to inhibit histamine release from rat peritoneal mast cells stimulated by anti-IgE in a dose dependent manner. The mode of action responsible for this antihistaminic property is different from that of either quercetin or sodium chromoglycate.[25]

A cytotoxic action for both a crude extract of feverfew and parthenolide has been demonstrated *in vitro*. They were found to inhibit mitogen-induced human mononuclear cell proliferation and interleukin 1 stimulated synovial cells.[26] In addition, sesquiterpene lactones, containing an alpha-methylenebutyrolactone unit, have been shown *in vitro* to exert a cytotoxic activity towards various cell lines. It has been suggested that this action is exerted by influencing DNA replication and synthesis.[21] However, since platelets do not possess DNA and feverfew has been shown to influence their function, it appears that the cytotoxic action may be more generalized.[6]

While numerous mechanisms of action for feverfew and some of its constituents have been identified *in vitro*, the relevance of these mechanisms to the use of feverfew leaf as a migraine prophylactic in humans is not at all clear. While most interest has been focused on the sesquiterpene lactones, notably parthenolide, it is possible that other constituents also exert a biological action. The possibility of a synergy between constituents has also been suggested.[5, 6]

MIGRAINE

Research into this indication was initiated primarily by a group of migraine sufferers in the late 1970s who used feverfew 'successfully' in the treatment of their conditions.[27, 28] The public demand led to two documented clinical trials in the 1980s. Following a survey of migraine sufferers in which it appeared that feverfew may be beneficial[29], a placebo controlled trial was performed. Volunteers (n=17) who had consumed fresh feverfew leaves daily (average of 2.44 leaves) for at least three months and had a history of migraines (common or classic) for two years with no more than 8 attacks per month were selected. One group (n=8) received 'freeze-dried' feverfew (50mg daily) and a second group (n=9) received placebo. Assessment was made by using diary cards scoring the visual symptoms, nausea, headache (including times of onset and relief and of any additional treatment taken) according to a predetermined scale. The group given the feverfew product reported no change in condition, while the group given the placebo noted both an increased frequency of attacks (3.43 attacks/month as compared to 1.22/month before) and increased severity of headache, nausea and vomiting over 6 periods of 4 months. The abrupt withdrawal of feverfew in two of the patients led to the recurrence of some symptoms.[30] The observations and conclusions drawn from this study have been questioned because of the poor methodology.[31]

The efficacy of feverfew in the prophylactic management of migraines was evaluated in a randomized double-blind placebo-controlled cross-over trial in 1988. Volunteers (n=76) who had suffered from migraines (classic or common) for 2 years or more (at least 1 attack per month) were selected. Following a one-month single-blind placebo run-in, the volunteers were given either 1 capsule of feverfew daily (mean weight 82mg equivalent to 2.19 μmol parthenolide) or placebo. The treatment was continued for 4 months and patients were then transferred to the other option. Conventional migraine medications were stopped at the beginning of the trial. A symptom diary was used to record number and duration of individual attacks, severity of headache and any associated symptoms. In addition, the overall impression of the patients was assessed by use of a visual analogue scale and the selection of a predefined 'descriptive' in order to describe the change in headache (much worse, worse, same, better, much better). Patients were assessed every 2 months during the double-blind portion of the study. Following treatment with feverfew, an improvement was noted in the number and severity of attacks, degree of vomiting and general improvement (visual analogue scale). There was no alteration in the duration of individual attacks.[32]

Another recent well-designed randomized double-blind placebo-controlled crossover trial of feverfew did not find such promising results.[33] Patients (n=50) were selected who had suffered from migraines since their youth and continued to suffer from at least one migraine, classic or common, at least once per month and had never taken feverfew in the past. The patients involved suffered serious migraines that were not receptive to conventional medication. While all migraine-related medications were stopped at the start of the trial, volunteers were permitted to treat any attacks acutely using conventional symptomatic drugs. After a one-month placebo phase, patients were treated with either a dried alcoholic extract of feverfew leaves containing 0.5mg of parthenolide or placebo. After four months the patients were crossed over to the opposing group. The severity of the migraine attacks was recorded according to a predetermined scale and the number of headaches during the period month 2 to 4 recorded. There was no significant difference in the number of migraines experienced between the groups. Of the group of 44 volunteers that completed the study, 7 in the feverfew group reported "using considerably fewer anti-migraine preparations." This study has been criticized on a number of points. The investigators noted that unlike the previous studies, the individuals selected had never used feverfew before. Also, the feverfew product used an alcoholic extract rather than dried feverfew leaves. While extracts used were standardized to parthenolide, other necessary active moities could be absent.[33] Concerns about the use of acute migraine drugs during the trial, and their effect on the assessment of the severity of the attacks, have also been raised.[34] In addition, the appropriateness of the criteria used by the investigators to measure changes in symptoms (the International Headache Society's scale) has been questioned.[34]

While the vast majority of feverfew users take feverfew prophylactically for the management of migraines, incidents of it proving useful in the symptomatic treatment of acute migraines have been documented.[4]

ARTHRITIS

While feverfew has been used in the management of various arthritic conditions, this claim is not supported by clinical research.[27] In a double-blind, placebo controlled study of female patients (n=41) suffering from rheumatoid arthritis, dried feverfew (70-86mg equivalent to 2-3μmol of parthenolide) taken once a day for 6 weeks was shown to offer no benefits over placebo. Patients were permitted to continue their conventional non-steroidal treatment throughout the study. Concerns were noted that the dose used might have been too low. The authors suggested that these findings did not exclude a benefit in the management of osteoarthritis or soft tissue damage.[35]

MISCELLANEOUS

Parthenolide has been shown to possess antimicrobial properties against a variety of Gram positive bacteria, fungi and dermatophytes.[3, 4, 36, 37] A weaker action has been noted against some Gram negative pathogens.[36] The clinical relevance of this is unknown.

ADVERSE EFFECTS

Adverse effects are greatly considered to be rare, primarily presenting as mouth ulceration and gastrointestinal upset.[6, 30] Mouth ulceration was noted in 12% and swelling of the lips in 7% of patients in one British clinical trial.[38] Mouth ulceration is due to a systemic rather than a direct irritant action; thus, encapsulation does not decrease its presentation.[30] Feverfew products may also cause inflammation of the mucous membranes of the buccal cavity resulting in inflammation of the lips/tongue and a loss of taste, which is likely to be reduced when the feverfew is taken as a tablet or capsule.[6] These adverse effects present usually within the first week, but may occur anytime in the first two months of treatment.[3, 6]

One study described a group of symptoms including nervousness, tension, fatigue and joint aches, which was associated with withdrawal of feverfew products. The phrase "Post Feverfew Syndrome" was coined to describe this finding.[30] No other reference to this syndrome could be found.

Numerous examples of contact dermatitis have been noted in individuals handling the fresh feverfew plant. The sesquiterpene lactone portion appears to be the component responsible. An appreciable cross sensitivity between feverfew and other plants containing these constituents has also been seen.[39-43]

In a comparative study between a group of migraine sufferers (n=30) who had been taking a variety of feverfew products (leaves, capsules or tablets of feverfew for at least 11 months) and a non-user control group, no significant chromosomal aberrations, sister chromatid exchanges or mutagenicity of urine (Ames test) were noted.[44]

CAUTIONS/CONTRAINDICATIONS

Feverfew is considered an emmenagogue and abortifacient and consequently its use is contraindicated in pregnancy.[45, 46] Feverfew should not be administered to children under 2 years of age.[9] Also, feverfew products should not be taken for more than 4 months without consulting a physician. This caution is due to the lack of long-term information regarding toxicity.[9]

Feverfew should not be taken by people with known hypersensitivity to other members of the sunflower (Asteraceae) family due to the potential allergenicity of the sesquiterpene lactones present.[43]

DRUG INTERACTIONS

No documented instances of drug interactions occurring with feverfew were found for this review.[6] However, it has been suggested that the effect of feverfew may be reduced when it is taken concurrently with non-steroidal anti-inflammatory drugs or corticosteroids.[35] Theoretically, feverfew may potentiate the action of anticoagulants such as warfarin (see pharmacology section).

DOSAGE REGIMENS

A daily dose of 125mg of dried Feverfew leaf preparation (*Tanacetum parthenium* L. Schultz Bip. containing at least 0.2% parthenolide) is considered useful in the prophylactic treatment of migraines by the Canadian Health Protection Branch.[9]

Although it has been argued that administration should be limited to standardized extracts, other dosage forms seen in clinical practice include:[33]

- 50-200mg of the dried aerial parts daily[47]
- 5 to 20 drops of tincture (1:5, 25% ethanol) daily[47]

For optimal results in the management of recurrent migraines, it is advisable that feverfew be taken continuously for a minimum of 4 to 6 weeks.[27]

Comparison Of Dosage Forms

In a very detailed review article, Awang discusses many concerns related to the practical use of feverfew preparations.[9] Many of the statements made by manufacturers regarding the superiority of a particular product (freeze-dried or certain extracts) cannot be substantiated.[9] The quality, with regard to parthenolide content, of commercial feverfew products has also been questioned. Investigation of commercially available feverfew products found that many did not contain the parthenolide content considered necessary for therapeutic efficacy.[38, 48-50] In addition, the parthenolide content of the dried feverfew leaf has been shown to decrease appreciably over time. This led to questions regarding effective shelf life and the need for more specific storage conditions.[4, 48, 51] Many factors, such as the season in which the feverfew is harvested and the growing conditions, can effect the sesquiterpene lactone content.[4] To further complicate matters, the bioactivity (ability to inhibit the release of serotonin from bovine blood platelets) appears to vary within and between samples. This variance can be independent of the geographical source of the sample of *T. pathenium.*[52] The Health Protection Branch of the Canadian Federal government granted a DIN (Drug Identification Number) to a British feverfew product, allowing it to claim that the product was effective in the prevention of migraine headaches.[7,9] They stipulated that the original harvested plant should have undergone independent "botanical certification" and that the feverfew leaf product should contain at least 0.2% pathenolide.[9] Medical claims can only be made legitimately in Canada for dried feverfew leaf products. Awang also made note that "there is no scientific evidence supporting either the superiority of wild traditional feverfew or effectiveness of non-traditional or cultivated variants." [9] In comparing capsule versus tablet formulations, Awang comments, "while there is no fundamental reason to reject tablets *per se*, it should be noted that their effectiveness would be dependent upon satisfactory disintegration/dissolution characteristics." [9]

Products marketed in France require that feverfew extracts be standardized to 0.1% parthenolide, extracted from both the leaves and stem.[7]

REFERENCES

1. Wren R. *Potter's New Encyclopaedia of Botanical Drugs and Preparations.* Saffron Walden: C.W Daniel Company; 1988:362.
2. Hutchens A. *Indian Herbology of North America.* Boston, MA: Shambhala Press; 1991:382.
3. Newall C, Anderson L, David Philipson J. *Herbal Medicines: A Guide for Health Care Professionals.* London: The Pharmaceutical Press; 1996:296.
4. Groenewegen W, Knight D, Heptinstall S. Progress in the Medicinal Chemistry of the Herb Feverfew. *Progress in Medicinal Chemistry*. 1992;29:217-238.
5. Awang D. Herbal Medicine, feverfew. *Canadian Pharmaceutical Journal*. 1989;122:266-270.
6. Berry M. Feverfew. *Pharmaceutical Journal*. 1994;253:806-8.
7. Leung A, Foster S. *Encyclopedia of Common Natural Ingredients Used in Food, Drugs and Cosmetics.* 2nd ed. New York, NY: John Wiley and Sons; 1996:649.
8. Berry M. Feverfew faces the future. *Pharmaceutical Journal*. 1984;232:611-14.
9. Awang D. Feverfew fever — a headache for the consumer. *Herbalgram*. 1993;29:34-36,66.
10. Wagner H, *et al.* New chlorine containing sesquiterpene lactones from *Chrysanthemum parthenium*. *Planta Medica*. 1988;54:171-2.
11. Marles RJ, Associate Professor, Department of Botany, Brandon University, Brandon, Manitoba. Review of Medicinal Plant Modules for CCNM; 1997.
12. Collier H, Butt N, McDonald-Gibson W, Saeed S. Extract of feverfew inhibits prostaglandin biosynthesis. *Lancet*. 1980;ii:922-73.
13. Capasso F. The effect of an aqueous extract of *Tanacetum parthenium* L. on arachidonic acid metabolism by rat peritoneal leucocytes. *Journal of Pharmacy and Pharmacology*. 1986;38:71-2.
14. Makheja A, Martyn Bailey J. The active principle in feverfew. *Lancet*. 1981;11:1054.
15. Makheja A, Bailery J. A platelet phospholipase inhibitor from the medicinal herb feverfew. *Prostaglandins, Leukotrienes Med*. 1982;8:653-660.
16. Sumner H, Salan U, Knight D, Hoult R. Inhibition of 5-lipoxygenase and cyclooxygenase in leukocytes by feverfew. *Biochemical Pharmacology*. 1992;43:2313-2320.
17. Groenewegen W, Heptinstall S. A comparison of the effects of an extract of feverfew and parthenolide, a component of feverfew, on human platelet activity *in vitro*. *Journal of Pharmacy and Pharmacology*. 1990;42(8):553-7.
18. Pugh W, Sambo K. Prostaglandin synthetase inhibitors in feverfew. *Journal of Pharmacy and Pharmacology*. 1988;40:743-745.
19. Heptinstall S, White A, Williamson L, *et al*. Extracts of feverfew inhibit granule secretion in blood platelets and polymorphonuclear leukocytes. *Lancet*. 1985;i(1071-1074).
20. Loesche W, Mazurov A, Voyno-Yasenetskaya A, *et al*. Feverfew — an antithrombotic drug. *Folia Haematol*. 1988;115(1-2):181-4.
21. Groenewegen W, Knight D, Heptinstall S. Compounds extracted from feverfew that have anti-secretory activity contain an alpha-methylene butyrolactone unit. *Journal of Pharmacy and Pharmacology*. 1986;38:709-12.
22. Losche W, Mitchel E, Heptinstall S, *et al.* Inhibition of the behaviour of human polynuclear leukocytes by an extract of *Chrysanthemum parthenium*. *Planta Medica*. 1988;54:381-384.
23. Heptinstall S, Groenewegen W, Spangenberg P, *et al*. Extracts of feverfew may inhibit platelet behaviour via

neutralization of sulphydryl groups. *Journal of Pharmacy and Pharmacology*. 1987;39:459-65.
24. Voyno-Yasenetskaya T, Loesche W, Hepistall S, *et al*. Effects of an extract of feverfew on endothelial cell integrity and on cAMP in rabbit perfused aorta. *Journal of Pharmacy and Pharmacology*. 1988;40(7):501-2.
25. Hayes N, Foreman J. The activity of compounds extracted from feverfew on histamine release from rat mast cells. *Journal of Pharmacy and Pharmacology.* 1987;39:466-70.
26. O'Neill L, Barrett M, Lewis G. Extracts of feverfew inhibit mitogen induced human peripheral blood mononuclear cell proliferation and cytokine mediated responses: a cytotoxic effect. *British Journal of Clinical Pharmacology*. 1987;23:81-3.
27. Brown D. *Herbal Prescriptions for Better Health.* Rocklin, CA: Prima Publishing; 1995:349.
28. Diamond S. Herbal therapy for migraine. An unconventional approach. *Postgraduate Medicine*. 1987;July:197-8.
29. Johnson E. Patients who chew chrysanthemum leaves. *MIMS Magazine*. 1983;May 15:32-5.
30. Johnson ES, Kadam NP, Hylands DM, Hylands PJ. Efficacy of feverfew as prophylactic treatment of migraine. *British Medical Journal*. 1985;291:569-73.
31. Waller P, Ramsay L. Efficacy of feverfew as prophylactic treatment of migraine. *British Medical Journal*. 1985;291:1128.
32. Murphy JJ, Hepinstall S, Mitchell JRA. Randomized double-blind placebo-controlled trial of feverfew in migraine prevention. *Lancet*. 1988;ii:189-92.
33. De Weerdt CJ, Bootsma HPR, Hendriks H. Herbal medicines in migraine prevention. *Phytomedicine*. 1996;3:225-30.
34. Brown D. Feverfew — disappointing results in migraine study. *Quarterly Review of Natural Medicine*. 1997;4(2):89-90.
35. Pattrick M, hepinstall S, Doherty M. Feverfew in rheumatoid arthritis: A double blind, placebo controlled study. *Ann Rheum Dis.* 1989;48:547-549.
36. Kalodera Z, Pepeljnjak S, Petrak T. The antimicrobial activity of *Tanacetum parthenium* extract. *Pharmazie*. 1996;51(12):995-6.
37. Blakeman J, Atkinson P. Antimicrobial properties and possible role in host pathogen interactions of parthenolide, a sesquiterpene lactone isolated from glands of *Chrysanthemum parthenium*. *Physiol Plant Pathol*. 1979;15:183-92.
38. Tyler V. *Herb's of Choice. The Therapeutic Use of Phytomedicinals.* Binghampton, NY: Pharmaceutical Products Press; 1994:208.
39. Schmidt R, Kingston T. Chrysanthemum dermatitis in South Wales; diagnosis by patch testing with feverfew (*Tanacetum parthenium*) extract. *Contact Dermatitis*. 1985;13:120-7.
40. Rodriguez E, Epstein W, Mitchell J. The role of sesquiterpene lactones in contact hypersensitivity to some North and South American species of Feverfew (*Parthenium-compositae*). *Contact Dermatitis*. 1977;3:155-162.
41. Mensing H, Kimming W, Hausen B. Airborne contact dermatitis. *Der Hautarzt*. 1985;36(7):398-402.
42. Hausen B. Occupational contact allergy to feverfew *Tanacetum pathenium*. *Dermatosen in Beruf and Umwelt*. 1981;29(1):18-21.
43. Hausen B, Osmundsen P. Contact allergy to parthenolide in *Tanacetum parthenium* schulz-Bip (feverfew, Asteraceae) and cross-reactions to related sesquiterpene lactone containing compositae species. *Acta Dermato-Venereologica*. 1983;63(4):308-14.
44. Anderson D, Jenkinson P, Dewdney R, Blowers S, Johnson E, Kadam N. Investigation of possible genotoxic effects of feverfew in migraine patients. *Human Toxicology*. 1987;6:533-4.
45. Lepik K. Safety of Herbal Medications in Pregnancy. *Canadian Pharmaceutical Journal*. 1997;130(3):29-33.
46. Farnsworth N, Bingel A, Cordell G, *et al*. Potential Value of Plants as Sources of New Antifertility Agents I. *Journal of Pharmaceutical Sciences.* 1975;64(4):535-598.
47. Bradley P. *British Herbal Compendium*. Bournemouth, UK: BHMA; 1992:239.
48. Heptinstall S, Awang DVC, Dawson BA, *et al*. Parthenolide content and bioactivity of feverfew (*Tanacetum parthenium*). Estimation of commercial and authenticated feverfew products. *Journal of Pharmaceutical Pharmacology*. 1992;44(5):391-5.
49. Awang D, Dawson B, Kindack D. Parthenolide content of Feverfew (*Tanacetum parthenium*) assessed by HPLC and H-NMR spectroscopy. *Journal of Natural Products*. 1991;Nov-Dec 54(6):1516-21.
50. Groenewegen W, Hepinstall S. Amounts of feverfew in commercial preparations of the herb. *Lancet*. 1986;ii:44-5.
51. Smith R, Burford M. Supercritical fluid extraction and gas chromatographic determination of the sesquiterpene lac tone parthenolide in the medicinal herb feverfew (*Tanacetum parthenium*). *Journal of Chromatography*. 1992;627:255-261.
52. Marles R, Heptinstall J, Kaminski J, *et al.* A bioassay for inhibition of serotonin release from bovine platelets. *Journal of Natural Products.* 1992;55(8):1044-56.

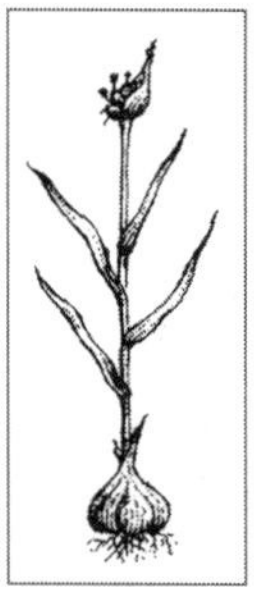

GARLIC

Allium sativum L.

THUMBNAIL SKETCH

Active Constituents

- A variety of sulfur-containing products including alliin, allicin, diallyl disulfide and ajoene

Common Uses

- Cardiovascular protective effects including: decreased cholesterol levels, decreased blood pressure, decreased platelet aggregation
- Anti-microbial
- Protection against cancer (especially stomach and colon cancer)

Adverse Effects

- Heartburn, flatulence, and gastro-intestinal upset (usually only at doses greater than 4 cloves daily)
- contact dermatitis (if the skin is exposed to raw garlic for an extensive period of time)
- post-operative bleeding

Cautions/Contraindications

- Garlic supplements should not be used by pregnant or lactating women; its use should be discontinued prior to surgery; caution should be exercised after organ transplants and individuals with pemphigus should avoid use of garlic.

Drug Interactions

- Anticoagulants
- Possibly antidiabetic therapy

Doses

- Doses range from 3-30 g fresh garlic (1 to 8 cloves) daily;
- 600-900 g of garlic powder (often in tablet or capsule formulations) daily in 3 divided doses

INTRODUCTION

Family: Liliaceae

Synonyms: Russian penicillin (Allicin)[1]

Garlic has been used medicinally since approximately 3000 BC. The Latin name *Allium* is derived from the Celtic word for pungent, hot and burning, properties common to all the *Allium* species.[1-3] The species name, *sativum*, means cultivated or planted, referring to the fact that garlic is no longer found in the wild. It was one of the earliest cultivated crops and continues to be extensively grown for both medicinal and culinary purposes.[2, 3]

Garlic has been described as an aphrodisiac, as well as a treatment for a large variety of other conditions, including colds, coughs, high blood pressure, hypertension, diarrhea, rheumatism, and snakebites.[2] In addition, garlic oil has been used to 'expel' round worms and was generally considered to be a good antiseptic. Traditionally, garlic was used to treat diabetes in Norway and Central Europe, and it was considered to be a heart remedy in traditional Ayurvedic medicine.[1] In Traditional Chinese Medicine (TCM), garlic was used in controlling dysentery, as an antiparasitic, antifebrile and stomachic.[2] More than 1300 papers have reported on the chemical constituents, mechanisms of action and clinical applications of garlic over the last 100 years,[3] making it one of the most extensively researched medicinal plants. Fenwick and Hanley (1985) provide an excellent review of many of these.[4-6]

The garlic bulb is the part used medicinally. When intact it is odorless; however, crushing the cells brings the enzyme alliinase into contact with the sulfur-containing compound alliin, converting it to allicin which produces the characteristic garlic odor. Allicin is relatively unstable and is converted to a variety of other active sulfur-containing compounds. Some people argue that the potency of a garlic product can be determined by its ability to produce allicin, which in turn yields many of the other active components. Some commercial products are now standardized to their allicin yield.[7]

Constituents [1-3, 8-10]

The biological action of garlic is generally thought to be due to its organosulfur compounds, specifically those containing the allyl CH2=CH-CH2- group.[1]

Enzymes:
- alliinase, peroxidase, myrosinase

Sulfur-containing Compounds:
- alliin (S-allyl cysteine sulfoxide)
- allicin (diallyl thiosulfinate) which is formed when the enzyme alliinase acts on alliin when the garlic clove is crushed
- allyl methanethiosulfinate
- diallyl disulfide (breakdown product of allicin)
- diallyl trisulfide
- allyl methyl trisulfide
- S-allyl-mercaptocysteine

- ajoene ($C_9H_{14}S_3O$) (formed by combining allicin and diallyl disulfide) which is considered to be unstable and may rearrange to a variety of polysulfides
- 2-vinyl-4H-1,3-dithiin
- 2-vinyl-4H-1,2-dithiin
- S-allylcysteine
- allixin

Miscellaneous:
- neutral lipids (predominant), phospholipids, glycolipids
- essential amino acids, of particular importance are those containing sulfur (i.e., cysteine and methionine) as well as arginine
- anthocyanins
- quercetin and its flavone aglycone analogues
- kaempferol glycosides
- scordinins (biologically active thioglycosides)
- tellurium compounds

Note: It has been estimated that one gram of fresh garlic will release 3.7 mg of allicin when crushed or chopped.[11]

THERAPEUTIC USES & RELEVANT PHARMACOLOGY

CARDIOVASCULAR

Cardiovascular Protective Effects

The German Commission E has approved garlic for the treatment of hyperlipoproteinemia in conjunction with other dietary measures and to prevent age-related arteriosclerosis.[12] The ability of garlic to decrease cholesterol, triglycerides and low-density lipoprotein in the blood has been documented by numerous studies.[13-31] However, studies reporting no lipid or cholesterol lowering effect have also been published.[32, 33]

Studies over the past 25 years have reported that the ingestion of garlic can decrease serum cholesterol, sometimes as much as 20%; however, the study designs, doses, forms (raw or powder), study populations and blinding mechanisms (the smell of garlic makes it very difficult to conduct blinded studies) vary widely, making it difficult to reach firm conclusions regarding the efficacy of garlic for this indication.[6, 16, 34-36] For example, Kleijnen *et al.* (1989) severely criticized both the quality of commercial garlic products and the methodological quality of the 13 controlled trials they reviewed.[15, 16, 32, 37-46] They concluded that while experiments with fresh garlic are consistent in showing that garlic lowers cholesterol levels, the doses required to achieve this effect are extremely high (a minimum of 7 cloves daily). In addition, it appeared that the effects of garlic ingestion lasted only a few hours. In response to this finding, several manufacturers began producing dehydrated garlic preparations (water accounts for up to 60% of the bulk of garlic) which are standardized to alliin content.

Other reviews of double-blind controlled studies have concluded that ingestion of garlic significantly decreases lipid and cholesterol levels.[47, 48] A meta-analysis of five placebo-controlled, randomized trials,[18-20,49,50] which assessed the effect of garlic on total serum cholesterol in individuals with cholesterol levels greater than 5.17 mmol/L (200 mg/dL) concluded that the oral ingestion of the equivalent of 1/2 to 1 clove of raw garlic daily significantly decreased serum cholesterol levels by approximately 9%.[48] The study suggests that these effects are possible with relatively low doses of garlic. However, problems with the low quality of the trials included in the analysis continues to be of concern. Another meta-analysis of 16 trials (952 subjects combined) found an overall 12% reduction in total serum cholesterol in those taking garlic compared to those taking placebo. This effect was apparent after approximately one month and persisted approximately six months after the therapy was discontinued. Garlic powders were also reported to reduce triglyceride levels by an average of 13%. However, the authors cautioned that more than half the trials reviewed were of poor quality.[51]

A double-blind, placebo-controlled, randomized cross-over clinical trial (n=28) of individuals with mild to moderate hypercholesterolemia (5.5 to 8.05 μmol/L) taking 300 mg of garlic powder tablets (Kwai®) or placebo three times daily for 12 weeks found no significant difference between the group taking the garlic and the group taking the placebo on outcome measures of: plasma cholesterol, LDL cholesterol, HDL cholesterol, plasma triglycerides, lipoprotein(a) or blood pressure.[52] Another double-blind, randomized study of 42 healthy adults with total serum cholesterol levels greater than 220 mg/dL who received the same product (300 mg three times daily) reported a significant decrease in total serum cholesterol and low-density lipoprotein cholesterol (LDL) in the garlic group when compared with the placebo group; however, there was no significant change in high density lipoprotein cholesterol (HDL), triglycerides, serum glucose or blood pressure.[53] Finally, a third double-blind crossover study comparing 7.2 g aged garlic daily with placebo (for 4 to 6 months) in 41 men (total serum cholesterol 220-290 mg/dL) reported statistically significant decreases in total serum cholesterol and LDL cholesterol in individuals treated with garlic.[27]

In one of the few studies comparing garlic to standard lipid-lowering products, garlic was compared in a double-blind clinical trial with bezafibrate in 98 patients. There was no significant difference in the outcome measures between the two groups – both groups had significant reductions in triglyceride, total cholesterol, and LDL levels, as well as increased HDL levels.[54]

Mechanism of Action

Several mechanisms of action have been postulated including: increased bile acid excretion;[55] reduced 3-hydroxy-3-methyl-glutaryl coenzyme A reductase activity;[56-58] and inhibition of squalene epoxidase, the final enzyme in the synthetic pathway of cholesterol by tellurium compounds found in garlic bulbs.[10] All these mechanisms decrease the hepatic production of cholesterol. It appears that components of garlic (e.g., allicin, diallyl disulfide, allyl mercaptan and the vinyldithiins) may all play a role in the interference of cholesterol biosynthesis although via a variety of different mechanisms.[59]

In addition, it is suggested that components of garlic may decrease the activity of lipogenic enzymes (e.g., glucose-6-phosphate dehydrogenase and malic dehydrogenase)[55,56] which leads to a decrease in fatty acid synthesis. Another hypothesis is that components of garlic may exert cardioprotective effects by decreasing the levels of glycosaminoglycans (GAGs). The amount of GAGs has been shown to be proportional to the susceptibility of different species to cholesterol induced athersclerosis. GAGs are able to bind to plasma lipoproteins and thus have been implicated in lipid accumulation in developing lesions.[26]

Of interest is the finding in several studies of an initial rise in cholesterol, triglycerides and LDL/Very Low-Density Lipoprotein (VLDL) blood levels during the first few months of garlic ingestion.[15, 50] Researchers have postulated that this initial increase could be due to the garlic causing tissue lipids to move into circulation.[3]

Platelet Aggregation Inhibitory Ability

The anti-thrombotic effects of garlic have been extensively studied.[17, 23, 24, 60-69] Garlic has been shown to inhibit platelet aggregation induced by epinephrine,[65] adenosine diphosphate (ADP),[65, 70] and collagen.[70] An excellent review of the inhibition of platelet aggregation by a variety of components of garlic is available in Agarwal 1996.[3]

Clinical Studies

A review of 13 trials, most rated as poor in quality, concluded that although fresh garlic reliably decreases platelet aggregation, it does so only at very high doses (greater than 7 cloves per day) and the effects appear to last for only a few hours.[36] Other studies have found decreased platelet aggregation at significantly lower doses.[70] For example, one double-blind, placebo-controlled, crossover study of 10 individuals randomized to receive either 900 mg (1.3% alliin) daily or placebo found no significant effects at 6 hours; however, at 7 and 14 days those taking the garlic had decreased platelet aggregation caused by ADP and decreased platelet aggregability in response to collagen.[70] In contrast, another clinical study of daily consumption of 600 mg garlic powder in tablet form (equal to 1.7 g of cloves) for 4 weeks found no inhibitory effects of platelet aggregation.[17]

A recent study suggests a slow build up of active constituents may occur, making higher doses necessary to achieve inhibition of platelet aggregation in a single dose, but lower doses of garlic are effective in long-term administration.[69]

Mechanism of Action

Both alliin and allicin have been shown to inhibit collagen-induced platelet aggregation; however, allicin is approximately fifteen times more active.[3] *In vitro* studies indicate that platelet cAMP, cyclooxygenase and thromboxane synthetase activity are not affected by either of these constituents of garlic.[63] It should be noted that the anti-thrombotic effects of allicin are destroyed above 56°C and at a pH greater than 8.5.[63] Several studies have noted decreased or complete lack of the antithrombotic action of garlic after it has been exposed to heat.[71, 72] The exact antithrombotic mechanism of action is unknown; however, raw garlic has been shown to: irreversibly inhibit cyclooxygenase activity in a dose-dependent manner[71] and decrease thromboxane B_2 levels.[30, 72] Thus, other constituents of garlic must play a role in this effect.

Although allicin is considered to be one of the most potent antiaggregation constituents in garlic, it is not found in the blood stream after oral ingestion of garlic. Shortly after it is absorbed into the blood stream, it is converted to allyl mercaptan.[3] Allicin may also be converted to ajoene, which has been identified as an active anti-thrombotic agent;[73, 74] however, ajoene is often not present in commercial garlic pills, or powders of steamed garlic distillates. Ajoene has been shown to inhibit platelet aggregation traditionally induced by a variety of stimulatory agents including: collagen, ADP, epinephrine, arachidonic acid, platelet-activating factor, and thrombin.[75-77] This activity is increased by prostcyclin (PGI_2), forskolin, indomethacin, and dipyridamole.[75, 77] Several mechanisms have been postulated for the anti-thrombotic activity of ajoene. It is thought to inhibit the exposure of fibrinogen receptors on platelet membranes.[78, 79] Other researchers have suggested that it may interact with a purified hemoprotein which in turn may play an important role in the activation of platelets.[80]

Other components of garlic have also been implicated as anti-thrombotic agents (e.g., diallyl disulfide and methyl allyl trisulfide); however, studies regarding their anti-thrombotic activity have been conflicting.[2] For example in one study, methyl allyl trisulfide was shown to be the agent responsible for the complete blockage of platelet aggregation in response to serotonin one hour post oral ingestion of fresh garlic (100-150 mg/kg). It should be noted that no inhibition was seen at 30 minutes or 2 hours post ingestion.[81] In addition, components of garlic may activate calcium-dependent nitric oxide synthase, producing increased amount of nitric acid by which the therapeutic actions of garlic may be exerted. This activation does not appear to be dependent upon the alliin-derived products or arginine.[65, 82]

Effect on Blood Pressure

Although several trials have demonstrated garlic's ability to decrease blood pressure,[17, 19, 20, 23, 24, 27] others have not been able to show such an effect.[3, 22, 53, 83] For example, a double-blind, placebo-controlled study of 42 patients getting 300 mg three times daily of standardized garlic powder in tablet form found no effects on blood pressure.[53] In contrast, a double-blind, placebo-controlled crossover study of 41 men (total serum cholesterol 220-290 mg/dL) taking 7.2 g of aged garlic or placebo daily for 4 to 6 months reported a 5.5% decrease in systolic blood pressure and a slight reduction in diastolic blood pressure in the group taking garlic.[27] In addition, a study of 47 patients with mild hypertension (mean diastolic blood pressure 102 mmHg) who took 600 mg dried garlic powder (Kwai®) daily (or placebo) for 12 weeks, reported that the supine diastolic blood pressure in the group taking the garlic was significantly lower at 8 weeks and 12 weeks than those in the control group.[19]
A meta-analysis which reviewed 8 randomized controlled trials[19, 20, 53, 54, 84-87] of a least 4 weeks in duration (all of which used Kwai® garlic powder) concluded that there is currently insufficient evidence to routinely recommend garlic use in patients with hypertension. Of the eight studies reviewed, only three were conducted in hypertensive subjects and only seven compared garlic to a placebo. Overall, three showed a significant reduction in systolic blood pressure and four showed a significant decrease in diastolic blood pressure.[88]

Mechanism of Action

The ability of garlic to decrease blood pressure may be due to its ability to inhibit adenosine deaminase, the enzyme which degrades adenosine to inosine, enhancing the physiological effects of adenosine.[89, 90]

ANTIMICROBIAL EFFECT

Garlic has been used as an antimicrobial for hundreds of years in a variety of cultures.[91] Allicin is considered to be the primary anti-bacterial constituent of garlic.[3, 92] Garlic has been shown to inhibit the growth of *Staphylococcus aureus, Streptococcus* (alpha- and beta-hemolytic), *Escherichia coli, Proteus vulgaris, Salmonella enteritidis, Citrobacter* sp., *Klebsiella pneumoniae*, *Mycobacteria*, and *Helicobacter pylori*.[91, 93-96] However, other researchers have been unable to demonstrate any inhibition of *Staphylococcus aureus*.[96]

In addition, garlic has been shown to have a significant anti-fungal effect, especially against fungal skin infections. Studies have demonstrated its effectiveness against *Microsporum, Epidermophyton, Trichophyton and Candida albicans*.[91, 97] In Asia, garlic preparations are used (alone or in combination with amphotericin B) to treat systemic fungal infections and cryptococcal meningitis. *In vitro* evidence supports garlic's fungistatic and fungicidal activity against *Cryptococcus neoforans*.[98]

CANCER PREVENTIVE EFFECT

Garlic has long had a reputation for providing protection from cancer. Much of the evidence that garlic may reduce cancer deaths comes from epidemiological studies.[99-102] Several good reviews of the evidence (or lack thereof) for this indication for garlic have been published over the last 10 years.[100, 103-106] The most recent of these (Ernst 1997) reviews nine epidemiological studies[107-115] of the association between garlic consumption and cancer. Of these studies, 4 reported that garlic had a protective effect against cancer (thyroid nodular disease, stomach cancer, cancer of the larynx, colon cancer); two found positive, but non-significant trends (gastric cardia, cancers of the nasal cavity and sinuses); and 3 found no protective effect for garlic (gastric cancer — 2 studies, stomach cancer). The authors conclude that "the hypothesis that regular consumption of *Allium* vegetables (including garlic, onions and leeks) reduces the risk of cancer is compelling and would seem to deserve testing in intervention trials."[106]

Two specific studies have garnered attention due to their more rigorous designs. The Iowa Women's Health Study followed 41,837 women aged 55 to 69 years for 5 years and found that garlic consumption was inversely associated with risk of colon cancer. The protective association with garlic was stronger than with any other nutrient analyzed in the study.[114] The second notable study followed 58,279 men and 62,573 women aged 55 to 69 for just over 3 years. This study found no protective effect against cancers of the stomach or breast from garlic.[105, 116]

Animal studies have shown garlic to be effective at inhibiting chemically-induced stomach and colon cancer;[117-119] suppressing the growth of human colon tumor cell xenografts in mice;[120] protecting against the clastogenic effects of known genotoxicants;[121, 122] both alone[118] and in combination with selenium[123-125] inhibiting induced mammary carcinogenesis; and inhibiting gamma-radiation-induced chromosomal damage.[126] In addition, diallyl disulfide has been shown to inhibit the proliferation of human tumor cells *in vitro*.[127] Lau (1990) and Dausch (1990) provide excellent reviews of the both *in vivo* and *in vitro* studies in this area.[100, 104]

It has been hypothesized that components of garlic may exert their anti-neoplastic effects by modulating gluthione S-transferase dependent detoxification enzymes.[126, 128-130] Other researchers have suggested that the sulfur components of garlic may inactivate endogenously formed nitrosamines.[131] In addition, the antibacterial effect of garlic (esp. against *Helicobacter pylori* which is a major risk factor for stomach cancer) may add to the protective effects.[95, 96] For example, it may limit the formation of potentially carcinogenic nitrosamines by bacterial conversion in the stomach.[114] One author identified ajoene as a primary antimutagenic compound based on his investigation using the Ames test.[132]

ANTIDIABETIC EFFECTS

Animal studies have demonstrated the hypoglycemic action of garlic.[133] Allicin has been shown to have a significant hypoglycemic action because it appears to compete with insulin for insulin-inactivating sites in the liver. This results in an increase in free insulin in the bloodstream.[134]

MISCELLANEOUS

HIV and AIDS

One small German study of 10 patients with advanced AIDS and severely low natural killer cell activity (all had opportunistic infections) involved the ingestion of 5 g of garlic (Kyolic brand) daily for six weeks, followed by 10 g daily for another six weeks. Three patients died before the trial was completed. All seven patients who completed the trial were reported to have normal natural killer cell activity by the completion of the trial. Symptoms from their opportunistic infections were also reported to have improved including: chronic diarrhea and genital herpes.[135]

Anti-aging Properties

Garlic has a reputation for an ability to prolong longevity and youthful appearance. However, few studies support these claims. Researchers report that ingestion of garlic was able to increase the survival of senscence-accelerated-prone mice (genetically bred to have shorter survival times), but did not affect the survival of another strain of mice bred to have longer survival times. Garlic appears to have improved the performance of mice in several models designed to test learning deficits, memory acquisition and memory deficits.[136, 137] The applicability of these findings to human physiological aging and age-related memory deficits is unknown.

Earaches

Garlic oil is a popular folk remedy for the relief of earaches.[138] Traditionally, raw garlic is inserted into the ear. Garlic's usefulness for this indication is thought to be related to the antibacterial action of allicin.

Ischemia

Aged garlic extracts have been shown to provide a protective action in a rat model of brain ischemia.[139, 140] The mechanism of action is hypothesized to be either an antioxidant action[139, 141] or an inhibitory action on arachidonic acid metabolism.[140]

Antioxidant Effects

Several *in vitro* studies have demonstrated the antioxidant activity of garlic.[141-143] This activity is thought to be related to the mechanisms of action of many of its clinical effects, including decreasing blood cholesterol levels and providing protection in ischemic attacks.

Protection from Acetaminophen-induced Hepatotoxicity

Two animal studies report that pre-treatment with garlic provides protection from acetaminophen-induced hepatoxicity in a time- and dose-dependent manner.[144, 145]

ADVERSE EFFECTS

Heartburn, flatulence, and gastro-intestinal upset have been noted, usually at doses equivalent to 5 or more cloves daily.[7, 36] In addition, the odor of garlic is noticeable in the milk of lactating women. This has been reported to cause colic in nursing children.

Contact dermatitis (caused by direct skin contact with raw garlic) is also possible, although most case reports occur in individuals (often young children) where crushed garlic pastes are applied to the skin for extended periods of time.[36, 146-153]

Several cases of post-operative bleeding associated with the ingestion of garlic have been reported.[154-156] A 72-year old man who had been taking garlic for "many years" experienced unusual bleeding following a transurethral resection procedure (TURP). Laboratory tests confirmed a decrease in platelet coagulation in the presence of collagen.[154] Another case involved a 32-year old women undergoing elective cosmetic surgery who also experienced increased bleeding post-operatively. Her heavy dietary garlic intake prior to surgery is suspected to have caused her increased blood clotting time.[155]

In animal studies, rats fed high concentrations of garlic for a prolonged period of time suffered from anemia, weight loss and failure to grow.[157]

Rats administered 500 mg/kg (equivalent to 10 cloves per day in humans) intraperitoneally once daily were reported to have extensive damage to the lungs (thickening of the alveolar walls) and liver (vacuolation especially near the organ surface). The same dose administered orally cause less damage and those fed low doses of garlic orally (50 mg/kg which is equivalent to 1 clove or 3-4 g in humans) daily had no significant lung or liver damage.[158]

CAUTIONS/CONTRAINDICATIONS

Garlic supplements should be used with caution by pregnant and lactating women.[159] In addition, they should be avoided before undergoing surgical procedures due to possible post-surgical bleeding.[156] One author also recommends caution after organ transplants because it has been reported that garlic enhances the activity of natural killer (NK) cells, which are largely responsible for tissue rejection.[135]

Finally, attacks of pemphigus, a relatively rare autoimmune disorder resulting in lesions of the mucous membranes and skin, may be induced by drugs which contain active thiol groups. This sulfur-containing group is found in garlic; thus, it is suggested that patients with this condition avoid garlic.[160]

DRUG INTERACTIONS

A possible interaction with warfarin has been reported.[161] In addition, it has been suggested that garlic may potentiate the anti-thrombotic effects of ASA[162] and may interfere with existing diabetic therapy.[159]

DOSAGE REGIMENS

- Suggested doses range from 3-30 g fresh garlic (1-8 cloves) daily.[12, 163]
- The German Commission E considers a daily dose equivalent to 4 g of fresh garlic to be therapeutically effective.[12]
- The British Herbal Compendium recommends the following: 2-5 mg of allicin, 2-5 mg of Garlic oil, 2-5 g of fresh air-dried garlic or 400-1200 mg of fully dried powder daily.[164]

Dried garlic contains no allicin, which appears to be the precursor for many of the major active constituents of garlic; however, it does contain both alliin and alliinase, and thus theoretically should be able to produce allicin. It should be noted that allinase is inactivated by acids and thus the conversion to allicin does not occur in the stomach. It has been suggested that dried garlic is most effective if it is ingested as an enteric coated formulation so that it is released in the alkaline medium of the intestine. In the intestine the conversion to allicin occurs rapidly and allicin is quickly combined with cysteine to produce 5-allylmercaptocysteine which prevents the distinctly odored allicin from being absorbed into the blood stream. Thus this form of garlic is relatively odorless and most likely still effective.[7]

Odorless garlic products may be also prepared by coarsely chopping, peeling and rapidly freeze-drying the cloves before powdering so that there is little opportunity for enzymatic conversion of the odorless alliin to the odoriferous allicin and related breakdown products.[165]

Oil-based products are less likely to be efficacious because allicin is unstable in an oil base. Similarly, in aqueous products, allicin suffers substantial degradation.[7] A 1992 German study investigating the allicin content of 18 German garlic products found that only 5 had an allicin yield equivalent to the 4g of fresh garlic (or more) that the German Commission E considers necessary for therapeutic activity.[7]

REFERENCES

1. Augusti KT. Therapeutic values of onion (*Allium cepa* L.) and garlic (*Allium sativum* L.). [Review]. *Indian Journal of Experimental Biology*. 1996;34(7):634-40.
2. Foster S. Garlic, *Allium sativum.* Austin, TX: The American Botanical Council; 1991.
3. Agarwal KC. Therapeutic actions of garlic constituents. [Review]. *Medicinal Research Reviews*. 1996;16(1):111-24.
4. Fenwick GR, Hanley AB. The Genus Allium Part 1. *CRC Critical Reviews in Food Science and Nutrition*. 1985;22:199.
5. Fenwick GR, Hanley AB. The Genus Allium Part 2. *CRC Critical Reviews in Food Science and Nutrition.* 1985;22:273.
6. Fenwick GR, Hanley AB. The Genus Allium Part 3. *CRC Critical Reviews in Food Science and Nutrition*. 1985;23:1.
7. Tyler VE. *Herbs of Choice. The Therapeutic Use of Phytomedicinals.* Binghamton, NY: Pharmaceutical Products Press; 1994:209.
8. Block E. The chemistry of garlic and onions. *Scientific American*. 1985;252(3):94-99.
9. Nagae S, Ushijima M, Hatono S, *et al.* Pharmacokinetics of the garlic compound S-allylcysteine. *Planta Medica*. 1994;60(3):214-7.
10. Larner AJ. How does garlic exert its hypocholesterolaemic action? The tellurium hypothesis. *Medical Hypotheses*. 1995;44(4):295-7.
11. Lawson LD, Wang Z, Hughes BG. Identification and HPLC quantiation of the sulfides and dralk(en)yl thoisulfinates in commercial garlic products. *Planta Medica*. 1991;57:263q.
12. Blumenthal M, Brusse WR, Goldberg A, *et al. The Complete German Commission E Monographs.* Austin, Texas: American Botanical Council; 1994.
13. Bordia A, Bansal HC. Essential oil of garlic in the prevention of athersclerosis. *Lancet*. 1973;II:1491-2.
14. Jain RC. Effect of garlic on serum lipids, coagulability, and fibrinolytic activity of blood. *American Journal of Clinical Nutrition*. 1977;30:1380-1.
15. Bordia A. Effect of garlic on blood lipids in patients with coronary heart disease. *American Journal of Clinical Nutrition*. 1981;34:2100-3.
16. Lau B, Adetumbia MA, Sanchez A. *Allium sativum* (Garlic) and athersclerosis: A review. *Nutrition Research*. 1983;3:119-28.
17. Harenberg J, Giese C, Zimmermann R. Effect of dried garlic on blood coagulation, fibrinolysis, platelet aggregation and serum cholesterol levels in patients with hyperlipoproteinemia. *Athersclerosis*. 1988;74:247-9.
18. Mader FH. Treatment of hyperlipidaemia with garlic powder tablets. Evidence from the German Association of General Practitioner's multicentric placebo-controlled double-blind study[German]. *Arzneimittelforschung*. 1990;40:1111-6.
19. Auer W, Eiber A, Hertkorn E, *et al.* Hypertension and hyperlipidemia: Garlic helps in mild cases. *British Journal of Clinical Practice*. 1990;44(8 (Supplement 69)):3-6.
20. Vorberg G, Schneider B. Therapy with garlic: Results of a placebo-controlled, double-blind study. *British Journal of Clinical Practice*. 1990;44(8 (Supplement 69)):7-11.
21. Brosche T, Platt D, Dorner H. The effect of a garlic preparation on the composition of plasma lipoproteins and erythrocyte membranes in geriatric subjects. *British Journal of Clinical Practice*. 1990;44(supplement 69):12-19.
22. Zimmermann W, Zimmerman B. Reduction in elevated blood lipids in hospitalized patients by a standardized garlic preparation. *British Journal of Clinical Practice*. 1990;44(supplement 69):20-3.
23. Mansell P, Reckless JPD. Garlic: effects on serum lipids, blood pressure, coagulation, platelet aggregation, and vasodilation. *British Medical Journal*. 1991;303:379-80.
24. Barrie SA, Wright JV, Pizzorno JE. Effects of garlic oil on platelet aggregation, serum lipids, and blood pressure in

humans. *Journal of Orthomolecular Medicine*. 1987;2:15-21.
25. Mathew BC, Daniel RS, Augusti KT. Hypolipidemic effect of garlic protein substituted for casein in diet of rats compared to those of garlic oil. *Indian Journal of Experimental Biology*. 1996;34(4):337-40.
26. Mathew BC, Augusti KT. Biochemical effects of garlic protein diet and garlic oil on glycosaminoglycan in cholesterol fed rats. *Indian Journal of Experimental Biology*. 1996;34(4):346-50.
27. Steiner M, Khan AH, Holbert D, Lin RI. A double-blind crossover study in moderately hypercholesterolemic men that compared the effects of aged garlic extract and placebo administration on blood lipids. *American Journal of Clinical Nutrition*. 1996;64(6):866-70.
28. Adler AJ, Holub BJ. Effect of garlic and fish-oil supplementation on serum lipid and lipoprotein concentrations in hypercholesterolemic men. [See comments]. *American Journal of Clinical Nutrition*. 1997;65(2):445-50.
29. Gupta NK. Modification of radiation induced changes in murine hepatic lipid profiles by garlic (*Allium sativum* Linn.) unsaturated oils. *Indian Journal of Experimental Biology*. 1996;34(9):851-3.
30. Ali M, Thomson M. Consumption of a garlic clove a day could be beneficial in preventing thrombosis. *Prostaglandins Leukotrienes and Essential Fatty Acids*. 1995;53(3):211-2.
31. Sainani GS, Desai DB, Gorhe NH, Nath SM, Pise DV, Sainani PG. Effect of dietary garlic and onion on serum lipid profile in Jain community. *Indian Journal of Medical Research*. 1979;69:776-80.
32. Luley C, Lehmann-Leo W, Moller B, Martin I, Schwartzkopff W. Lack of efficacy of dried garlic in patients with hyperlipoproteinemia. *Arzneimittelforschung*. 1986;36:766-8.
33. Arora RC, Arora S, Gupta RK. The long-term use of garlic in ischemic heart disease. *Atherosclerosis*. 1981;40:175-9.
34. Ernst E. Cardiovascular effects of garlic (*Allium stivum*): A review. *Pharmatherapeutica*. 1987;5(2):83-9.
35. Kendler BS. Garlic (*Allium sativum*) and onion (*Allium cepa*): A review of their relationship to cardiovascular disease. *Preventative Medicine*. 1987;16:670-85.
36. Kleijnen J, Knipschild P, ter Riet G. Garlic, onions and cardiovascular risk factors. A review of the evidence from human experiments with emphasis on commercially available preparations. *British Journal of Clinical Pharmacology*. 1989;28:535-44.
37. Bordai A, Bansal HC, Arora SK, Singh SV. Effect of the essential oils of garlic and onion on alimentary hyper lipemia. *Atherosclerosis*. 1975;21:15-19.
38. Bordia A, Joshi HK, Sanadhya YK, Bhu N. Effect of essential oil of garlic on serum fibrinolytic activity in patients with coronary artery disease. *Atherosclerosis*. 1977;28:155-9.
39. Bordia A, Sharma KD, Parmar YK, Verma SK. Protective effect of garlic oil on the changes produced by 3 weeks of fatty diet on serum cholesterol, serum triglycerides, fibrinolytic activity and platelet adhesiveness in man. *Indian Heart Journal*. 1982;34:86-8.
40. Bhushan S, Sharma SP, Singh SP, *et al*. Effect of garlic on normal blood cholesterol level. Indian *Journal of Physiology and. Pharmacology*. 1979;23:211-4.
41. Sucur M. Effect of garlic on serum lipids and lipoproteins in patients suffering from hyperlipoproteinemia. *Diabetologia Croatica*. 1980;9:323-8.
42. Chutani SK, Bordia A. The effect of fried versus raw garlic on fibinolytic activity in man. *Atherosclerosis*. 1981;38:417-21.
43. Arora RC, Arora S. Comparative effect of clofibrate, garlic and onion on alimentary hyperlipemia. *Atherosclerosis*. 1981;39:447-52.
44. Lutomski J. Klinische untersuchungen zur therapeutischen wirksamkeit von ilja rogoff knoblauchpillen mit rutin. *Zeitschrift fur Phytotherapie*. 1984;5:938-42.
45. Ernst E, Weihmayr T, Matrai A. Garlic and blood lipids. *British Medical Journal*. 1985;291:139.
46. Sitprija S, Plengvidhya C, Kangkaya V, *et al*. Garlic and diabetes mellitus phase II clinical trial. *Journal of the Medical Association of Thailand*. 1987;70(supplement #2):223-7.
47. Turner M. Garlic and circulatory disorders. *Journal of the Royal Society of Health*. 1990;110:90-3.
48. Warshafsky S, Kamer RS, Sivak SL. Effect of garlic on total serum cholesterol. A meta-analysis. [See comments]. *Annals of Internal Medicine*. 1993;119(7 Pt 1):599-605.
49. Plengvidhya C, Sitprija S, Chinayon S, *et al*. Effects of spray dried garlic preparation on primary hyper lipoproteinemia. *Journal of the Medical Association of Thailand*. 1988;71:248-52.
50. Lau BH, Lam F, Wang-Cheng R. Effect of an odor modified garlic preparation on blood lipids. *Nutrition Research*. 1987;7:139-49.
51. Silagy C, Neil A. Garlic as a lipid lowering agent — a meta-analysis. *Journal of the Royal College of Physicians of London*. 1994;28(1):2-8.

52. Simons LA, Balasubramaniam S, von Konigsmark M, *et al*. On the effect of garlic on plasma lipids and lipoproteins in mild hypercholesterolaemia. *Atherosclerosis*. 1995;113(2):219-25.
53. Jain AK, Vargas R, Gotzkowsky S, McMahon FG. Can garlic reduce levels of serum lipids? A controlled clinical study. *American Journal of Medicine*. 1993;94(6):632-5.
54. Holzgartner H, Schmidt U, Kuhn U. Comparison of the efficacy and tolerance of a garlic preparation vs. bezafibrate. *Arzneimittelforschung*. 1992;42:1473-7.
55. Chi MS, Koh ET, Steward TJ. Effects if garlic on lipid metabolism in rats fed cholesterol or lard. *Journal of Nutrition*. 1982;112:241-8.
56. Qureshi AA, Din ZZ, Abuirmeileh N, *et al*. Suppression of avian hepatic lipid metabolism by solvent extracts of garlic: Impact on serum lipids. *Journal of Nutrition*. 1983;113:1746-55.
57. Qureshi AA, Crenshaw TD, Abuirmeileh N, *et al*. Influence of minor plant constituents on porcine hepatic lipid metabolism. Impact on serum lipids. *Atherosclerosis*. 1987;64:109-115.
58. Qureshi AA, Abuirmeileh N, Din ZZ, *et al*. Inhibition of cholesterol and fatty acid biosynthesis in liver enzymes and chicken hepatocytes by polar fractions of garlic. *Lipids*. 1983;18:343-8.
59. Gebhardt R, Beck H. Differential inhibitory effects of garlic-derived organosulfur compounds on cholesterol biosynthesis in primary rat hepatocyte cultures. *Lipids*. 1996;31(12):1269-76.
60. Bordia A. Effect of garlic on human platelet aggregation *in vitro*. *Atherosclerosis*. 1978;30:355-60.
61. Vanderhoek JY, Makheja AN, Bailey JM.Inhibition of fatty acid oxygenases by onion and garlic oils. Evidence for mechanism by which these oils inhibit platelet aggregation. *Biochemical Pharmacology*. 1980;29:3169-73.
62. Samson RR. Effects of dietary garlic and temporal drift on platelet aggregation. *Atherosclerosis*. 1982;44:199-20.
63. Mohammad SM, Woodward SC. Characterization of a potent inhibitor of platelet aggregation and release reaction isolated from *allium sativum (garlic)*. *Thrombosis Research*. 1986;44:793-806.
64. Lawson LD, Ransom DK, Hughes BG. Inhibition of whole blood platelet-aggregation by compounds in garlic clove extracts and commercial garlic products. *Thrombosis Research*. 1992;65:141-56.
65. Das I, Khan NS, Sooranna SR. Potent activation of nitric oxide synthase by garlic: a basis for its therapeutic applications. *Current Medical Research & Opinion*. 1995;13(5):257-63.
66. Makeja AN, Bailey JM. Antiplatelet constituents of garlic and onions. *Agents and Actions*. 1990;29:360-3.
67. Kiesewetter H, Jung F, Mrowietz C, Wenzel E. Hemorrheological and circulatory effects of Gincosan. *International Journal of Clinical Pharmacology, Therapy and Toxicology*. 1992.
68. Kiesewetter H, Jung F, Jung EM, *et al*. Effect of garlic on platelet aggregation in patients with increased risk of juvenile ischaemic attack. *European Journal of Clinical Pharmacology*. 1993;45(4):333-6.
69. Bordia A, Verma SK, Srivastava KC. Effect of garlic on platelet aggregation in humans: a study in healthy subjects and patients with coronary artery disease. *Prostaglandins Leukotrienes and Essential Fatty Acids*. 1996;55(3):201-5.
70. Legnani C, Frascaro M, Guazzaloca G, *et al*. Effects of a dried garlic preparation on fibrinolysis and platelet aggregation in healthy subjects. *Arzneimittelforshung*. 1993;43(2):119-22.
71. A\li M. Mechanism by which garlic (*Allium sativum*) inhibits cyclooxygenase activity. Effect of raw versus boiled garlic extract on the synthesis of prostanoids. *Prostaglandins Leukotrienes and Essential Fatty Acids*. 1995.
72. Bordia T, Mohammed N, Thomson M, Ali M. An evaluation of garlic and onion as antithrombotic agents. *Prostaglandins Leukotrienes and Essential Fatty Acids*. 1996;54(3):183-6.
73. Block E, Ahmad S, Jain MK, Crecely RW, Apitz-Castro R, Ross MR. *American Journal of Clinical Nutrition*. 1984;34:2100-3.
74. Villar R, Alvarino MT, Flores R. Inhibition by ajoene of protein tyrosine phosphatase activity in human platelets. *Biochimica et Biophysica Acta*. 1997;1337(2):233-40.
75. Apitz-Castro R, Escalante J, Vargas R, Jain MK. Ajoene, the autiplatelet principle of garlic, synergistically potentiates the antiaggregatory action of prostacyclin, forskolin, indomethancin and dypiridamole on human platelets. *Thrombosis Research*. 1986;42:303-11.
76. Apitz-Castro R, Badimon JJ, Badimon L. A garlic derivative, ajoene, inhibits platelet deposition on severely damaged vessel wall in an *in vivo* porcine experimental model. *Thrombosis Research*. 1994;75(3):243-9.
77. Jain MK, Apitz-Castro R. *Trends Biol Sci*. 1987;12:252.
78. Block E. Antithrombotic agent of garlic: A lesson from 5,000 years of folk medicine. In: Steiner RP, ed *Folk Medicine: The Art and the Science*. Washington, D.C.: American Chemical Society; 1986:125-38.
79. Jain MK. Apitz-Castro R. Garlic — a product of spilled ambrosia. *Current Science*. 1993;65:148-156.
80. Jamaluddin MP, Krishnan LK, Thomas A. Ajoene ingibition of platelet aggregation: Possible mediation by a

hemo-protein. *Biochemical and Biophysical Research Communications*. 1988;153:479.
81. Boullin DJ.Garlic as a platelet inhibitor. *Lancet*. 1981;I:776-7.
82. Das I, Hirani J, Sooranna S. Arginine is not responsible for the activation of nitric oxide synthase by garlic. *Journal of Ethnopharmacology*. 1996;53(1):5-9.
83. Pantoja CV, Norris BC, Contreras CM. Diuretic and natriuretic effects of chromatographically purified fraction of garlic (*Allium sativum*). *Journal of Ethnopharmacology*. 1996;52(2):101-5.
84. Kandziora J. Antihypertensive effectiveness and tolerance of a garlic medication. [German]. *Arzliche Forschung*. 1988;1:1-8.
85. Kandziora J. The blood pressure lowering and lipid lowering effect of a garlic preparation in combination with a diuretic. *Arzliche Forschung*. 1988;3:1-8.
86. Kiesewetter H, Jung F, Pinder G, *et al*. Effect of garlic on thrombocyte aggregation, microcirculation, and other risk factors. *International Journal of Clinical Pharmacology Therapy and Toxicology*. 1991;29:151-5.
87. Santos OS, Grunwald J. Effect of garlic powder tablets on blood lipids and blood pressure. A six month placebo-controlled double-blind study. *British Journal of Clinical Research*. 1993;4:37-44.
88. Silagy CA, Neil HA. A meta-analysis of the effect of garlic on blood pressure. *Journal of Hypertension*. 1994;12(4):463-8.
89. Melzig MF, Krause E, Franke S. Inhibition of adenosine deaminase activity of aortic endothelial cells by extracts of garlic (*Allium sativum* L.). *Pharmazie*. 1995;50(5):359-61.
90. Koch HP, Jager W, Hysek J, Korpert B. *Phytotherapy Research*. 1992;6:50.
91. Adetumbi MA, Lau BH. *Allium sativum* (garlic) — A natural antibiotic. *Medical Hypotheses*. 1983;12:227-37.
92. Fulder S. Scorn not Garlicke. *Pharmacy Update*. 1988;October:327-9.
93. Sharma VD, Sethi MS, Kumar PS, Rarotra JR. Antibacterial property of *Allium sativum* Linn.: *in vivo* and *in vitro* studies. *Indian Journal of Experimental Biology*. 1977;15:466-8.
94. Elnima EI, Ahmed SA, Mekkawi A, Mossa JS. The antimicrobial activity of garlic and onion extracts. *Pharmazie*. 1983;38:747-8.
95. Cellini L, Di Campli E, Masulli M, *et al*. Inhibition of Helicobacter pylori by garlic extract (*Allium sativum*). *FEMS Immunology and Medical Microbiology*. 1996;13(4):273-7.
96. Sivam GP, Lampe JW, Ulness B, *et al*. Helicobacter pylori — *in vitro* susceptibility to garlic (*Allium sativum*) extract. *Nutrition and Cancer*. 1997;27(2):118-21.
97. Amer M, Taha M, Tosson Z. The effect of aqueous garlic extract on the growth of dermatophytes. *International Journal of Dermatology*. 1980;19:285-7.
98. Davis LE, Shen J, Royer RE. *In vitro* synergism of concentrated *Allium sativum* extract and amphotericin B against *Cryptococcus neoformans*. *Planta Medica*. 1994;60(6):546-9.
99. You WC, Blot WJ, Chang YS, *et al.* Diet and high risk of stomach cancer in Shandoug, China. *Cancer Research*. 1988;48:3518-23.
100. Dausch JG, Nixon DW. Garlic: A review of its relationship to malignant disease. *Preventive Medicine*. 1990;19:346-61.
101. Buiatti E, Palli D, Decarli A, *et al.* A case-control study of gastric cancer and diet in Italy. *International Journal of Cancer*. 1989;44:611-6.
102. Haenszel W, Kurihara M, Segi M. Stomach cancer among Japanese in Hawaii. *Journal of the National Cancer Institute*. 1972;49:969-88.
103. Sumiyoshi H, Wargovich MJ. Garlic (Allium sativum): A review of its relationship to cancer. *Asia Pacific Journal of Pharmacology*. 1989;4:133-140.
104. Lau BHS, Tadi PP, Tosk JM. *Allium sativum* (garlic) and cancer prevention. *Nutrition Research*. 1990;10:937-48.
105. Dorant E, van den Brandt PA, Goldbohm RA, *et al*. Garlic and its significance for the prevention of cancer in humans: a critical review. [Review]. *British Journal of Cancer*. 1993;67(3):424-9.
106. Ernst E. Can Allium vegetables prevent cancer? *Phytomedicine*. 1997;4(1):79-83.
107. Wang Z, Boice JD, Wei L, *et al.* Thyroid nodularity and chromosone aberrations among women in areas of high background radiation in China. *Journal of the National Cancer Institute*. 1990;82:478-85.
108. You W, Blot WJ, Chang Y, *et al.* Allium vegetables and reduced risk of stomach cancer. *Journal of the National Cancer Institute*. 1989;81:162-4.
109. Palli D, Bianchi S, Decarli A, *et al.* A case-control study of cancer of the gastric cardia in Italy. *British Journal of Cancer*. 1992;65:263-6.
110. Tuyns AJ, Kaaks R, Haelterman M, Riboli E. Diet and gastric cancer. A case control study in Belgium. *International Journal of Cancer.* 1992;51:1-6.

111. Zheng W, Blot WJ, Shu X-O, *et al.* A population-based case-control study of cancers of the nasal cavity and paranasal sinuses in Shanghai. *International Journal of Cancer*. 1992;52:557-61.
112. Zheng W, Blot WJ, Shu X-O, *et al.* Diet and other risk factors for laryngeal cancer in Shanghai. *American Journal of Epidemiology*. 1992;136:178-91.
113. Hasson LE. Diet and risk of cancer. A population-based case-control study in Sweden. *International Journal of Cancer*. 1993;55:181-9.
114. Steinmetz KA, Kushi LH, Bostick RM, Folsom AR, Potter JD. Vegetables, fruit, and colon cancer in the Iowa Women's Health Study. [See comments]. *American Journal of Epidemiology*. 1994;139(1):1-15.
115. Dorant E, van den Brandt PA, Goldbohm RA. A prospective cohort study on the relationship between onion and leek consumption, garlic supplement use and the risk of colorectal carcinoma in The Netherlands. *Carcinogenesis*. 1996;17(3):477-84.
116. Dorant E, van den Brandt PA, Goldbohm RA. Allium vegetable consumption, garlic supplement intake, and female breast carcinoma incidence. *Breast Cancer Research and Treatment*. 1995;33(2):163-70.
117. Belman S. Onion and garlic oils inhibit tumour progression. *Carcinogenesis*. 1983;4:1063-5.
118. Schaffer EM, Liu JZ, Green J, *et al*. Garlic and associated allyl sulfur components inhibit N-methyl-N- nitrosourea induced rat mammary carcinogenesis. *Cancer Letters*. 1996;102(1-2):199-204.
119. Cheng JY, Meng CL, Tzeng CC, Lin JC. Optimal dose of garlic to inhibit dimethylhydrazine-induced colon cancer. *World Journal of Surgery.* 1995;19(4):621-5.
120. Sundaram SG, Milner JA. Diallyl disulfide suppresses the growth of human colon tumor cell xenografts in athymic nude mice. *Journal of Nutrition*. 1996;126(5):1355-61.
121. Das T, Choudhury AR, Sharma A, Talukder G. Effects of crude garlic extract on mouse chromosomes *in vivo*. Food and *Chemical Toxicology*. 1996;34(1):43-7.
122. RoyChoudhury A, Das T, Sharma A, Talukder G. Dietary garlic extract in modifying clastogenic effects of inorganic arsenic in mice: Two-generation studies. *Mutation Research*. 1996;359(3):165-70.
123. Ip C, Lisk DJ, Thompson HJ. Selenium-enriched garlic inhibits the early stage but not the late stage of mammary carcinogenesis. *Carcinogenesis*. 1996;17(9):1979-82.
124. Schaffer EM, Liu JZ, Milner JA. Garlic powder and allyl sulfur compounds enhance the ability of dietary selenite to inhibit 7,12-dimethylbenz [a]anthracene-induced mammary DNA adducts. *Nutrition and Cancer*. 1997;27(2):162-8.
125. Amagase H, Schaffer EM, Milner JA. Dietary components modify the ability of garlic to suppress 7, 12-dimethylbenz(a) anthracene-induced mammary DNA adducts. *Journal of Nutrition*. 1996;126(4):817-24.
126. Singh SP, Abraham SK, Kesavan PC. *in vivo* radioprotection with garlic extract. *Mutation Research*. 1995;345 (3-4):147-53.
127. Sundaram SG, Milner JA. Diallyl disulfide inhibits the proliferation of human tumor cells in culture. *Biochimica et Biophysica Acta*. 1996;1315(1):15-20.
128. Maurya AK, Singh SV. Differential induction of glutathione transferase isoenzymes of mice stomach by diallyl sulfide, a naturally occurring anticarcinogen. *Cancer Letters*. 1991;57:121-9.
129. Hatono S, Jimenez A, Wargovich MJ. Chemopreventive effect of S-allylcysteine and its relationship to the detoxification enzyme glutathione S-transferase. *Carcinogenesis*. 1996;17(5):1041-4.
130. Hu X, Benson PJ, Srivastava SK, *et al.* Glutathione S-transferases of female A/J mouse liver and forestomach and their differential induction by anti-carcinogenic organosulfides from garlic. *Archives of Biochemistry and Biophysics*. 1996;336(2):199-214.
131. Shenoy NR, Choughuley ASU. Inhibitory effect of diet related sulphydryl compounds on the formation of carcinogenic nitrosamines. *Cancer Letters*. 1992;65:227-32.
132. Ishikawa K, Naganawa R, Yoshida H, *et al.* Antimutagenic effects of ajoene, an organosulfur compound derived from garlic. *Bioscience, Biotechnology and Biochemistry*. 1996;60(12):2086-8.
133. Sheela CG, Kumud K, Augusti KT. Anti-diabetic effects of onion and garlic sulfoxide amino acids in rats. [Letter]. *Planta Medica*. 1995;61(4):356-7
134. Bever BO, Zahnd GR. Plants with oral hypoglycemic action. *Quarterly Journal of Crude Drug Research*. 1979;17:139-96.
135. Abdullah TH, Kirkpatrick DV, Carter J. Enhancement of natural killer cell activity in AIDS with garlic .[German]. *Deutsche Zeitschrift Onkologie (German Journal of Oncology)*. 1989;21:52-3.
136 Moriguchi T, Saito H, Nishiyama N. Aged garlic extract prolongs longevity and improves spatial memory deficit in senescence-accelerated mouse. *Biological and Pharmaceutical Bulletin*. 1996;19(2):305-7.
137. Moriguchi T, Takashina K, Chu PJ, Saito H, Nishiyama N. Prolongation of life span and improved learning in the

senescence accelerated mouse produced by aged garlic extract. *Biological and Pharmaceutical Bulletin*. 1994;17(12):1589-94.

138. Wei-cheng H. Garlic slice in repairing eardrum perforation. *Chinese Medical Journal.* 1977;3:204-5.
139. Numagami Y, Sato S, Ohnishi ST. Attenuation of rat ischemic brain damage by aged garlic extracts: A possible protecting mechanism as antioxidants. *Neurochemistry International*. 1996;29(2):135-43.
140. Batirel HF, Aktan S, Aykut C, *et al*. The effect of aqueous garlic extract on the levels of arachidonic acid metabolites (leukotriene C4 and prostaglandin E2) in rat forebrain after ischemia-reperfusion injury. *Prostaglandins Leukotrienes and Essential Fatty Acids*. 1996;54(4):289-92.
141. Prasad K, Laxdal VA, Yu M, Raney BL. Evaluation of hydroxyl radical-scavenging property of garlic. *Molecular and Cellular Biochemistry*. 1996;154(1):55-63.
142. Prasad K, Laxdal VA, Yu M, Raney BL. Antioxidant activity of allicin, an active principle in garlic. *Molecular and Cellular Biochemistry*. 1995;148(2):183-9.
143. Rekka EA, Kourounakis PN. Investigation of the molecular mechanism of the antioxidant activity of some *Allium sativum* ingredients. *Pharmazie*. 1994;49(7):539-40.
144. Wang EJ, Li Y, Lin M, *et al.* Protective effects of garlic and related organosulfur compounds on acetaminophen-induced hepato toxicity in mice. *Toxicology and Applied Pharmacology*. 1996;136(1):146-54.
145. Hu JJ, Yoo JS, Lin M, *et al*. Protective effects of diallyl sulfide on acetaminophen-induced toxicities. *Food and Chemical Toxicology*. 1996;34(10):963-9.
146. Burden AD, Wilkinson SM, Beck MH, Chalmers RJ. Garlic-induced systemic contact dermatitis. *Contact Dermatitis*. 1994;30(5):299-300.
147. Garty BZ. Garlic burns. *Pediatrics*. 1993;91(3):658-9.
148. Lembo G, Balato N, Patruno C, *et al*. Allergic contact dermatitis due to garlic (*Allium sativum*). *Contact Dermatitis*. 1991;25(5):330-1.
149. McFadden JP, White IR, Rycroft RJ. Allergic contact dermatitis from garlic. *Contact Dermatitis*. 1992;27(5):333-4.
150. Farrell AM, Staughton RC. Garlic burns mimicking herpes zoster. [Letter]. *Lancet*. 1996;347(9009):1195.
151. Parish RA, McIntire S, Heimbach DM. Garlic burns: A naturopathic remedy gone awry. *Pediatric Emergency Care.* 1987;3:258-60.
152. Kaplan B, Schewach-Miller M, Yorav S. Factitial dermatitis induced by application of garlic. *International Journal of Dermatology*. 1990;29:75-6.
153. Canduela V, Mongil I, Carrascosa M, Docio S, Cagigas P. Garlic: always good for the health? [Letter]. *British Journal of Dermatology*. 1995;132(1):161-2.
154. German K, Kumar U, Blackford HN. Garlic and the risk of TURP bleeding. *British Journal of Urology*. 1995;76(4):518.
155. Burnham BE. Garlic as a possible risk for postoperative bleeding. [Letter; see comments]. *Plastic and Reconstructive Surgery*. 1995;95(1):213.
156. Petry JJ. Garlic and postoperative bleeding. [Letter; comment]. *Plastic & Reconstructive Surgery*. 1995;96(2):483-4.
157. Brewster JL, Rabinowitch. *Onions and Allied Crops.* Boca, Florida: CRC Press, Inc.; 1990.
158. Alnaqeeb MA, Thomson M, Bordia T, Ali M. Histopathological effects of garlic on liver and lung of rats. *Toxicology Letters*. 1996;85(3):157-64.
159. Newall CA, Anderson LA, Phillipson JD. *Herbal Medicines: A Guide for Health Care Professionals.* London: The Pharmaceutical Press; 1996:296.
160. Brenner S, Wolf R. Possible nutritional factors in induced pemphigus. [Review]. *Dermatology*. 1994;189(4):337-9.
161. Sunter W. Warfarin and garlic. *Pharmaceutical Journal*. 1991;246:72.
162. Fulder S. Garlic and the prevention of cardiovascular disease. *Cardiology in Practice*. 1989;March:30,34-5.
163. Murray MT. *The Healing Power of Herbs.* Rocklin, CA: Prima Publishing; 1992:246.
164. Bradley P. *British Herbal Compendium*. Bournemouth, UK: The British Herbal Medical Association; 1992:239.
165. Marles RJ, Associate Professor, Department of Botany, Brandon University, Brandon, Manitoba. Review of Medicinal Plant Modules for CCNM; 1997.

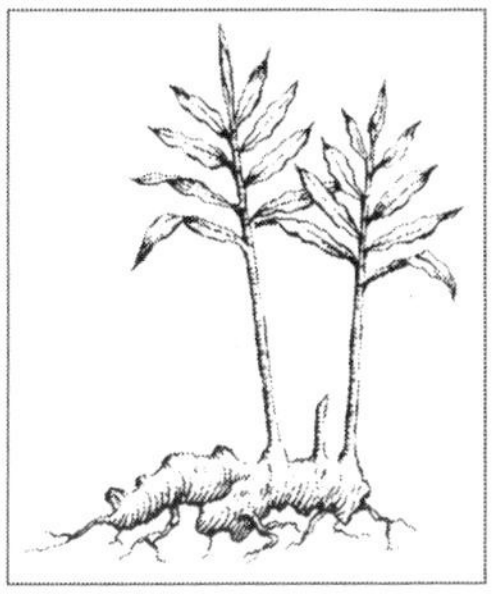

GINGER

Zingiber officinale Roscoe

THUMBNAIL SKETCH

Active Constituents

- Components of the oleoresin portion, notably the gingerols and shogaols

Common Uses

- Digestive aid in dyspepsia and gastrointestinal upset
- Management of motion sickness
- Management of nausea following anaesthesia
- Management of nausea and vomiting due to pregnancy (see adverse effects section)
- Management of inflammatory conditions such as osteoarthritis, rheumatoid arthritis and myalgias

Adverse Effects

- Rare; limited to heartburn and digestive upset

Cautions/Contraindications

- Ginger should only be used under medical supervision in cases of gallstones.
- Doses greater than 1 g daily should only be used in pregnancy when the patient is under medical supervision

Drug Interactions

- None noted when ginger is taken at the suggested therapeutic doses

Doses

- General Use: 0.25-1g powdered rhizome three times daily
- For motion sickness: 2-4 g daily in divided doses
- As an antiemetic: 1-2 g as a single dose

INTRODUCTION

Family: Zingiberaceae

Synonyms: Zingiber, Gan-jiang[1, 2]

Very few herbs have more of a medicinal history than ginger.[3] Its use originated in the healing models of the Orient and quickly spread to the ancient cultures of Europe and the Middle East. It was introduced to North America during the exploration of the "New World" in the 16th century.[4] Historically, it was used for numerous conditions ranging from dyspepsia and vomiting to cholera and malaria.[2]

While native to southern Asia, ginger is one of the most widely used spices in the world and is now cultivated throughout India, Australia, the Caribbean (notably Jamaica) and parts of West Africa. The plant is an erect perennial growing up to 1m in height. The rhizome (underground stem), which is often referred to as the 'root', is the part used medicinally.[5] Once the rhizomes are harvested, they can be used fresh (green ginger); syruped (candied ginger); dried (ginger as a spice); or as extracts (e.g., volatile oil).[4]

Constituents [1, 4-6]

- Oleoresin: pungent principles notably gingerols, shogaols and zingerone. (Proportion of shogaols increases upon drying; these compounds are largely absent in the fresh plant).
- Volatile Oils: complex mixture of various hydrocarbons including: beta-bisabolene, zin giberene, zingiberol, various alcohols and aldehydes
- Lipids: free fatty acids, triglycerides, phosphatidic acids and lecithins.
- Carbohydrates: up to 50% starch
- Miscellaneous: various amino acids, proteins and vitamins

THERAPEUTIC USES & RELEVANT PHARMACOLOGY

DIGESTIVE ACTION

Ginger has long been praised in the management of digestive conditions. It is classically described as a 'stimulating carminative', both aiding digestive function as well as tonifing the gastrointestinal system.[7] Like many other spices, it has traditionally been used to enhance digestion by those who believed it increased salivary flow and gastric acid secretion.[8]

Gastroprotective Action

Historical wisdom suggests that spices promote and/or irritate gastric ulcers.[9] However, several animal studies have demonstrated that ginger has potential gastroprotective properties.[10-12] In these studies, extracts of ginger were administered orally to rats in doses ranging from 500 to 1000 mg/kg resulting in significant decreases in the incidence of stress-induced gastric ulcers initiated by various experimental protocols (including HCl/ethanol, and NSAID). Acetone extracts of ginger compared favourably to cimetidine and misoprostol in one animal study.[12] Whilst an exact mechanism of action has yet to be ascertained, it is suggested that certain components (esp. zingiberene and 6-gingerol) may be influencing the activation of a cellular protective action.[10]

In addition, several studies have demonstrated that extracts of ginger increased gastric pH and decreased gastric secretions.[9, 13] In one study with rabbits, the effect of an aqueous extract of ginger (dose 169 mg/kg) on gastric secretion 3 hours after oral administration was comparable to an oral dose of 50 mg/kg of cimetidine.[13] Another study found that the increase in gastric pH due to the ginger extract was very slight when compared to cimetidine.[9] These actions may play a role in the gastroprotective action noted above.

Digestive Aid

Animal studies have shown that dried ginger added to the diet results in increased digestive enzyme action, especially lipase activity.[8] Other studies have reported that an acetone extract of ginger caused an increase in bile secretion.[14] These studies support the historical use of ginger to aid in the digestion of fatty meals.

HAEMATOLOGY

Inhibition of Platelet Aggregation

Several studies have found that ginger inhibits platelet aggregation induced by various means, including adenosine diphosphate (ADP) and epinephrine.[15, 16] In one randomized study, volunteers (n =20) ingested 10 g of dried ginger or placebo in addition to 100 g of butter daily for 7 days. Although serum lipids remained unchanged in both groups, platelet aggregation was significantly decreased in the group ingesting ginger.[15] An *in vitro* study of an aqueous extract of fresh ginger found a dose-dependent inhibition of platelet aggregation. However, a recent randomized, double-blind trial (n=8) in the United Kingdom suggests that this effect may be limited to doses greater than 2 g of dried ginger daily or doses of fresh ginger.[17] As with the anti-inflammatory mechanism described below, the anti-aggregation activity of ginger may be due to its influence on prostaglandin and thromboxane synthesis.

Anti-hypercholestermic Effect

It has been suggested that ginger may be useful in the management of patients with elevated cholesterol levels. In 1978, a study of cholesterol fed rats concluded that oral administration of ginger oleoresin (1.5 mg/kg) resulted in significantly lowered serum and hepatic cholesterol levels as well as increased fecal cholesterol excretion.[18] These findings have been only partially supported by more recent studies. A 1984 study found that oral ingestion of 1 g of fresh ginger by rats offered no immediate protection against a cholesterol rich diet. While ginger, was shown to have an anti-hypercholesterolemic effect, their results suggested that it must be ingested for several days before this action is manifested.[19] A recent report of the isolation and identification of a specific compound (ZT) from ginger, which is assumed to be an HMG-CoA reductase inhibitor, found that ZT exerted an inhibitory effect on cholesterol biosynthesis.[20]

MUSCULOSKELETAL

Ginger has historically been used for its anti-inflammatory properties in many Asian healing models notably in the Ayurvedic (Indian subcontinent) and Karpo (Japanese) systems of medicine.[21] Attempts have been made to investigate this action in both animal models and human subjects.[22-24]

In two reviews of case studies (n=7 and n=56), patients suffering from a variety of arthritic conditions and mylagias were investigated.[22, 23] When ginger was ingested, an appreciable decrease in pain and swelling was noted in the majority of cases. The daily doses ingested by these patients ranged from 3-7g of powdered ginger, with one individual ingesting 50 g of raw ginger daily. No adverse reactions were reported in any of these patients who had taken ginger from periods ranging for 3 months to 2.5 years. Relief was normally noted within 1-3 months and remained for as long as the ingestion of ginger continued. Symptoms returned when the therapy was discontinued, usually within two weeks. It should be noted that these reports were not clinical trials but case studies and no attempt was made to standardize the therapeutic protocols. However, a recent experiment using a rat model of inflammation found that ginger oil (33 mg/kg) given orally for 26 days caused a significant suppression of both paw and joint swelling.[24]

While no exact mechanism of action is known, the anti-inflammatory action of ginger could be due in part to its influence on eicasonoid production and other inflammatory mediators.[23, 25] Constituents of the oleoresin portion (especially the gingerols) are thought to decrease levels of inflammatory mediators produced from lipid membranes. It has been suggested that by inhibiting cyclooxygenase and 5-lipoxygense, respectively, the production of both inflammatory prostaglandins and leukotrienes could be prevented. In addition, aromatic components of ginger may inhibit the inflammatory action initiated by pyrogens such as interleukin 1.[26]

NAUSEA

Motion Sickness

Of all its modern-day applications, ginger is perhaps best known for its suggested use in the management of motion sickness. While many clinical trials have been conducted, their results have often been conflicting. In 1982, Mowrey and Clayson reported that 940 mg powdered ginger was superior to 100 mg dimenhydrinate in preventing symptoms of motion sickness in blindfolded subjects (n=36) placed in a tilted, rotating chair.[27] This study has been critiqued because all subjects were selected because of their self-reported high susceptibility to motion sickness and because the main outcome measure was the patients' self-assessment of gastrointestinal discomfort.[28] Another double-blind, randomized, placebo-controlled trial found that 1 g of powdered ginger ingested every hour for four hours reduced the tendency to vomiting and cold sweating significantly better than placebo in seasickness. The authors also noted that fewer symptoms of nausea and vertigo were reported after ginger ingestion, but that this difference was not statistically significant.[29] This study has also been critiqued because the difference between the effect of ginger and the placebo did not reach statistical significance until the fourth hour of the trial;[28] however, it is also important to note that this is currently the only study carried out in field conditions. In 1988, a second trial using a rotating chair model of motion sickness found that 1000 mg of fresh ginger, 500 mg and 1000 mg of dried ginger given 2 hours before the test were all no more effective than the placebo.[30] The design of this study differed from the study conducted by Mowrey and Clayson because: 1) a Latin square design allowed each participant to serve as his/her own control; 2) participants were not blind folded; 3) the ginger was ingested 2 hours prior to the test (rather than 20-25 minutes as in the previous trial); and 4) standardized N.A.S.A. outcome measures were used. Finally, a third trial of the efficacy of ginger for the prevention of the symptoms of motion sickness in a revolving chair model was conducted in 1991. In this study, participants were blindfolded and ingested the ginger (500 mg or 1000 mg of powdered or 1000 mg of fresh) one hour prior to the test. The authors concluded that ginger does not possess antimotion sickness activity.

It is interesting to note that the majority of the negative trials have been conducted in North America, leading some to suggest that the quality of ginger and ginger preparations locally available may be influencing the outcome.[31, 32] Also of interest is the fact that irrespective of the negative trials, the Commission E, a German government advisory body, has approved the use of ginger in the management of motion sickness. Their suggested dosage of 2-4g daily is higher than those used in the majority of the studies.[31] In addition, many practitioners suggest that for the prevention of motion sickness, ginger must be ingested for a prolonged period of time starting several days before the journey commences.[32] In conclusion, while ginger is a long established treatment for motion sickness in complementary health-care circles, its efficacy has yet to be conclusively confirmed by clinical trials.

Nausea Associated with Anaesthesia

Many antiemetics commonly used to control nausea and vomiting following surgery have adverse effects, which has led to a search for a less toxic agent. Studies of the use of ginger for the prevention of nausea and vomiting post-operatively have been conflicting. One study of 60 women who had major gynaecological surgery found that 500 mg of powdered ginger given 1.5 hours prior to surgery was superior to placebo and comparable to metoclopramide in decreasing the number of incidences of nausea post-operatively.[33] This study was supported by a study of 120 women following laparoscopic gynaecological surgery which found that 1 g of powdered ginger given 1 hour prior to induction of anaesthesia reduced the incidence of nausea and vomiting comparably to metoclopramide and significantly more than a placebo.[34] However, a more recent Australian study of 108 women undergoing laparoscopic gynaecological surgery found that the ingestion of 500 mg or 1000 mg of powdered ginger one hour prior to surgery slightly, but not significantly increased the incidence of nausea and vomiting post-operatively.[35]

Nausea Associated with Pregnancy

The use of ginger as an antiemetic during pregnancy is controversial. To date, only one study provides direct evidence on this issue. In a double-blind, randomized, cross-over, placebo-controlled trial of women diagnosed with hyperemesis gravidarum (n=30), 250 mg of powdered ginger ingested four times daily was found to be significantly more effective in relieving symptoms than a placebo. No adverse effects were observed.[36] It should be noted that it is difficult to generalize the results of this study to those which may be expected if ginger is ingested for the relief of routine morning sickness due to the severity of the symptoms associated with hyperemesis gravidarum.

Drug-induced Nausea

A single animal study found that an acetone extract of ginger (150 mg/kg) ingested orally by rats was comparable to metoclopramide (25 mg/kg) when administered 60 minutes prior to cyclophosphamide (300 mg/kg s.c.). Both provided complete protection from vomiting episodes. The authors suggest that this warrants further investigation.[37]

Mechanism of Action

The exact mechanism responsible for the antiemetic effects of ginger is unknown. It appears that this is primarily due to a gastrointestinal action, rather than one mediated through the central nervous system.[38] However, several studies have concluded that ingestion of ginger does not affect the gastric emptying rate, as has been hypothesized by many investigators.[28, 34] More recently it has been suggested that ginger exerts a more generalized action on the entire gastrointestinal tract. In addition, the lack of centrally-mediated action is being questioned.[39, 40] For example, ginger has been reported to antagonize 5-HT3 receptors, which are found in both the wall of the gastrointestinal tract and the brain. Antagonism of these receptors produces anti-emetic effects.[41]

MISCELLANEOUS

Cardiotonic

Ginger has long been praised within many healing models as an effective circulatory stimulant.[42] While clinical evidence confirming its influence on the cardiovascular system is limited, it has been shown that the gingerol portion exerts an inotropic effect on isolated guinea pig atria.[43]

Migraines

Given its proposed anti-emetic action and the fact that the treatment of headaches is one of ginger's traditional uses, some have suggested that it may play a role in the management of migraines. The evidence to support this is limited to a single published paper reviewing one case history. In this case, 500-600 mg of powdered ginger was ingested by the patient at the first sign of an aura and then every four hours for three to four days thereafter. The development of the migraine was halted within thirty minutes. Subsequently the patient began adding ginger to her diet, which resulted in a decreased incidence of migraines over the next thirteen months.[44]

Antimicrobial Action

Certain constituents of ginger, notably the shogaols and zingerone, appear to exert an antimicrobial action against specific pathogens, including *Salmonella typhi, Vibrio cholerae,* and *Tricophyton violaceum in vitro*. The clinical relevance of this property is unknown.[45]

ADVERSE EFFECTS

Adverse effects of ginger appear to be so rare that the majority of Western European pharmacopoeias fail to mention any observed cases at all. In practice, unwanted adverse effects appear to be limited to gastric burning and dyspepsia.[7] This is found more often when unencapsulated preparations are taken and the individual lies down soon after taking the preparation.[28] While some have cautioned against the prolonged use of ginger due to its anticoagulant properties (see haemotology section), the use of ginger for culinary purposes or at therapeutic doses less than 1 g daily do not appear to be associated with any adverse affects.[17]

CAUTIONS/CONTRAINDICATIONS

Pregnancy

The use of ginger in pregnancy has been questioned. This concern arises from two sources: (1) the use of ginger is 'contraindicated' during pregnancy within the Traditional Chinese Medical (TCM) model; and (2) several animal studies performed in the eighties suggested that large doses of the gingerol portion may exert a mutagenic action *in vitro*.[7, 46, 47] When considering the first source of concern, it should be noted that the doses given within TCM therapeutic protocols are normally far higher (approximately 9 g daily) than those suggested for therapeutic purposes in North America (1-2 g daily).[7] Regarding the second source, while it was shown that 6-gingerol possessed mutagenic properties, it should be noted that antimutagenic components were also found to be present in the total ginger extract.[47] In addition, in the only study in pregnant women (with hyperemesis gravidarum) no teratagenic effects nor increased rates of abortion were observed. Ginger has also been shown in animal studies to be devoid of any spermatoxic qualities.[48]

While the Commission E monographs does caution against the use of ginger in pregnancy, this concern is not shared by the other major pharmacopeias such as the British Herbal Compendium.[7] Consequently, it is reasonable to conclude that ginger can be taken during pregnancy in doses within the North American standard therapeutic range for a limited period of time.[7]

MISCELLANEOUS

Concerns have been raised over the possibility of increased bleeding time following surgery if the patient is taking ginger preparations due to the reported inhibition of thromboxane synthetase.[49] It appears unlikely that this presents a problem when the plant is taken in standard North American therapeutic doses as described in the management of post-surgical nausea.[17]

Given ginger's cholagogic properties some authors suggest against its use in cases of gall stones without medical supervision.[50]

DRUG INTERACTIONS

No specific interactions could be found between ginger and any conventional medications. Given the described pharmacological actions of ginger, it should be used with caution in situations of concurrent conventional cardiac, diabetic and anticoagulant therapy.[1]

DOSAGE REGIMENS

General Use

- Dried rhizome 0.25-1.0 g taken orally as a capsule, tablet, powder or decoction three times daily[6]
- Weak Ginger Tincture BP (1:5, 90% ethanol) 1.5 -3ml three times daily[6]
- Strong Ginger Tincture BP (1:2, 90% ethanol) 0.25-0.5 mL[6]

- As a general antiemetic, single dose of powdered rhizome, 1-2 g[6]
- Motion Sickness, 2-4g daily of powdered rhizome[31]

REFERENCES

1. Newall CA, Anderson LA, Phillipson JD. *Herbal Medicines: A Guide for Health Care Professionals.* London: The Pharmaceutical Press; 1996:296.
2. Foster S, Chongxi Y. *Herbal Emissaries. Bringing Chinese Herbs to the West.* Rochester, VT: Healing Arts Press; 1992:356.
3. Mascolo N, Jain R, Jain SC, Capasso F. Ethnopharmacologic investigation of ginger (*Zingiber officinalis*). *Journal of Ethnopharmacology*. 1989;27:129-40.
4. Awang DVC. Ginger. *Canadian Pharmaceutical Journal*. 1992;125:309-11.
5. Leung AY, Foster S. *Encyclopedia of Common Natural Ingredients Used in Food, Drugs, and Cosmetics.* 2nd ed. New York, NY: John Wiley and Sons Inc; 1996:649.
6. Bradley P. *British Herbal Compendium*. Bournemouth, UK: The British Herbal Medical Association; 1992:239.
7. Fulder S, Tenne M. Ginger as anti-nausea remedy in pregnancy. The issue of safety. *Herbalgram*. 1996;38:47-50.
8. Platel K, Srinivasan K. Influence of dietary spices or their active principles on digestive enzymes of small intestinal mucosa in rats. International *Journal of Food Sciences & Nutrition*. 1996;47(1):55-9.

9. Pengelly A. Ginger extracts prevent ulcers. *Australian Journal of Medical Herbalism*. 1993;59(2):73.
10. Yamahara J, Mochizuki M, Rong HQ, *et al*. The anti-ulcer effect in rats of ginger constituents. *Journal of Ethnopharmacology*. 1988;23:299-304.
11. Al-Yahya MA, Rafatullah S, Mossa JS, *et al*. Gastroprotective activity of ginger *Zingiber officinale* Rosc., in albino rats. *American Journal of Chinese Medicine*. 1989;17(1-2):51-6.
12. Sertie J, Basile A, Oshiro T, Mazella A. Preventative anti-ulcer activity of the rhizome extract of *Zingiber officinale*. *Fitoterapia*. 1992;63:55-9.
13. Sakai K, Miyazaki Y, Yamane T, *et al*. Effect of extracts of Zingiberaceae herbs on gastric secretion in rabbits. *Chemical and Pharmaceutical Bulletin*. 1989;37(1):215-7.
14. Yamahara J, Miki K, Chisaka T, *et al*. Cholagogic effect of ginger and its active constituents. *Journal of Ethnopharmacology*. 1985;13:217-25.
15. Verma S, Singh J, Khamesra R, Bordia A. Effect of ginger on platelet aggregation in man. *Indian Journal of Medical Research*. 1993;98:240-2.
16. Srivastava KC. Effects of aqueous extracts of onion, garlic and ginger on the platelet aggregation and metabolism of arachidonic acid in the blood vascular system: *In vitro* study. *Prostaglandins, Leukotrienes and Medicine*. 1984;13:277-35.
17. Lumb AB. Effect of dried ginger on human platelet function. *Thrombosis & Haemostasis*. 1994;71(1):110-1.
18. Gujral S, Bhumra H, Swaroop M. Effect of ginger (*Zingiber officinale* roscoe) oleoresin on serum and hepatic cholesterol levels in cholesterol fed rats. *Nutr Rep Intl.* 1978;17:183-9.
19. Giri J, Devi STK, Meerarani S. Effect of ginger on serum cholesterol levels. *The Indian Journal of Nutrition and Dietetics*. 1984;21:433-6.
20. Tanabe M, Chen Y-D, Saito K-i, Kano Y. Cholesterol biosynthesis inhibitory component from *Zingiber officinale* Roscoe. *Chemical & Pharmaceutical Bulletin*. 1993;41(4):710-3.
21. Brown D. Anti-Inflammatory potential of ginger. *Quarterly Review of Natural Medicine*. 1993;Spring:17.
22. Srivastava KC, Mustafa T. Ginger (*Zingiber officinale*) and rheumatic disorders. *Medical Hypotheses*. 1989;29:25-8.
23. Srivastava KC, Mustafa T. Ginger (*Zingiber officinale*) in rheumatism and musculoskeletal disorders. *Medical Hypotheses*. 1992;39:342-8.
24. Sharma JN, Srivastava KC, Gan EK. Suppressive effects of eugenol and ginger oil on arthritic rats. *Pharmacology*. 1994;49(5):314-8.
25. Kiuchi F, Shibuyu M, Sankawa U. Inhibitors of prostaglandin biosynthesis from ginger. *Chemical and Pharmaceutical Bulletin.* 1982;30:754-7.
26. McCaleb R. Ginger and atractylodes as an anti-inflammatory. *Herbalgram*. 1993;29:19.
27. Mowrey DB, Clayson DE. Motion sickness, ginger, and psychophysics. *Lancet*. 1982;I:655-7.
28. Stewart JJ, Wood MJ, D. WC, Mims ME. Effects of ginger on motion sickness susceptibility and gastric function. *Pharmacology*. 1991;42:111-20.
29. Grøntved A, Brask T, Kambskard J, Hentzer E. Ginger root against seasickness. A controlled trial on the open sea. *Acta Otolaryngologica* (Stockholm). 1988;105(1-2):45-9.
30. Wood CD, Manno JE, Wood MJ, *et al*. Comparison of efficacy of ginger with various antimotion sickness drugs. *Clinical Research Practices and Drug Regulatory Affairs*. 1988;6(2):129-36.
31. Tyler VE. *Herbs of Choice. The Therapeutic Use of Phytomedicinals.* Binghamton, NY: Pharmaceutical Products Press; 1994:209.
32. Brown D. Antimotion sickness action of ginger questioned. *Quarterly Review of Natural Medicine*. 1993;Spring:15-6.
33. Bone ME, Wilkinson DJ, Young JR, *et al*. Ginger Root — A new antiemetic. The effect of ginger root on postoperative nausea and vomiting after major gynaecological surgery. *Anaesthesia*. 1990;45(8):669-71.
34. Phillips S, Ruggier R, Hutchinson S. *Zingiber officinale* (ginger) — an antiemetic for day case surgery. *Anaesthesia*. 1993;48(8):715-7.
35. Arfeen Z, Owen H, Plummer J, *et al*. A double-blind randomized controlled trial of ginger for the prevention of postoperative nausea and vomiting. *Anaesthesia & Intensive Care*. 1995;23(4):449-52.
36. Fischer-Rasmussen W, Kjaer SK, Dahl C, Asping U. Ginger treatment of hyperemesis gravidarum. *European Journal of Obstetrics and Gynecology and Reproductive Biology*. 1990;38:19-24.
37. Yamahara J, Rong HQ, Naitoh Y, *et al*. Inhibition of cytotoxic drug-induced vomitting in suncus by a ginger constituent. *Journal of Ethnopharmacology*. 1989;27:353-5.
38. Holtmann S, Clarke AH, Scherer H, Hohn M. The anti-motion sickness mechanism of ginger. A comparative

study with placebo and Dimenhydrinate. *Acta Oto-Laryngologica* (Stockholm). 1989;198(3-4):168-74.
39. Kawai T, Kinosita K. Antiemetic principle of *Magnolia obovata* and *Zingiber officinale* rhizome. *Planta Medica*. 1994;60:17-20.
40. Lumb A. Mechanism of antiemetic effect of ginger. [Letter; comment]. *Anaesthesia*. 1993;48(12):1118.
41. Yamahara J, Rong H, Iwamoto M, *et al* Active components of ginger exhibiting antiserotonergic action. *Phytotherapy Research*. 1989;3(2):70-1.
42. Mills S. *Essential Book of Herbal Medicine.* London: Penguin; 1991:677.
43. Shoji N, Iwasa A, Takemoto T, Ishida Y, Ohizumi Y. Cardiotonic principles of ginger (Zingiber officiniale Roscoe). *Journal of Pharmaceutical Sciences*. 1982;71(10):1174-5.
44. Mustafa T, Srivastava KC. Ginger (*Zingiber officinale*) in migraine headaches. *Journal of Ethnopharmacology*. 1990;29(3):267-73.
45. Chang HM, But PPH. *Pharmacology and Application of Chinese Materia Medica*. Hong Kong: World Scientific Publishing; 1987:1320.
46. Nagabhushan M, Amonkar AJ, Bhide SV. Mutagenicity of gingerol and shogaol and antimutagenicity of zingerone in salmonella microsome assay. *Cancer Letters*. 1987;36:221-33.
47. Nakamura H, Yamamoto T. Mutagen and anti-mutagen in ginger, *Zingiber officinale*. *Mutation Research*. 1982;103:119-26.
48. Qureshi S, Shah AH, Tariq M, Ageel AM. Studies on herbal aphrodisiacs used in Arab system of medicine. *American Journal of Chinese Medicine*. 1989;17(1-2):57-63.
49. Backon J. Ginger as an antiemetic: Possible side effects due to its thromboxane synthetase activity [Letter/comment]. *Anaesthesia*. 1991;46(8):669-71.
50. Brown D. *Herbal Prescriptions for Better Health.* Rocklin, CA: Prima Publishing; 1996:349.

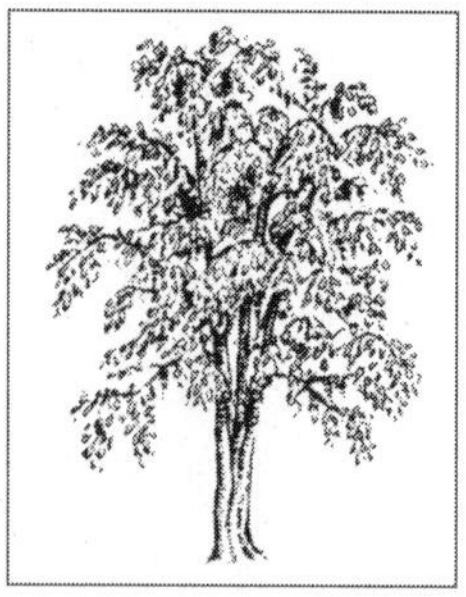

GINKGO

Ginkgo biloba L.

THUMBNAIL SKETCH

Active Constituents
- Ginkolides
- Bilobides
- Flavone glycosides

Common Uses
- Cerebral insufficiency
- Intermittent claudication
- Raynaud's syndrome
- Memory impairment/dementia
- Tinnitus
- Vertigo

Adverse Effects
- Extremely infrequent, but include: gastrointestinal disturbances and headache; very rarely spontaneous bleeding

Cautions /Contraindications
- Safety not established in nursing and pregnant women

Drug Interactions
- May potentiate the effect of anticoagulants (theoretical)

Doses
- 40 mg GBE (standardized extract) three times daily (standardized to 24% ginkgo-flavone glycosides and 6% terpenoids)
- 300 mg of dried leaves daily

INTRODUCTION

Family: Ginkgoaceae[1]

Synonyms: Maidenhair-tree[2-4]

It has been estimated that the ginkgo tree has existed for more than 200 million years, making it the oldest known tree species on earth.[5, 6] A given tree may live for 1000 years, growing to a height of 30 m and up to 120 cm in diameter. The leaves, which are the part used medicinally in North America, fan out from short, horizontal branches. The foul-smelling fruit is inedible, but contains an edible seed which resembles an almond.[4] Ginkgo trees are now extensively cultivated to meet the growing medicinal demand and they continue to be favored by city planners because they flourish in adverse conditions such as urban environments.[7]

Although ginkgo has been used in Traditional Chinese Medicine (TCM) for such indications as: 'benefiting the brain,' astringent to the lungs, and for the relief of asthma symptoms and coughs,[7-9] it is not generally regarded as a particularly important herb in TCM. Currently, ginkgo is considered a conventional drug in Europe, where annual sales are estimated at over US $500 million. Today *Ginkgo biloba* products are used for a variety of conditions, many associated with aging, including: peripheral vascular disease, tinnitus, eye disease, heart disease, dementia, cases of trauma to the brain and "chronic cerebral insufficiency".[7, 8] Products standardized to 24% flavone glycosides and 6% terpenoids have been available for several decades as non-prescription agents.[8] To date, the majority of the research has been conducted using one specific extract of ginkgo: EGb 761; however, several trials using a similar extract (LI 1370) are also reviewed here.

Constituents[1-4, 9-14]

Leaves:

- Terpenes: diterpene ginkgolides (A, B, C, J and M); sesquiterpenes (bilobalides)
- Flavonoids: ginkgo-flavone glycosides (e.g., bilobetin, gikgetin, isoginkgetin, sciadopitysin); glycosides of quercetin, and kaempferol; isorhamnetin derivatives
- Organic acids: 6-hydroxykynurenic acid, kynurenic acid, shikimic acid, protocatechic acid, vanillic acid, *p*-hydroxybenzoic acid
- Essential oils
- Tannins

Sticher provides an excellent review of the quality control and standardization of ginkgo preparations.[12]

THERAPEUTIC USES & RELEVANT PHARMACOLOGY

CARDIOVASCULAR

Mechanism of Action/Pharmacology

Many studies have demonstrated the ability of extracts of ginkgo (EGb 761) to increase blood flow.[3, 15-17] Egb 761 has been shown to: increase skin perfusion;[3] decrease blood viscosity;[3] decrease blood vessel elasticity;[3] increase blood flow in nail-fold capillaries;[15] decrease erythrocyte aggregation;[15] increase coronary blood flow (in isolated guinea pig heart);[18] and increase cerebral blood flow.[19] However, plasma viscosity,[3, 15] packed cell volume;[15] haematocrit[15] and thrombocyte aggregation[15] do not appear to be affected by this ginkgo extract. The specific compounds in the ginkgo extract responsible for these effects have not yet been identified, although much attention has been focused on the flavonoids and the ginkolides.[20, 21]

Ginkgo extracts (e.g., EGb 761) appear to have the ability to relax blood vessels in spasm and constrict those that are abnormally dilated by increasing their tone.[22-25] Several authors have noted the ability of GBE (*Ginkgo biloba* extract) to produce dose-dependent relaxation of the aorta in animal models.[26] This relaxant effect appears to be at least partially mediated by a factor(s) that is released from endothelial cells.[26] Other studies report a dose-dependent contractile effect on rabbit isolated aorta[27, 28] and vena cava.[29] It is suggested that ginkgo extracts cause contracted blood vessels to relax by prolonging the half-life of endothelium-derived relaxing factor.[30, 31] The flavonoids are thought to be primarily responsible for this action.

Another important mechanism of action is the competitive antagonism of platelet activating factor (PAF).[10, 21, 32-45] Braquet and Smith provide excellent reviews of this action.[10, 21] Ginkgo extracts have been shown to: decrease platelet aggregation;[39] decrease microvascular permeability; cause bronchodilation; and inhibit thromboformation *in vitro*[40, 46] and *in vivo* to a degree comparable to ASA.[46, 47] It is thought that the ginkgolides (especially ginkgolide B) are responsible for this action. However, several researchers have reported that ginkgo extracts do not affect coagulation or skin bleeding time.[39]

Interestingly, gingko seems to act preferentially at ischemic sites.[48-56] For example, administration of extracts of ginkgo in animals subjected to cerebral ischemia increased glucose consumption;[49] normalized mitochondrial respiration;[50] diminished cerebral edema;[50] preserved neurological function;[50] and decreased the accumulation of free polyunsaturated fatty acids.[55] In an animal study, *Ginkgo biloba* extract was found to be comparable to methylprednisone and more effective than thyroid releasing hormone at providing a protective effect against ischaemic spinal cord injury. This effect was thought to be due to its antioxidant actions.[52]

In addition, ginkgo has been shown to protect healthy volunteers from the effects of hypoxia.[57] Animal studies have confirmed this finding.[58-60] One study reported that both *Ginkgo biloba* extract and bilobalide alone were able to inhibit a hypoxia-induced decrease in ATP content and increase in total lactate production in endothelial cells *in vitro*.[61]

The flavonoid components of *Ginkgo biloba* extract are also reported to possess potent antioxidant activity.[62-68] Ginkgo's activity as an antioxidant is thought to play a role in many of its therapeutic actions, especially its postulated neuroprotective effect and its protection from ischemia-reperfusion damage.[64, 66-71] Several studies have demonstrated that the ginkgo extract EGb 761 has both hydroxyl radical scavenging and superoxide dismutase-like activity.[30, 71, 72]

Cerebral Insufficiency

A variety of studies report the effectiveness of ginkgo in the treatment of "chronic cerebral insufficiency".[73-78] Symptoms typical of "cerebral insufficiency" include: memory loss; difficulty concentrating; confusion; fatigue; decreased physical strength; anxiety; dizziness; tinnitus; headache and depressive mood. It is hypothesized that these symptoms may be associated with some impairment of the cerebral circulation.[3] Kleijnen and Knipschild reviewed 40 controlled trials studying the use of *Ginkgo biloba* in cases of "cerebral insufficiency,"[3] concluding that although only 8 trials[78-85] were of "good quality," all the trials reviewed, except one,[86] showed clinically-relevant positive effects for ginkgo when compared with a placebo. For example, in an open trial of 112 patients suffering from symptoms of "chronic cerebral insufficiency" (mean age 71 years) taking 40 mg *Ginkgo biloba* extract three times daily for one year, significant improvements in short-term memory, alertness, mood disturbances, vertigo, headaches and tinnitus were reported.[78] A more recent double-blind, placebo-controlled trial of 90 patients suffering from "cerebral insufficiency" found that those taking ginkgo scored significantly higher on a variety of tests of cognitive function.[87]

Intermittent Claudication

Kleijnen and Knipschild also reviewed 15 placebo-controlled trials which investigated the use of ginkgo extracts in the treatment of intermittent claudication.[3] They report that only two[88, 89] were of "acceptable" quality, and that all fifteen indicated positive effects for treatment with ginkgo. Bauer's double-blind, placebo-controlled study of 79 patients given either ginkgo (40 mg) or placebo three times daily for 1 year reported reduction in pain that was 4 times greater in the ginkgo group ($p<0.001$).[88] Given the overall poor quality of trials in this area Kleijnen and Knipschild recommend further research into the use of ginkgo extract for this indication.[3] A more recent double-blind, placebo-controlled trial with 20 patients suffering from stage II claudicating arterial occlusive disease provides some further evidence that ginkgo may useful in the management of this condition. Each patient ingested 160 mg *Ginkgo biloba* extract (EGb 761) or placebo twice daily for four weeks. The main outcome measure of this trial was measurement of the transcutaneous partial pressure of oxygen both at rest and after a treadmill test. The areas of ischemia decreased by 38% in the ginkgo group, but did not change in the placebo group ($p<0.04$). It should be noted that this trial used a much higher dose of ginkgo than most other reports in the literature.[90]

A double-blind, randomized study of 36 patients with arteritis found that those treated with *Ginkgo biloba* for 6 months experienced significantly greater pain relief and walking tolerance than those taking placebo. These benefits persisted when the ginkgo treatment was continued in an open trial for a total of 65 weeks.[91]

Ischemic Heart Disease

It is suggested that *Ginkgo biloba* extract may have a protective effect against cardiac-reperfusion injury.[70, 92] One study reports that EGb 761 improved cardiac mechanical recovery, suppressed leakage of lactate dehydrogenase and diminished the decrease of myocardial ascorbate during reperfusion.[93] It is hypothesized that this action of ginkgo may be attributed to its antioxidant properties.[70] In addition, ginkgolide B has been shown to have dose-related protection against dysrrhythmias induced by ischemia (comparable to diltiazem and superior to metoprolol) which the authors hypothesize may be related to an antagonism of an increase in slow calcium influx induced by PAF in myocardial cells.[94] This study noted that gingkolide B did not produce any changes in heart function, even in when given in high doses.

NEUROLOGY

Mechanism of Action / Pharmacology

Animal studies have shown that extracts of *Ginkgo biloba* can influence neuron metabolism and have a positive effect on neurotransmitter disturbances.[23] It appears to increase the production of dopamine and noradrenaline, as well as increasing the number of acetylcholine and serotonin receptors.[95-99] In addition, one study demonstrated that chronic oral treatment with ginkgo prevented decline in muscarinic (cholinergic) receptor density in the hippocampus of rats as they aged.[100] *In vitro and in vivo* studies indicate that the *Ginkgo biloba* extract EGb 761 increases synaptosomal uptake of 5-hydroxytryptamine[101] and decreases the synaptosomal uptake of dopamine and serotonin.[98]

It has been suggested that the bilobalides may aid in the regrowth of damaged neurons in the central nervous system; however, an exact mechanism of action has yet to be proposed.[9, 102] *Ginkgo biloba* extract (EGb 761) was also reported to prevent dopaminergic neurotoxicity in an animal study.[103] Amri and colleagues suggest that the neuroprotective effects of ginkgo are caused by its effect on glucocorticoid biosynthesis: it appears to decrease glucocorticoid levels and increase ACTH release. They described this mechanism of action in detail.[104] Other possible mechanisms for the neuroprotective properties associated with ginkgo have been described by many other authors.[10, 20, 105-107]

The effect of ginkgo on cerebral glucose utilization continues to be controversial, some studies reporting increases in cerebral glucose utilization;[23, 48, 108-110] some reporting no change;[19] and others reporting decreases.[111]

Dementia

A variety of studies indicate that ginkgo may be useful in the treatment of vascular dementia or dementia of the Alzheimer type.[75, 77, 82, 112-118] One of the most convincing is a prospective, randomized, double-blind, placebo-controlled, multi-center trial of the efficacy of *Gingko biloba* extract (EGb 761) in which 216 outpatients diagnosed with mild to moderate pre-senile, senile primary degenerative dementia of the Alzheimer type and multi-infarct dementia ingested either EGb 761 or placebo for 24 weeks. Ginkgo was found to be more effective than placebo ($p<.005$). The three primary outcome measures in this study were: the Clinical Global Impressions (CBI) for psychopathological assessment; the Syndrom-Kurztest (SKT) for assessment of memory and attention and the Nurnberger Alters-Beobachtungsskala (NAB) for assessment of behavior during the activities of daily life.[114] These results confirm the findings of an earlier, smaller (n=40) double-blind, placebo-controlled trial.[116]

A recent North American multi-center, randomized, controlled trial that followed 309 outpatients who had been diagnosed with mild to severe Alzheimer disease or multi-infarct dementia for 52 weeks reported similar results. *Ginkgo biloba* extract (EGb 761) at a dose of 40 mg three times daily was compared with placebo on the following outcome measures: the Alzheimer's Disease Assessment Scale — Cognitive subscale (ADAS-Cog); the Geriatric Evaluation by Relative's Rating Instrument (GERRI); and the Clinical Global Impression of Change Scale (CGIC). The investigators used an intention-to-treat analysis and reported that the treatment group scored significantly higher on both the ADAS-Cog and the GERRI; however, there was no difference between the placebo group and the ginkgo group with respect to the CGIC scores. Although the changes in patients taking ginkgo were considered modest by the investigators, they were of sufficient magnitude as to be identified by the caregivers as measured by the GERRI.[118]

Another longitudinal, multi-center, double-blind, placebo controlled study (n = 166) of ginkgo extract for the treatment of a variety of cerebral disorders due to ageing found that those on ginkgo for more than 3 months showed significantly higher scores (as compared to the placebo group) on a specially designed geriatric clinical evaluation scale. This difference continued to increase in subsequent months.[82]

Memory Impairment

Studies on the effectiveness of *Ginkgo biloba* in the treatment of memory impairment and as an agent of memory enhancement have been conflicting.[85, 115, 119-126] Generally, ginkgo preparations appear to enhance memory in cases where significant memory impairment exists (often associated with increasing age), but have no effect on those whose memory is unimpaired. For example, one study found that aged rats (22-24 months old) treated with 100 mg/kg of ginkgo extract EGb 761 daily for three weeks had improved short-term memory measured by avoidance latency after adverse stimulus ($p<.05$); however, no significant effects were seen in young (3 months old) or middle-aged (12 month old) rats.[125] In addition, in a study of 40 volunteers (57-77 years), those with initially low scores on tests of vigilance and reaction time showed significant improvement when taking ginkgo as compared to placebo, while those with initially normal scores on these tests showed no improvement when taking ginkgo when compared to the placebo group.[127] In another double-blind, placebo-controlled study, 31 patients over the age of 50 with mild to moderate memory impairment were given 40 mg of *Ginkgo biloba* extract or placebo three times daily for 6 months. The results indicate that those taking ginkgo had improved performance on the Kendrick digit copying task, and the median reaction time for the classification task; however, no statistical difference was found with the Kendrick object learning task and a decrease in performance on the digit recall task was noted. The authors suggest that more significant results may be expected if the subjects had more severe memory impairment at baseline.[119] Finally, a double-blind, placebo-controlled, cross-over study of 18 elderly men and women diagnosed with slight age-related memory impairment suggests that ingestion of 320 or 600 mg of ginkgo (EGb 761) one hour before performing a dual-coding test is associated with an improvement in the speed of information processing.[120] It should be noted that this is considered a relatively large dose of *Ginkgo biloba*.

Although improvement of short-term memory[121, 122] and simple reaction time[76] in young, healthy volunteers and improved retention of learned behavior in healthy rats have also been reported,[123, 126, 128] the evidence supporting these effects is limited and controversial. In one double-blind, randomized, crossover human study, 8 women (mean age 32 years) were given *Ginkgo biloba* extract at a variety of doses (120 mg, 240 mg and 600 mg) or placebo and asked to perform the following four psychological tests one hour later: critical flicker fusion (CFF); choice reaction time (CRT); subjective ratings of drug effects (LARS) and Sternberg memory scanning test. The only significant difference between placebo and ginkgo was found in the results of the Sternberg memory scanning test (which measures reaction time) at doses of 120 mg and 600 mg (but not at 240 mg).[121]

Depression

One randomized, placebo-controlled trial with 40 patients diagnosed with resistant depression (aged 51 to 78 years) found that *Ginkgo biloba* extract (EGb 761) was significantly more effective than placebo. Patients in the trial had shown insufficient improvement on tri- and/or tetracyclic antidepressants for a minimum of three months prior to being enrolled in the trial. During the trial, patients continued to take anti-depressant therapy, but were also given either EGb 761 (80 mg) or placebo three times daily. The main outcome measure was the sum score of the Hamilton Depression Scale (HAMD). After four weeks, a 50% decrease in the severity of depression for the EGb 761 group (compared to a 10% decrease in the placebo group) was noted ($p<.01$). A further decrease in the HAMD scores was noted after 8 weeks for the ginkgo group.($p<.01$).[129]

Animal studies have suggested that ginkgo extracts may reduce the emotional and behavioural consequences of stress.[128, 130] One study found that extracts of ginkgo leaves caused reversible inhibition of rat brain MAO-A and MAO-B, suggesting a mechanism for reported anti-stress and anxiolytic activities of *Ginkgo biloba*.[131]

Trauma to the Brain

Numerous animal studies have suggested that gingkolide B has a protective effect against neuronal damage following trauma, probably related to its PAF antagonist action.[55] A study with rats suggests that treatment with *Ginkgo biloba* extract (GBE) reduced the extent of brain swelling in response to injury (bilateral frontal cortex lesions) and was associated with less impairment following the injury.[132] In addition, it has been shown in rat experiments that EGb 761 treatment prior to electroconvulsive shock (ECS) treatment reduces the extent and duration of the remodelling of membrane phospholipids which traditionally results from seizures.[133]

OPHTHALMOLOGY

Ginkgo biloba extract is believed to protect the eye from damage by reducing free-radical damage to the retina.[134, 135] Animal studies suggest that ginkgo may be useful in the prevention of retinal damage in diabetes[134, 136] and in cases of lesions, inflammations or degenerative insults of the retina.[137] In addition, a double-blind trial (n =10) with senile macular degeneration, found ginkgo to be significantly better than placebo at improving long-distance visual acuity.[138]

OTOLOGY

The effects on the ear appear to be related to the ability of ginkgo to increase cochlear blood flow (CBF). One study of *Ginkgo biloba* extract (EGb 761) in guinea pigs demonstrated that after 4 to 6 weeks of treatment, EGb 761 partly counteracted sodium salicylate-induced decreases in CBF. [139] In a double-blind trial of ginkgo for the treatment of acute cochlear deafness, ginkgo was found to be more effective than nicergoline (an alpha-blocker), but significant improvement was seen with both treatments.[140]

Tinnitus

Studies of *Ginkgo biloba* for the treatment of tinnitus have reported conflicting results.[81, 141-143] One double-blind study (n=103) reported "marked improvement" in 40% of patients on ginkgo and 24% of patients on placebo, concluding ginkgo was an effective treatment.[81] In contrast, an uncontrolled trial (n=21) noted only slight improvement and the authors concluded that the treatment was ineffective.[142] A double-blind, crossover trial in 20 individuals who reported that ginkgo had improved their tinnitus previously found that *Ginkgo biloba* extract (29.2 mg daily for two weeks) was no more effective than placebo.[143] Although this study was well-designed, it should be noted that this is a very low dose of ginkgo. Additional trials are needed in this area.

Vertigo

Several animal studies have demonstrated that the administration of ginkgo extracts speeds vestibular compensation.[144, 145] For example, accelerated postural, locomotor balance recovery, spontaneous neck muscle activity, vestibulo-collic reflexes, and spontaneous firing rates of vestibular units on the lesioned side were noted in unilateral vestibular neurectomized cats.[144] One clinical study of patients with recent-onset idiopathic vertigo found that ginkgo significantly decreased the intensity, frequency and duration of symptoms of vertigo when compared with placebo.[83]

UROLOGY

Impotence

Ginkgo biloba extract has been suggested in the treatment of impotence. One study of 60 patients with proven arterial erectile dysfunction who had not responded to papaverine injections were given 60 mg/day of ginkgo extract for 12-18 months. Improvement in blood flow (as measured by duplex sonography) was noted after 6 to 8 weeks and 50% of the men gained potency after 6 months. In another 20% of the sample, a new trial with papaverine proved successful.[146] This trial was not blinded and given the large psychological component of impotence, the placebo-controlled, blinded study currently underway by the same authors is needed to confirm these results. In another study it was found that fractions of *Ginkgo biloba* extract had a relaxing effect on corpus cavernosum tissue *in vitro*.[147]

RESPIROLOGY

Asthma

Several preliminary studies suggest that *Ginkgo biloba* extracts may have a beneficial effect in patients with asthma.[8, 38, 42] A study of the smooth muscle relaxant activity of *Ginkgo biloba* on the guinea pig trachea noted a concentration-dependent relaxation *in vitro* and an antagonism of bronchoconstriction induced by various agonists *in vivo*.[25] One single-blind, randomized crossover study in 10 patients found that ingestion of 240 mg of *Ginkgo biloba* extract (BN 52063) 1 hour prior to induction of bronchoconstriction by hyperventilation with dry cold air did not result in any reduction in bronchoconstriction. However, an inhibition of PAF- induced platelet aggregation was noted after oral administration of BN 52063. On the third day of treatment with either BN 52063 or placebo, asthma was induced by exercise in these patients. There was no effect on the initial bronchoconstriction of those receiving ginkgo; however, the prolonged reduction of peak expiratory flow was attenuated. The rise in plasma concentrations of platelet factor 4 and beta-thromboglobin seen in the placebo group was inhibited in the group treated with ginkgo extract ($p<.01$).[36]

MISCELLANEOUS

Ginkgolide B (BN 52021) administered i.v. (120 mg twice daily for 4 days) was found to be useful as an adjunct to standard intensive care support in the treatment of patients with severe Gram-negative bacterial sepsis, as determined by a randomized, double-blind, placebo-controlled, multicentre phase III clinical trial. There was a significant reduction in mortality of patients treated with ginkolide B compared with those taking the placebo. The authors suggest that this was due to its ability to prevent a systemic inflammatory response to infection through platelet-activating factor (PAF) antagonism, inhibition of amplification of sepsis-induced tumor necrosis factor and thromboxane B_2 release, plasma trypsin-like activity and several other steps of the immuno-inflammatory cascade associated with gram negative bacterial sepsis.[45]

Persons irradiated (either for therapeutic reasons or accidentally) have clastogenic factors in their plasma. Thirty workers accidentally exposed to radiation were given 40 mg of *Ginkgo biloba* extract (EGb 761) three times daily for two months, at which time the clastogenic activity of their plasma had returned to the same level as controls. This effect persisted for at least 7 months.[148] This anticlastogenic effect was also demonstrated *in vitro*.[149] Another study demonstrates the ability of ginkgo to protect microsomal fatty acids and proteins from UV-C radiation-induced peroxidative degradation.[150]

Ginkgo biloba extract was shown to inhibit cyclosporin A-induced peroxidation in human liver microsomes in a dose-dependent manner. Thus, it may have some use in the prevention of damage to human membranes caused by cyclosporin A.[151]

Several components isolated from *Ginkgo biloba* have been reported to have anti-tumor activity.[152]

Ginkgo is reported to have beneficial effects in cases of cyclic edema. The flavonoids are thought to normalize excessive capillary permeability and one clinical study found complete elimination of edema in 3 patients and partial elimination of the edema in 6 patients.[153] Ginkgo has also been reported to be effective against the "congestive" symptoms of premenstrual symptom (PMS) (esp. breast symptoms).[154]

ADVERSE EFFECTS

Most sources suggest that adverse effects from *Ginkgo biloba* are extremely infrequent, but include: gastrointestinal disturbances, headache, and allergic skin reactions.[1, 8, 9, 23] Skin reactions appear to be caused only by direct contact with the fruit of the ginkgo tree,[155, 156] which is not the part used medicinally. Kleijnen and Knipschild report no serious side effects in any trial they reviewed.[3] Headaches, although relatively rare, appear to be the most common adverse effect.[80] Some authors have suggested that these adverse effects may be decreased by slowly increasing to the therapeutic dose level.

Although researchers have warned against hypothetical problems due to the potential increase in blood clotting time, no clinical reports supported this hypothesis until recently. In one case report, a healthy 33-year-old women with a long term history of use of *Ginkgo biloba* (60 mg twice daily for 2 years) was reported to have an increased bleeding time and suffered bilateral subdural hematomas. Her bleeding times had returned to normal 35 days after discontinuation of Ginkgo ingestion.[157] In another case, a 70-year-old man presented with spontaneous bleeding from the iris into the anterior chamber of the eye one week after beginning treatment with 40 mg *Ginkgo biloba* extract daily. The patient had also been taking acetylsalicyclic acid (ASA) (325 mg) daily for three years.[158] Given the large number of individuals ingesting *Ginkgo biloba* world-wide, this appears to be a relatively rare phenomenon.

CAUTIONS/CONTRAINDICATIONS

Safety in pregnant and nursing mothers has yet to be established.[8, 9, 13]

DRUG INTERACTIONS

Most authors suggest that there are no known drug interactions.[3, 8, 9, 78] Although there is little clinical evidence, theoretically *Ginkgo biloba* may potentiate the action of anticoagulants.

DOSAGE REGIMENS

- 40 mg GBE (standardized extract) three times daily[1, 8]
- 300 mg of dried leaves daily[9]

Almost all the research has been conducted using a standardized extract (SE): ginkgo-flavone glycosides (24%) and terpenoids (6%).[3] A recent pharmacokinetic study found no significant differences between the bioavailability of three different formulations of *Ginkgo biloba* (capsules, drops and tablets).[159]

Treatment for many conditions must be continued for 1 to 3 months before positive results can be expected.[3, 8, 9]

REFERENCES

1. Tyler VE. *Herbs of Choice. The Therapeutic Use of Phytomedicinals.* Binghamton, NY: Pharmaceutical Products Press; 1994:209-362.
2. Wren RC. *Potter's New Encyclopaedia of Botanical Drugs and Preparations.* Saffron Waldon, UK: C.W. Daniel Company; 1988:362.
3. Kleijnen J, Knipschild P. *Ginkgo biloba*. *Lancet*. 1992;340:1136-9.
4. Murray MT. *The Healing Power of Herbs.* Rocklin, CA: Prima Publishing; 1992:246.
5. Michel PF. The doyen of trees: the *Ginkgo biloba*. [French]. *Presse Medicale*. 1986;15(31):1450-4.
6. Major RT. The ginkgo, the most ancient living tree. *Science*. 1967;157:1270-3.
7. Foster S. Ginkgo, *Ginkgo biloba*. Austin, Texas: American Botanical Council; 1990:7.
8. Gaby AR. *Ginkgo biloba* extract: A review. *Alternative Medicine Review*. 1996;1(4):236-42.
9. Houghton PJ. Ginkgo. *Pharmacy Journal*. 1994;253:122-3.
10. Braquet P. The ginkgolides: potent platelet-activating afactor antagonists isolated from *Ginkgo biloba* L.: Chemistry, pharmacology and clinical applications. *Drugs of the Future*. 1987;12:643-99.
11. van Beek TA, Rantio HA, Melger WC, Lelyveld GP. Determination of ginkolides and bilobalide in *Ginkgo biloba* leaves and phytopharmaceuticals. *Journal of Chromotography*. 1991;543:375-87.
12. Sticher O. Quality of Ginkgo preparations. [Review]. *Planta Medica*. 1993;59(1):2-11.
13. Newall CA, Anderson LA, Phillipson JD. *Herbal Medicines: A Guide for Health Care Professionals*. London: The Pharmaceutical Press; 1996:296.
14. Briancon-Scheid F, *et al.* HPLC separation and quantitative determination of biflavones in leaves from Ginkgo biloba. *Planta Medica*. 1983;49:204-20.
15. Jung F, Mrowietz C, Kiesewetter H, Wenzel E. Effect of *Ginkgo biloba* on fluidity of blood and peripheral microcirculation in volunteers. *Arzneimittelforschung*. 1990;40(5):589-93.
16. Liberti. Ginkgo. *The Lawrence Review of Natural Products*. 1988;February.
17. Le Poncin Lafitte M, Rapin J, Rapin JR. Effects of *Ginkgo Biloba* on changes induced by quantitative cerebral microembolization in rats. *Archives Internationales de Pharmacodynamie et de Therapie*. 1980.
18. Chatterjee SS, *et al.* Studies on the mechanism of action of an extract of *Ginkgo biloba*, a drug used for treatment of ischemic vascular disease. *Arch Pharmacol*. 1988;320:R52.
19. Krieglstein J, Beck T, Seibert A. Influence of an extract of *Ginkgo biloba* on cerebral blood flow and metabolism. *Life Sciences*. 1986;39(24):2327-34.
20. Tighilet B, Lacour M. Pharmacological activity of the *Ginkgo biloba* extract (EGb 761) on equilibrium function recovery in the unilateral vestibular neurectomized cat. *Journal of Vestibular Research*. 1995;5(3):187-200.
21. Smith PF, Maclennan K, Darlington CL. The neuroprotective properties of the *Ginkgo biloba* leaf: A review of the possible relationship to platelet-activating factor (PAF). [Review]. *Journal of Ethnopharmacology*. 1996;50(3):131-9.
22. Stucker O, Pons C, Duverger JP, Drieu K. Effects of *Ginkgo biloba* extract (EGb 761) on arteriolar spasm in a rat cremaster muscle preparation. *International Journal of Microcirculation: Clinical & Experimental*. 1996.
23. DeFeudis FV. *Ginkgo Biloba Extract (EGb 761): Pharamacological Activities and Clinical Applications.* Paris: Elsevier; 1991:3-5.
24. Vilain B, DeFeudis FV, Clostre F. Effect of an extract of *Ginkgo biloba* on the isolated ileum of the guinea pig. *General Pharmacology*. 1982;13(5):401-5.
25. Puglisi L, Salvadori S, Gabrielli G, Pasargiklian R. Pharmacology of natural compounds. I. Smooth muscle relaxant activity induced by a *Ginkgo biloba* L. extract on guinea-pig trachea. *Pharmacological Research Communications*. 1988;20(7):573-89.
26. Delaflotte S, Auguet M, DeFeudis FV, *et al.* Endothelium-dependent relaxations of rabbit isolated aorta produced by carbachol and by *Ginkgo biloba* extract. *Biomedica Biochimica Acta*. 1984;43(8-9):S212-6.

27. Auguet M, DeFeudis FV, Clostre F. Effects of *Ginkgo biloba* on arterial smooth muscle responses to vasoactive stimuli. *General Pharmacology*. 1982;13(2):169-71.
28. Auguet M, DeFeudis FV, Clostre F, Deghenghi R. Effects of an extract of *Ginkgo biloba* on rabbit isolated aorta. *General Pharmacology*. 1982;13(3):225-30.
29. Hellegouarch A, Baranes J, Clostre F, *et al.* Comparison of the contractile effects of an extract of *Ginkgo biloba* and some neurotransmitters on rabbit isolated vena cava. *General Pharmacology*. 1985;16(2):129-32.
30. Pincemail J, Dupuis M, Nasr C, *et al.* Superoxide anion scavenging effect and superoxide dismutase activity of *Ginkgo biloba* extract. *Experientia*. 1989;45(8):708-12.
31. Robak J, Gryglewski RJ. Flavonoids are scavengers of superoxide anions. *Biochemical Pharmacology*. 1988;37:837-41.
32. Chung KF. Effect of a ginkgolide mixture (BN 52063) in antagonising skin and platelet responses to platelet activating factor in man. *Lancet*. 1987;i:248-51.
33. Braquet P. Proofs of involvement of PAF-acether in various immune disorders using BN 52021 (ginkgolide B): A powerful PAF-acether antagonist isolated from *Ginkgo biloba* L. *Advances in Prostaglandin, Thromboxane, and Leukotriene Research*. 1986;16.
34. Braquet P, Hosford D. Ethnopharmacology and the development of natural PAF antagonists as therapeutic agents. *Journal of Ethnopharmacology*. 1991;32:135-9.
35. Markey AC, Baker JN, Archer CB, *et al.* Platelet activating factor-induced clinical and histopathologic responses in atopic skin and their modification by the platelet activating factor antagonist BN52063. *Journal of the American Academy of Dermatology*. 1990;23(2):263-268.
36. Wilkens JH, Uffmann J, *et al.* Effects of a PAF-antagonist (BN 52063) on bronchoconstriction and platelet activation during exercise induced asthma. *British Journal of Clinical Pharmacology*. 1990;29(1):85-91.
37. Guinot P, Braquet P, Duchier J, Cournot A, *et al.* Inhibition of PAF-acether induced wheal and flare reaction in man by a specific PAF antagonist. *Prostaglandins*. 1986;32(1):160-3.
38. Guinot P, Brambilla C, Duchier J, *et al.* Effect of BN 52063, a specific PAF-acether antagonist, on bronchial provocation test to allergens in asthmatic patients. A preliminary study. *Prostaglandins*. 1987;34(5):723-31.
39. Guinot P, Coffrey E, Lamb R, Darragh A. Tanakan inhibits platelet-activating-factor-induced platelet aggregation in healthy male volunteers. *Haemostasis*. 1989;19(4):219-223.
40. Bourgain RH, Andries R, Braquet P. Effect of ginkgolide PAF-acether antagonists on arterial thrombosis. *Advances in Prostaglandin, Thromboxane, & Leukotriene Research*. 1987.
41. Koltai M, Lepran K, Szekeres L, *et al.* Effect of BN 52021, a specific PAF-acether antagonist, on cardiac anaphylax is in langendorff hearts isolated from passively sensitized guinea pigs. *European Journal of Pharmacology*. 1986;130:133-6.
42. Kurihara K, Wardlaw AJ, Moqbel R, Kay AB. Inhibition of platelet-activating factor (PAF)-induced chemotaxis and PAF binding to human eosinophils and neutrophils by the specific ginkgolide-derived PAF antagonist, BN 52021. *Journal of Allergy and Clinical Immunology*. 1989;83(1):83-90.
43. Lamant V, Mauco G, Braquet P, *et al.* Inhibition of the metabolism of platelet activating factor (PAF-acether) by three specific antagonists from *Ginkgo biloba*. *Biochemical Pharmacology*. 1987;36:2749-2752.
44. Harczy M, Maclouf J, Pradelles P, *et al.* Inhibitory effects of a novel platelet activating factor (PAF) antagonist (BN 52021) on antigen-induced prostaglandin and thromboxane formation by the guinea pig lung. *Pharmacological Research Communications*. 1986;18:111-7.
45. Dhainaut J-FA, Tenaillon A, Le Tulzo Y, *et al.* Platelet activating factor receptor antagonist BN 52021 in treatment of severe spepsis: A randomized, double-blind, placebo-controlled, multicentre clinical trial. *Critical Care Medicine*. 1994;22(11):1720-8.
46. Bourgain RH, Maes L, Andries R, Braquet P. Thrombus induction by endogenic paf-acether and its inhibition by *Ginkgo biloba* extracts in the guinea pig. *Prostaglandins*. 1986;32(1):142-4.
47. Belougne E, Aguejouf O, Imbault P, *et al.* Experimental thrombosis model induced by laser beam. Application of aspirin and an extract of *Ginkgo biloba*: EGb 761. *Thrombosis Research*. 1996;82(5):453-8.
48. Clostre F. From the body to the cell membrane: The different levels of pharmacological action of *Ginkgo biloba* extract. [Review] [French]. *Presse Medicale*. 1986;15(31):1529-38.
49. Rapin JR, Le Poncin Lafitte M. Cerebral glucose consumption. The effect of *Ginkgo biloba* extract. [French]. *Presse Medicale*. 1986;15(31):1494-7.
50. Spinnewyn B, Blavet N, Clostre F. Effects of *Ginkgo biloba* extract on a cerebral ischemia model in gerbils. [French]. *Presse Medicale*. 1986;15(31):1511-5.
51. Spinnewyn B, Blavet N, Clostre F, *et al.* Involvement of platelet-activating factor (PAF) in cerebral post-ischemic

phase in Mongolian gerbils. *Prostaglandins*. 1987;34(3):337-49.
52. Koc RK, Akdemir H, Kurtsoy A, *et al.* Lipid peroxidation in experimental spinal cord injury. Comparison of treatment with *Ginkgo biloba*, TRH and methylprednisolone. *Research in Experimental Medicine*. 1995;195(2):117-23.
53. Otamiri T, Tagesson C. *Ginkgo biloba* extract prevents mucosal damage associated with small-intestinal ischaemia. *Scandinavian Journal of Gastroenterology*. 1989;24(6):666-70.
54. Seif-El-Nasr M, El-Fattah AA. Lipid peroxide, phospholipids, glutathione levels and superoxide dismutase activity in the rat brain after ischemia: Effect of ginkgo biloba extract. *Pharmacological Research*. 1995;32(5):273-8.
55. Birkle DL, Kurian P, Braquet P, Bazan NG. Platelet-activating factor antagonist BN52021 decreases accumulation of free polyunsaturated fatty acid in mouse brain during ischemia and electroconvulsive shock. *Journal of Neurochemistry*. 1988;51:1900-5.
56. Panetta T, Marcheselli VL, Braquet P, *et al*. Effects of a platelet activating factor antagonist (BN 52021) on free fatty acids, dicylglycerols, polyphosphoinositides and blood flow in the gerbil brain: inhibition of ischemia-reperfusion induced cerebral injury. *Biochemical and Biophysical Research Communications*. 1987;149:580-7.
57. Schaffler K, Reeh PW. Double blind study of the hypoxia protective effect of a standardized *Ginkgo biloba* preparation after repeated administration in healthy subjects [German]. *Arzneimittelforschung*. 1985;35(8):1283-6.
58. Oberpichler H, Beck T, Abdel-Rahman MM, Bielenberg GW, Krieglstein J. Effects of *Ginkgo biloba* constituents related to protection against brain damage caused by hypoxia. *Pharmacological Research Communications*. 1988;20(5):349-68.
59. Karcher L, Zagermann P, Krieglstein J. Effect of an extract of *Ginkgo biloba* on rat brain energy metabolism in hypoxia. *Naunyn Schmiedebergs Archives of Pharmacology*. 1984;327(1):31-5.
60. Punkt K, Welt K, Schaffranietz L. Changes of enzyme activities in the rat myocardium caused by experimental hypoxia with and without *Ginkgo biloba* extract EGb 761 pretreatment. A cytophotometrical study. *Acta Histochemica*. 1995;97(1):67-79.
61. Janssens D, Michiels C, Delaive E, Eliaers F, Drieu K, Remacle J. Protection of hypoxia-induced ATP decrease in endothelial cells by *Ginkgo biloba* extract and bilobalide. *Biochemical Pharmacology*. 1995;50(7):991-9.
62. Kose K, Dogan P. Lipoperoxidation induced by hydrogen peroxide in human erythrocyte membranes. 2. Comparison of the antioxidant effect of *Ginkgo biloba* extract (EGb 761) with those of water-soluble and lipid-soluble antioxidants. *Journal of International Medical Research*. 1995;23(1):9-18.
63. Kose K, Dogan P. Lipoperoxidation induced by hydrogen peroxide in human erythrocyte membranes. 1. Protective effect of *Ginkgo biloba* extract (EGb 761). *Journal of International Medical Research*. 1995;23(1):1-8.
64. Maitra I, Marcocci L, Droy-Lefaix MT, Packer L. Peroxyl radical scavenging activity of *Ginkgo biloba* extract EGb 761. *Biochemical Pharmacology*. 1995;49(11):1649-55.
65. Ni Y, Zhao B, Hou J, Xin W. Preventive effect of *Ginkgo biloba* extract on apoptosis in rat cerebellar neuronal cells induced by hydroxyl radicals. *Neuroscience Letters*. 1996;214(2-3):115-8.
66. Oyama Y, Fuchs PA, Katayama N, Noda K. Myricetin and quercetin, the flavonoid constituents of *Ginkgo biloba* extract, greatly reduce oxidative metabolism in both resting and Ca(2+) - loaded brain neurons. *Brain Research*. 1994;635(1-2):125-9.
67. Oyama Y, Chikahisa L, Ueha T, *et al*. *Ginkgo biloba* extract protects brain neurons against oxidative stress induces by hydrogen peroxide. *Brain Research*. 1996;712(2):349-52.
68. Rong Y, Geng Z, Lau BH. *Ginkgo biloba* attenuates oxidative stress in macrophages and endothelial cells. *Free Radical Biology & Medicine*. 1996;20(1):121-7.
69. Haramaki N, Aggarwal S, Kawabata T, Droy-Lefaix MT, Packer L. Effects of natural antioxidant *Ginkgo biloba* extract (EGB 761) on myocardial ischemia-reperfusion injury. *Free Radical Biology & Medicine*. 1994;16:789-94.
70. Shen JG, Zhou DY. Efficiency of *Ginkgo biloba* extract (EGb 761) in antioxidant protection against myocardial ischemia and reperfusion injury. *Biochemistry & Molecular Biology International*. 1995;35(1):125-34.
71. Szabo ME, Droy-Lefaix MT, Doly M, Braquet P. Free radical-mediated effects in reperfusion injury: a histologic study with superoxide dismutase and EGb 761 in rat retina. *Ophthalmic Research*. 1991;23(4):225-34.
72. Pincemail J, Deby C. Antiradical properties of *Ginkgo biloba* extract. [French]. *Presse Medicale*. 1986;15(31):1475-9.
73. Arrigo A, Cattaneo S. Clinical and psychometric evaluation of *Ginkgo biloba* extract in chronic cerebro-vascular diseases. In: Agnoli A, *et al.*, eds. *Effects of Ginkgo biloba Extracts on Organic Cerebral Impairment*: John Libbey Eurotext Ltd.; 1985:71-6.
74. Augustin P. *Ginkgo biloba* extract in geriatrics. Clinical and psychometric study of 189 patients. [French]. *Psychologie Mediacale*. 1976;8:123-130.

75. Eckmann VF, Schlag H. Knotrollierte doppelblind-studie zum wirksamkeitsnachweis von Tebonin forte bei patien ten mit zerebrovakularer insuffizienz. *Fortschritte der Medizin*. 1982;31:1474-8.
76. Gessner B, Voelp A, Klasser M. Study of the long-term action of a *Ginkgo biloba* extract on vigilance and mental performance as determined by means of quantitative pharmaco-EEG and psychometric measurements. *Arzneimittel Forschung*. 1985;35(9):1459-65.
77. Hofferberth B. The effect of *Ginkgo biloba* extract on neurophysiological and psychometric measurement results in patients with psychotic organic brain syndrome. A double-blind study against placebo. [German]. *Arzneimittel Forschung*. 1989;39(8):918-22.
78. Vorberg G. *Ginkgo biloba* extract (GBE): A long term study of cerebral insufficiency in geriatric patients. *Clinical Trials Journal*. 1985;22(149-157).
79. Schmidt U, Rabinovici K, Lande S. EifluB eines *Ginkgo-biloba*-spezialextraktes auf die befindlichkeit bei zerebraler insufizienz. *Munch Med Wochenschr*. 1991;133(Supplement 1):S15-8.
80. Bruchert E, Heinrich SE, Ruf-Kohler P. Wirksamkeit von LI 1370 bei alteren patienten mit hirnleistungsschwache. Multizentrische doppelblindstudie des fachverbandes deutscher allgemeinarzte. *Munch Med Wochenschr*. 1991;133(Supplement 1):S9-14.
81. Meyer B. Multicenter randomized double-blind drug vs. placebo study of the treatment of tinnitus with *Ginkgo biloba* extract. [French]. *Presse Medicale*. 1986;15(31):1562-4.
82. Taillander J, Ammar A, Rabourdin JP, *et al*. *Ginkgo biloba* extract in the treatment of cerebral disorders due to aging. A longitudinal multicenter double-blind drug vs. placebo study [French]. *Presse Medicale*. 1986;15(31): 1583-1587.
83. Haguenauer JP, Cantenot F, Koskas H, Pierart H. Treatment of equilibrium disorders with *Ginkgo biloba* extract. A multicenter double-blind drug vs. placebo study. [French]. *Presse Medicale*. 1986;15(31):1569-72.
84. Eckmann F. Cerebral insufficiency—treatment with *Ginkgo biloba* extract. Time of onset of effect in a double-blind study with 60 inpatients. [German]. *Fortschritte der Medizin*. 1990;108(29):557-60.
85. Wesnes K, *et al*. A double-blind placebo-controlled trial of *Gingko biloba* extract in the treatment of idiopathic cognitive impairment in the elderly. *Human Psychopharmacology*. 1987;2:159-169.
86. Hartmann A, Frick M. Wirkung eines Ginkgo-spezialextraktes auf psychometrische parameter bei patienten mit caskular bedingter demenz. *Munch Med Wochenschr*. 1991;133(Supplement 1):S23-5.
87. Vesper J, Hansgen KD. Efficacy of *Ginkgo biloba* in 90 outpatients with cerebral insufficiency caused by old age. Results of a placebo-controlled double-blind trial. *Phytomedicine*. 1994;1:9-16.
88. Bauer U. 6-Month double-blind randomised clinical trial of *Ginkgo biloba* extract versus placebo in two parallel groups in patients suffering from peripheral arterial insufficiency. *Arzneimittel Forschung*. 1984;34(6):716-20.
89. Saudreau F, Serise JM, Pillet J, *et al*. Efficacy of an extract of *Ginkgo biloba* in the treatment of chronic obliterating arteriopahies of the lower limbs in stage III of Fontaine's classification. [French]. *Journal des Maladies Vasculaires*. 1989;14(3):177-82.
90. Mouren X, Calliard PH, Schwarz F. Study of the anti-ischemic action of EGb 761 in the treatment of peripheral arterial occlusive disease by TcPO2 determination. *Angiology*. 1994;45:413-17.
91. Bauer U. *Ginkgo biloba* extract in the treatment of arteriopathy of the lower extremities. A 65-week trial. [French]. *Presse Medicale*. 1986;15(31):1546-9.
92. Tosaki A, Engelman DT, Pali T, *et al*. Ginkgo biloba extract (EGb 761) improves postischemic function in isolated preconditioned working rat hearts. *Coronary Artery Disease*. 1994;5(5):443-50.
93. Haramaki N, Aggarwal S, Kawabata T, *et al*. Effects of natural antioxidant *Ginkgo biloba* extract (EGB 761) on myocardial ischemia-reperfusion injury. *Free Radical Biology & Medicine*. 1994;16(6):789-94.
94. Koltai M, Tosaki A, Hosford D, Braquet P. Ginkgolide B protects isolated hearts against arrhythmias induced by ischaemia but not reperfusion. *European Journal of Pharmacology*. 1989;164:293-302.
95. Huguet F, Drieu K, Piriou A. Decreased cerebral 5-HT1A receptors during aging: reversal by *Ginkgo biloba* extract (EGb761). *Journal of Pharmaceutical Pharmacology*. 1994;46:316-318.
96. Racagni G, Brunello N, Paoletti R. Neuromediator changes during cerebral aging. The effect of *Ginkgo biloba* extract. [Review] [French]. *Presse Medicale*. 1986;15(31):1488-90.
97. Huguet F, Tarrade T. Alpha 2-adrenoceptor changes during cerebral ageing. The effect of *Ginkgo biloba* extract. *Journal of Pharmacy & Pharmacology*. 1992;44(1):24-7.
98. Ramassamy C, Naudin B, Christen Y, *et al*. Prevention by *Ginkgo biloba* extract (EGb 761) and trolox C of the decrease in synaptosomal dopamine or serotonin uptake following incubation. *Biochemical Pharmacology*. 1992;44(12): 2395-401.

99. Brunello N, Racagni G, Clostre F, *et al*. Effects of an extract of *Ginkgo biloba* on noradrenergic systems of rat cerebral cortex. *Pharmacological Research Communications*. 1985;17(11):1063-72.
100. Taylor JE. Neuromediator binding to receptors in the rat brain. The effect of chronic administration of *Ginkgo biloba* extract. [French]. *Presse Medicale*. 1986;15(31):1491-3.
101. Ramassamy C, Christen Y, Clostre F, Costentin J. The *Ginkgo biloba* extract, EGb761, increases synaptosomal uptake of 5-hydroxytryptamine: *in-vitro* and *ex-vivo* studies. *Journal of Pharmacy & Pharmacology*. 1992;44(11):943-5.
102. Bruno C, Cuppini R, Sartini S, *et al*. Regeneration of motor nerves in bilobalide-treated rats. *Planta Medica*. 1993;59(4):302-7.
103. Ramassamy C, Clostre F, Christen Y, Costentin J. Prevention by a *Ginkgo biloba* extract (GBE 761) of the dopaminergic neurotoxicity of MPTP. *Journal of Pharmacy & Pharmacology*. 1990;42(11):785-9.
104. Amri H, Ogwuegbu SO, Boujrad N, Drieu K, Papadopoulos V. *in vivo* regulation of peripheral-type benzodiazepine receptor and glucocorticoid synthesis by *Ginkgo biloba* extract EGb 761 and isolated ginkgolides. *Endocrinology*. 1996;137(12):5707-18.
105. Braquet P, Bourgain RH. Anti-anaphylactic properties of BN52021: A potent platelet activating factor antagonist. *Advances in Experimental Medicine and Biology*. 1987;215:215-33.
106. Brailowsky S, Montiel T, Medina-Ceja L. Acceleration of functional recovery from motor cortex ablation by two *Ginkgo biloba* extracts in rats. *Restorative Neurology and Neuroscience*. 1995;8:163-7.
107. Sancesario G, Kreutzberg GW. Stimulation of astrocytes affects cytotoxic brain edema. *Acta Neuropathologica*. 1986;72(1):3-14.
108. Auguet M, Delaflotte S, Hellegouarch A, Clostre F. Pharmacological bases of the vascular impact of *Ginkgo biloba* extract. [Review] [French]. *Presse Medicale*. 1986;15(31):1524-8.
109. Drieu K. Preparation and definition of *Ginkgo biloba* extract. [French]. *Presse Medicale*. 1986;15(31):1455-7.
110. Bruel A, Gardette J, Berrou E, Droy-Lefaix MT, Picard J. Effects of *Ginkgo biloba* extract on glucose transport and glycogen synthesis of cultured smooth muscle cells from pig aorata. *Pharmacological Research*. 1989;21(4):421-9.
111. Duverger D, DeFeudis FV, Drieu K. Effects of repeated treatments with an extract of *Ginkgo biloba* (EGb 761) on cerebral glucose utilization in the rat: an autoradiographic study. *General Pharmacology*. 1995;26(6):1375-83.
112. Weitbrecht WU, Jansen W. Primary degenerative dementia: Therapy with *Ginkgo biloba* extract. Placebo-controlled double-blind and comparative study. [German]. *Fortschritte der Medizin*. 1986;104(9):199-202.
113. Halama P, Bartsch G, Meng G. Disturbances in cerebral performance of vascular origin. Randomized, double blind study on the efficacy of *Ginkgo biloba* extract [German]. *Fortschritte der Medizin*. 1988;106:408-12.
114. Kanowski S, Herrman WM, Stephan K, *et al.* Proof of efficacy of the *Ginkgo biloba* special extract EGb 761 in out patients suffering from mild to moderate primary degenerative dementia of the Alzheimer type or multi-infarct dementia. *Pharmacopsychiatry*. 1996;29:47-56.
115. Warburton DM. Clinical psychopharmacology of *Ginkgo biloba* extract. [Review] [French]. *Presse Medicale*. 1986;15(31): 1595-604.
116. Hofferberth B. The efficacy of EGb 761 in patients with senile dementia of the Alzheimer type — a double-blind, placebo-controlled study on different levels of investigation. *Human Psychopharmacology*. 1994;9:215-22.
117. Funfgeld EW. A natural and broad spectrum nootropic substance for treatment of SDAT - the *Ginkgo biloba* extract. *Progress in Clinical & Biological Research*. 1989;317:1247-60.
118. Le Bars PL, Katz MM, Berman N, *et al.* A placebo-controlled, double-blind, randomized trail of an extract of *Ginkgo biloba* for dementia. *Journal of the American Medical Association*. 1997;278:1327-32.
119. Rai GS, Shovlin C, Wesnes KA. A double-blind, placebo controlled study of *Ginkgo biloba* extract ('tanakan') in elderly outpatients with mild to moderate memory impairment. *Current Medical Research & Opinion*. 1991;12(6):350-5.
120. Allain H, Raoul P, Lieury A, LeCoz F, Gandon JM, d'Arbigny P. Effect of two doses of *ginkgo biloba* extract (EGb 761) on the dual-coding test in elderly subjects. *Clinical Therapeutics*. 1993;15(3):549-58.
121. Subhan Z, Hindmarch I. The psychopharmacological effects of *Ginkgo biloba* extract in normal healthy volunteers. *International Journal of Clinical Pharmacology Research*. 1984;4(2):89-93.
122. Hindmarch I. Activity of *Ginkgo biloba* extract on short-term memory. [French]. *Presse Medicale*. 1986;15(31):1592-4.
123. Petkov VD, Kehayov R, Belcheva S, *et al.* Memory effects of standardized extracts of *Panax ginseng* (G115), *Ginkgo biloba* (GK 501) and their combination Gincosan (PHL-00701). *Planta Medica*. 1993;59(2):106-14.
124. Semlitsch HV, Anderer P, Saletu B, *et al*. Cognitive psychophysiology in nootropic drug research: Effects of *Ginkgo*

biloba on event-related potentials (P300) in age-associated memory impairment. *Pharmacopsychiatry*. 1995;28(4): 134-42.

125. Stoll S, Scheuer K, Pohl O, Muller WE. *Ginkgo biloba* extract (EGb 761) independently improves changes in passive avoidance learning and brain membrane fluidity in the aging mouse. *Pharmacopsychiatry*. 1996;29(4):144-9.
126. Winter E. Effects of an extract of *Ginkgo biloba* on learning and memory in mice. *Pharmacology, Biochemistry & Behavior*. 1991;38(1):109-14.
127. Gessner B, Voelp A, Klasser M. Study of the long-term action of a *Ginkgo biloba* extract on vigilance and mental performance as determined by means of quantitative pharamaco-EEG and psychometric measurements. *Arzneimittel Forschung*. 1985;35:1459-65.
128. Porsolt RD, Martin P, Lenegre A, *et al*. Effects of an extract of *Ginkgo Biloba* (EGB 761) on "learned helplessness" and other models of stress in rodents. *Pharmacology, Biochemistry & Behavior*. 1990;36(4):963-71.
129. Schubert H, Halama P. Depressive episode primarily unresponsive to therapy in elderly patients: Efficacy of *Ginkgo biloba* extract (EGb 761) in combination with antidepressants. *Geriatric Forschung*. 1993;3:45-53.
130. Rodriguez de Turco EB, Droy-Lefaix MT, Bazan NG. EGb 761 inhibits stress-induced polydipsia in rats. *Physiology & Behavior*. 1993;53(5):1001-2.
131. White HL, Scates PW, Cooper BR. Extracts of *Ginkgo biloba* leaves inhibit monoamine oxidase. *Life Sciences*. 1996;58(16):1315-21.
132. Attella MJ, Hoffman SW, Stasio MJ, Stein DG. *Ginkgo biloba* extract facilitates recovery from penetrating brain injury in adult male rats. *Experimental Neurology*. 1989;105(1):62-71.
133. Rodriguez de Turco EB, Droy-Lefaix MT, Bazan NG. Decreased electroconvulsive shock-induced diacylglycerols and free fatty acid accumulation in the rat brain by *Ginkgo biloba* extract (EGb 761): Selective effect in hippocampus as compared with cerebral cortex. *Journal of Neurochemistry*. 1993;61(4):1438-44.
134. Doly M, Braquet P, Droy MT, *et al*. Effects of oxygenated free radicals on the electrophysiological activity of the isolated retina of the rat. [French]. *Journal Français d Ophtalmologie*. 1985;8(3):273-7.
135. Droy-Lefaix MT, Bonhomme B, Doly M. Protective effect of *Ginkgo biloba* extract (EGB 761) on free radical-induced changes in the electroretinogram of isolated rat retina. *Drugs Under Experimental & Clinical Research*. 1991;17(12):571-4.
136. Apaydin C, Oguz Y, Agar A, *et al*. Visual evoked potentials and optic nerve histopathology in normal and diabetic rats and effect of *Ginkgo biloba* extract. *Acta Ophthalmologica*. 1993;71(5):623-8.
137. Pritz-Hohmeier S, Chao TI, Krenzlin J, Reichenbach A. Effect of *in vivo* application of the *Ginkgo biloba* extract EGb 761(Rokan) on the susceptibility of mammalian retinal cells to proteolytic enzymes. *Ophthalmic Research*. 1994;26(2):80-6.
138. Lebuisson DA, Leroy L, Rigal G. Treatment of senile macular degeneration with *Ginkgo biloba* extract. A preliminary double-blind drug vs. placebo study. [French]. *Presse Medicale*. 1986;15(31):1556-8.
139. Didier A, Droy-Lefaix MT, Aurousseau C, Cazals Y. Effects of *Ginkgo biloba* extract (EGb 761) on cochlear vasculature in the guinea pig: morphometric measurements and laser Doppler flowmetry. *European Archives of Oto Rhino Laryngology*. 1996;253(1-2):25-30.
140. Dubreuil C. Therapeutic trial in acute cochlear deafness. A comparative study of *Ginkgo biloba* extract and nicergoline. [French]. *Presse Medicale*. 1986;15(31):1559-61.
141. Sprenger FH. Gute therapie ergebnissemet *Ginkgo biloba*. *Arztlich Praxis*. 1986;12:938-40.
142. Coles R. Trial of an extract of *Ginkgo biloba* (EGB) for tinnitus and hearing loss .[Letter]. *Clinical Otolaryngology*. 1988;13(6): 501-2.
143. Holgers KM, Axelsson A, Pringle I. *Ginkgo biloba* extract for the treatment of tinnitus. *Audiology*. 1994;33(2):85-92.
144. Lacour M, Ez-Zaher L, Raymond J. Plasticity mechanisms in vestibular compensation in the cat are improved by an extract of *Ginkgo biloba* (EGb 761). *Pharmacology, Biochemistry & Behavior*. 1991;40(2):367-79.
145. Yabe T, Chat M, Malherbe E, Vidal PP. Effects of *Ginkgo biloba* extract (EGb 761) on the guinea pig vestibular system. *Pharmacology, Biochemistry & Behavior*. 1992;42(4):595-604.
146. Sikora R, Sohn M, *et al. Ginkgo biloba* extract in the therapy of erectile dysfunction. *Journal of Urology*. 1989;141:Abstract 73.
147. Paick JS, Lee JH. An experimental study of the effect of *Ginkgo biloba* extract on the human and rabbit corpus cavernosus tissue. *Journal of Urology*. 1996;156(5):1876-80.
148. Emerit I, Oganesian N, Sarkisian T, *et al.* Clastogenic factors in the plasma of Chernobyl accident recovery workers: anticlastogenic effect of *Ginkgo biloba* extract. *Radiation Research*. 1995;144(2):198-205.
149. Emerit I, Arutyunyan R, Oganesian N, *et al.* Radiation-induced clastogenic factors: anticlastogenic effect of *Ginkgo*

biloba extract. *Free Radical Biology & Medicine*. 1995;18(6):985-91.

150. Dumont E, Petit E, Tarrade T, Nouvelot A. UV-C irradiation-induced peroxidative degradation of microsomal fatty acids: protection by an extract of *Ginkgo biloba* (EGb 761). *Free Radical Biology & Medicine*. 1992;13(3):197-203.
151. Barth SA, Inselmann G, Engemann R, Heidemann HT. Influences of *Ginkgo biloba* on cyclosporin A induced lipid peroxidation in human liver microsomes in comparison to vitamin E, gluthathione and N-acetylcysteine. *Biochemical Pharmacology*. 1991;41(10):1521-6.
152. Itokawa H, Totsuka N, Nakahara K, *et al*. Antitumor principles from *Ginkgo biloba* L. *Chemical & Pharmaceutical Bulletin*. 1987;35(7):3016-20.
153. Lagrue G, Behar A, Kazandjian M, Rahbar K. Idiopathic cyclic edema. The role of capillary hyperpermeability and its correction by *Ginkgo biloba* extract. [French]. *Presse Medicale*. 1986;15(31):1550-3.
154. Tamborini A, Taurelle R. Value of standardized *Ginkgo biloba* extract (EGb 761) in the management of congestive symptoms of premenstrual syndrome. [French]. *Revue Francaise de Gynecologie et d Obstetrique*. 1993.
155. Lepoittevin JP, Benezra C, Asakawa Y. Allergic contact dermatitis to *Ginkgo biloba* L.: relationship with urushiol. *Archives of Dermatological Research*. 1989;281(4):227-30.
156. Mitchell JC, Maibach HI, Guin J. Leaves of *Ginkgo biloba* not allergenic for Toxicodendron-sensitive subjects. *Contact Dermatitis*. 1981;7(1):47-8.
157. Rowin J, Lewis SL. Spontaneous bilateral subdural hematomas associated with chronic *Ginkgo biloba* ingestion. *Neurology*. 1996;46(6):1775-6.
158. Rosenblatt M, Mindel J. Spontaneous hyphema associated with ingestion of *Ginkgo biloba* extract. [Letter]. *New England Journal of Medicine*. 1997;336(15):1108.
159. Wojcicki J, Gawronska-Szklarz B, Bieganowski W, *et al.* Comparative pharmacokinetics and bioavailability of flavonoid glycosides of *Ginkgo biloba* after a single oral administration of three formulations to healthy volunteers. *Materia Medica Polona*. 1995;27(4):141-6.

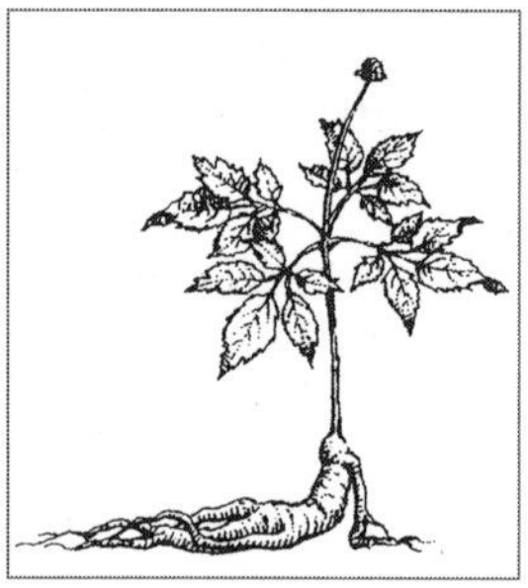

GINSENG, ASIAN

Panax ginseng C.A. Meyer; *Panax quinquefolius*

THUMBNAIL SKETCH

Active Constituents
- Ginsenosides
- Panaxans

Common Uses
- Stress and fatigue, both physical and mental
- Increase endurance and performance during exercise
- Strengthen the immune system in cases of inadequate resistance to infection (also to aid in convalescence)
- As an adjunct in the treatment of mild hyperglycemia

Adverse Effects
- Insomnia most common
- Others include hypertension, diarrhea, restlessness, nervousness, euphoria, and skin eruptions

Cautions/Contraindications
- Caution should be used with the following conditions: hypertension, acute illness, premenopausal women with unstable hormonal cycles, controlled diabetics and concomitant use of stimulants. Safety has not been established for use in children, pregnancy or lactation.

Drug Interactions
- Possible with many centrally-acting drugs (e.g., phenalzine, pentobarbital and haloperiol) and stimulants including caffeine

Doses
- Range from 100 mg to 500 mg of standardized extract (4% to 8% ginsenosides) daily in two or three divided doses

INTRODUCTION

Family: Araliaceae

Synonyms:[1-3]

- *Panax ginseng*: Asian ginseng, Chinese ginseng, Ginseng, Korean ginseng, *Panax schinseng* Nees, Asiatic ginseng, Oriental ginseng
- *Panax quinquefolius*: American ginseng, Canadian ginseng

Although many different kinds of 'ginseng' may be sold in Canadian and American retail outlets, two species are commonly seen in pharmacy practice: *Panax Ginseng* C.A. Meyer (also called Panax, Ginseng, Chinese ginseng, Korean ginseng or Oriental ginseng) and *Panax quinquefolius* (also called American or Canadian ginseng). Other closely related species include: *Panax pseudoginseng* Wallich var. *japonicus* (C.A. Meyer) G.Hoo & C. J. Tseng (Japanese ginseng), *Panax pseudoginseng* Wallich var. *notoginseng* (Burkill) G. Hoo & C.J. Tseng (Sanchi ginseng) and *Panax trilolius* L. (Canadian dwarf ginseng); however, these three species are rarely seen. Another product widely available is *Eleutherococcus senticosus* (Rupr. & Maxim.) Maxim. (Siberian ginseng or eleuthero), which is in the same family (Araliaceae) but is not a true ginseng (member of the *Panax* genus). *Panax ginseng* (Chinese/Korean ginseng) and *Panax quinquefolius* (Canadian/American ginseng) will be discussed in this monograph, while *Eleutehrococcus senticosus* (Siberian ginseng) will be reviewed in the following monograph.

Panax is derived from the Greek roots *pan* meaning "all" and *akos* meaning "cure" and refers to the "cure all" or "panacea" quality generally attributed to the herb.[4] The name ginseng means "essence of the earth in the form of a man," and refers to the resemblance of the root to a human form.[5] *Panax ginseng* C.A. Meyer is the most widely used and most extensively studied species of ginseng.[6, 7] It is native to (and is now widely cultivated in) both Korea and China. The shrub grows to a height of 60 to 70 cm and produces light-red berries which are approximately 1 cm in diameter. The roots from 4 to 6 year old plants are harvested in September or October and used medicinally. Fully grown roots are approximately 2 cm in diameter and 8 to 20 cm long. Many ginseng products available in Canada are made from *Panax ginseng* grown in the Orient. In contrast, *Panax quinquefolius* is native to eastern North America and is cultivated to be sold primarily for medicinal products in the Orient. *Panax quinquefolius* tastes sweeter and is considered to be more "yin" in the traditional Chinese medicine paradigm than *Panax ginseng*.[4]

Ginseng has been an important part of traditional Chinese medicine for over five thousand years. It is considered to be a bitter-sweet herb with a warming character. Within traditional Chinese medicine, ginseng was used to restore "yang" quality and to treat general weakness, deficient qi (chi) patterns, anemia, lack of appetite, nervous agitation, thirst and impotence.[5] It is classified as an adaptogen, which is thought to increase non-specific resistance to adverse influences such as stress and infection. Traditionally it was used as a tonic to "increase strength, increase blood volume, promote life and appetite, quiet the spirit, and give wisdom."[5] It was generally thought to improve vitality.

In Canada and America, ginseng is commonly sold in two forms: white and red, which represent different processing procedures. White ginseng is obtained by drying the root, often peeling the external skin in the process. In contrast, red ginseng root is steamed, which produces a caramel-like color.[7] According to traditional Chinese medicine philosophy, red ginseng is more 'heating' (more 'yang' in nature) than white ginseng.

Constituents

Panax ginseng [6-9]

- Triterpenoid glycosides (saponins):[10]
  ginsenosides Rb1, Rb2 = panaquilin B, panaxoside E
  ginsenoside Rc= panaquilin C, panaxoside D
  ginsenoside Rd= panaquilin D, panaquilin E_2, ganaxoside C, ginsenoside Re_2
  ginsenoside Re= panaquilin E_3, panaxoside B, ginsenoside Re_3
  ginsenoside Rg_1= panaquilin G_1, panaxoside A
  ginsenoside Rg_2= panaquilin G_2
  ginsenoside Ra= panaxoside F
- Other ginsensides: Ra_1, Ra_2, Rb_3, Rf, Rh_1, Rh_4, Ro
- Peptidoglycans: panaxans
- Volatile oil: panacene
- Polysaccharides
- Vitamins (e.g. thiamin, riboflavin, B12, nicotinic acid, pantothenic acid, and biotin)

Panax quinquefolius[4]

- Triterpenoid glycosides (saponins): ginsenosides (also called panaxosides) including: Rb_1, Rb_2, Rb_3, Rc, Rd, Re, Rg_1, Rg_2, Ro, which produce 20-S-protopanaxadiol and 20-S-protopanaxatriol in alkaline conditions

Note: There are both qualitative and quantitative differences in the ginsenoside content of various species and varieties, allowing easy verification of the identity and quality of commercial ginseng products by high performance liquid chromotography.

THERAPEUTIC USES & RELEVANT PHARMACOLOGY

Although hundreds of studies since the 1950s have attempted to separate factual therapeutic properties from fictitious ones, there are many inconsistencies among the results (primarily due to different extraction procedures, use of different plants, adulterants and lack of quality control).[11, 12] To compound this problem, very few of the studies involve the use of human subjects.[12, 13] Most of the studies reviewed here are animal studies, many of which examine the effects of a single ginsenoside; thus it is not possible to extrapolate the results to the human ingestion of commercial ginseng products. Unless noted otherwise, all studies discussed were completed with *Panax ginseng*, which is by far the most well-research Panax species.

ADAPTOGENIC ACTIVITY

Historically, ginseng has been used as a general tonic, relying on its adaptogenic action. An adaptogen is thought to work in a non-specific manner, drawing the patient toward normal function, irrespective of the direction of the pathologic state.[7, 8] For example, ginseng has been found to increase blood pressure in cases of hypotension or shock, but restored blood pressure to normal in cases of hypertension.[14] Other researchers have noted that there are at least 3 components of *Panax ginseng* root which can depress CNS activity and at least 2 other constituents that stimulate the central nervous system (CNS).[8] It appears that different constituents of *Panax ginseng* have opposing action, generally stimulating or sedating, respectively.[14-16] Thus different doses of ginseng can have opposite effects clinically and the same dose of ginseng given to individuals with differing physiological states can have different clinical actions. This is a defining feature of an adaptogenic herb.

Anti-stress Activity

Ginseng has been reported to enhance one's ability to cope with various mental and physical stressors (e.g., exposure to heat or cold,[17] environmental toxins, physical trauma and emotional responses to various stimuli).[11] One of the few double-blind clinical studies to date investigated the effects of taking a multivitamin and taking ginseng in addition to the same multivitamin on the quality of life of 501 city-dwellers. After 4 months, the study found that those ingesting both the ginseng and multivitamin had a significant improvement in all 11 quality-of-life measures, while those ingesting the vitamins alone had no significant improvement.[18]

Ginseng's anti-stress effects have been linked primarily to its effects on the adrenal glands.[19, 20] It has been suggested rather than a direct stimulation, ginseng influences the higher control centers including the hypothalamus and pituitary gland, which in turn influence the adrenals.[21] Studies suggest that *Panax ginseng* has the ability to increase both ascorbic acid and cholesterol stores in the adrenal gland, while decreasing the 17-ketosterol and increasing ACTH excreted in the urine.[14-16, 20] An increase in plasma ACTH and corticosteroids following administration of ginseng is well-documented.[20, 22, 23] All of these effects are blocked by the administration of dexamethasone. It is hypothesized that the end-organ effects of the ACTH and related substances, whose release ginseng stimulates, can explain many of its antistress and antifatigue actions.

Anti-fatigue – Physical

An extensive review concludes that there is currently insufficient scientific evidence to demonstrate enhancement of physical performance by ginseng due to poor methodological quality, conflicting results and the use of 10 to 100 times the usual human dose in many animal studies.[8] Animal studies report mice who were shown to: swim longer,[24] run up a seemingly endless rope for a longer period of time[25] and run on a treadmill longer,[26] when taking ginseng. Other animal experiments found no significant anti-fatigue action for ginseng compared to placebo.[27, 28] The majority of the animal trials in this area were not blinded or placebo-controlled.

Several clinical experiments with humans have also been published. One found that nurses (n=12) switching from day to night duty reported improvement in 11 of 16 mood variables and 8 of 14 somatic symptoms while taking 1.2 g of Korean ginseng as opposed to placebo; however, contrary to the description of this study in many lay publications, none of these differences were statistically significant.[29] It has been suggested that the lack of significant results in this study was due to the relatively low dose and short study period. Another study comparing army cadets (n=11) ingesting 2 g of *Panax ginseng* daily for 4 weeks found no difference in performance during heavy, prolonged exercise when compared with cadets taking a placebo.[30] In contrast, a double-blind, placebo-controlled, cross-over study with 50 male sports teachers found that total work load, and maximal oxygen uptake were increased, while plasma lactate levels, carbon dioxide production and heart rate were all significantly lower when the individuals were ingesting ginseng than when they were taking the placebo.[31] Another double-blind, placebo controlled trial with 43 male triathletes taking either 200 mg of ginseng or placebo twice daily found no significant differences in the physical fitness of the two groups after 10 weeks; however, at a follow up 10 weeks later, the group taking the ginseng had significantly better maximal oxygen uptake which suggested that ginseng may retard the loss of physical fitness.[32]

Several mechanisms of action have been postulated for ginseng's anti-fatigue effects including: stimulation of nerve impulses;[14] an ability to affect the hypothalamus/pituitary/adrenal axis;[11, 20, 26] an ability to spare glycogen utilization in exercising muscle[19, 33] and improved oxygen utilization.[31] Biochemical studies have noted increased blood glucose levels and decreased levels of both lactic acid and pyruvic acid in ginseng-treated animals after exercise when compared to saline controls (no differences were noted at rest).[34] However, much of this work has been criticized due to lack of proper control animals and little attempt to guarantee the purity and quality of the ginseng products tested.[8]

Anti-fatigue – Mental

Several much-quoted studies have reported that ginseng enhances mental activity and decreases mental fatigue. For example, radio operators who ingested ginseng extract were reported to transmit text faster and make fewer errors than those on placebo;[35] and university students in Italy were reported to perform better on a series of mental tests (including attention, mental arithmetic, logical deduction, integrated sensory-motor function and auditory reaction time) while taking ginseng in comparison to those on placebo.[36] However, a closer look at the second study reveals that although positive trends were noted in the some of the other tests, the only test in which the ginseng-treated group performed significantly (statistically) better than the control group was the mental arithmetic test and no difference at all was found between the placebo and the ginseng group on three other tests: pure motor function; recognition and visual reaction time. Animal studies have demonstrated the ability of ginseng to: modify brain-wave tracings;[37] improve metabolic activity in the brain;[38] affect the hypothalamus/pituitary/adrenal axis;[11, 20] and have favorable effects on learning and memory.[39]

Anti-aging Effects

Ginseng's "anti-aging" effects have yet to be proven; however, it does appear to exert an action on cellular function.[40] It appears to stimulate protein synthesis and decrease cellular destruction.[11] As well, it promotes Kupffer cell activity, which increases hepatic detoxification and thus may decrease cellular damage caused by external pollutants.[11]

Hepatic Effects

Many of the adaptogenic effects of ginseng appear to be related to its effects on the liver. Ginseng has been reported to: enhance the activity of the Kupffer cells (hepatic macrophages), which are primarily responsible for detoxification of the blood;[11] provide protection against carbon tetrachloride-induced hepatotoxicity in rats;[41, 42] induce tyrosine aminotransferase gene expression *in vitro*;[43] and decrease AST and ALT levels in dexamethasone-treated rats.[44] Ginseng has been reported to increase protein synthesis in the liver of animal models.[45, 46] This has yet to be confirmed in clinical trials. In addition, ginseng is thought to have a significant antihepatotoxic action.[47]

CARDIOVASCULAR EFFECTS

Blood Pressure

It appears that ginseng has a dose-related action on blood pressure. In low doses it slightly increases blood pressure and in high doses it appears to decrease blood pressure in animal models.[48, 49] One study of dogs given 10-20 mg/kg of ginseng intravenously reported an initial increase in blood pressure, which was followed by slight decrease in blood pressure.[50] Another study of 40 mg/kg of ginseng extracts administered intravenously to dogs reported significant decreases in mean arterial pressure, cardiac output, stroke volume and central venous pressure.[51] The applicability of these results to humans has been questioned because it is not known if oral ingestion of commercial ginseng products will produce ginseng blood levels high enough to produce such effects. Clinically, increased blood pressure has been reported as a adverse effect.[52]

Platelet Aggregation

Several *in vitro* and *in vivo* studies have noted ginseng's ability to decrease platelet aggregation.[53-57] Ginsenosides Rg2 and Ro were found to significantly inhibit the conversion of fibrinogen to fibrin induced by thrombin in experimental models.[55, 57] Other studies suggest that components of ginseng inhibit thromboxane A2.[58] However, the clinical effects of oral ingestion of commercial ginseng products by humans is unknown. Prolonged thrombin time (TT) and activated partial thromoboplastin time (APTT) have been reported in animal studies.[57] Decreases in blood-clotting time in humans do not appear to have been reported in the literature.

Other Cardiovascular Effects

Ginseng has also been reported to cause vasodilation of the coronary vessels,[50] and to have a cardioprotective action against catecholamine tachycardia.[14, 16] Under experimental conditions, *Panax ginseng* was found to delay induced heart mitochondrial impairment and muscle contraction deterioration.[59] When administered to patients with hyperlipidemia, ginseng has been shown to increase serum HDL-cholesterol levels while at the same time decreasing total serum cholesterol, triglyceride and fatty acid levels.[60] Other studies have found that *Panax ginseng* may protect against myocardial ischemia/reperfusion damage[61] and cerebral damage caused by ischemia.[62, 63] It has been suggested that the cardioprotective effects of ginseng may be mediated by the release of nitric oxide, a potent antioxidant.[61]

IMMUNOSTIMULATING EFFECTS

Ginseng appears to enhance antibody response;[64] increase natural killer cell activity;[64, 65] stimulate macrophage activity;[66, 67] stimulate lymphocytes *in vitro*;[68, 69] stimulate the reticuloendothelial system (RES);[70, 71] increase proliferation of T cells and B cells;[69] and increase the production of interferon.[72, 73] In laboratory animals, ginseng has been shown to reduce the incidence of viral infections.[74] This finding was recently confirmed by a multicenter, double-blind, randomized, placebo-controlled trial in 227 individuals.[64] Each participant was given 100 mg of Ginsana® daily for 12 weeks, while receiving an anti-influenza polyvalent vaccination at week 4. In the placebo group 42 cases of colds or flus were reported in the final 8 weeks of the trial in comparison with 15 reports in the ginseng group, which represents a statistically significant difference. In addition, the group receiving ginseng had significantly higher antibody titres, and natural killer activity levels.[64] However, at high doses there is *in vitro* evidence that ginseng may inhibit some immune functions including lymphocyte proliferation.[73, 75-77]

NEUROLOGICAL EFFECTS

Treatment of Emotional Disorders

Although *Panax ginseng* has reportedly been used in the treatment of a variety of emotional conditions, this clinical application is supported by very little research. Ginsenoside Rb_1 has been shown to decrease aggressive behavior (between resident and intruder mice) when given to the resident mouse at doses of 25 to 100 mg of ginsenoside/kg intraperitoneally (IP). However, when ginsenoside Rb_1 was given to the intruder mouse, no change in activity was noted. In addition, ginsenoside Rg_1 produced no change in behaviour when given to either mouse.[78] Another study reported that a crude extract of ginseng (50 and 100 mg/kg) and ginsenoside Rb_1 (2.5 and 5 mg/kg) given IP significantly decreased maternal aggression in female mice without causing motor dysfunction; however, ginsenoside Rg_1 appeared to increase maternal aggression.[79] None of these studies were blinded and there have been no studies reporting similar effects in humans.

A study of *Panax ginseng* 50 mg/kg showed that it was as effective as diazepam 1 mg/kg in decreasing experimentally-induced anxiety in mice.[80] However, another study using 50 to 100 mg/kg given orally to mice found no effect on the pentobarbital sleep of psychologically stressed mice.[81] This is supported by an additional study which also found no effect on pentobarbital sleep induction.[82]

Several animal studies have investigated the effects of ginseng on the development of tolerance to and dependence on a variety of narcotics, including morphine,[83, 84] cocaine,[85, 86] and methamphetamine.[85-87]

Other *in vitro* studies have reported the ability of ginsenoside Rb1 to potentiate nerve growth[88] and of ginsenosides Rg_1, Rb_2, Rd, Re and Rf to protect cerebellum growth *in vivo*.[89] Another *in vivo* study suggests that ginsenosides directly affect the activity-dependent synaptic plasticity in the brain.[90]

MISCELLANEOUS EFFECTS

Diabetes

Ginseng has had a long history of folk-use in the treatment of diabetes. One study reported that ginseng reduced serum cortisol (which antagonizes insulin) levels in patients with diabetes, but increased them in non-diabetic individuals. Another found that a fraction isolated from ginseng (DPG-3-2) stimulated insulin secretion, but only in diabetic mice and non-diabetic controls who had been loaded with glucose. There was no effect on insulin secretion in non-diabetic mice on a standard diet.[91] These findings reinforce the adaptogenic character of ginseng – an ability to restore balance. One double-blind, placebo-controlled study of 36 non-insulin dependent diabetics ingesting 200 mg of ginseng daily for 8 weeks found that those in the ginseng treatment group reported elevated mood, and reduced fasting blood glucose although complete statistical analyses were not provided.[92] Research suggests that the ginseng components responsible for these effects include: Panaxans A, B,C,D,E; adenosine; and a fraction designated DPG-3-2.[91, 93-95]

Reproductive Effects

Although ginseng has a reputation as an aphrodisiac, no human studies support this belief. However, *Panax spp.* have been shown to: increase the formation of sperm and the growth of the testes in rabbits;[96] enhance ovulation and the growth of the ovaries in frogs; stimulate egg-laying in hens and increase the mating activity in male rats.[7, 11] Ginseng has been shown to increase sperm count and motility in men, as well as increasing plasma total and free testosterone, DHT, FSH and

LH levels.[97] An *in vitro* study suggests that extracts from *Panax ginseng* may relax the corpus cavernosum by releasing nitric oxide.[98]

In addition, the estrogenic action of ginseng has been demonstrated in post-menopausal women who experienced reduced atrophy and dryness of the vaginal epithelium.[99] It should be noted that breast tenderness has been reported in women taking ginseng.[100, 101]

Anticancer Properties

Ginseng has been reported to decrease the incidence of some human cancers and to have a protective effect against the adverse effects of radiation;[102, 103] however, studies in humans were not found. Other studies have reported that components of *Panax ginseng* caused inhibition of lung metastasis of B16-BL6 melanoma and colon 26-M3.1 carcinoma in mice;[104, 105] inhibition of the growth of human ovarian cancer cells in mice;[106] and induction of differentiation in teratocarcinoma cells *in vitro*.[107] Two case-control epidemiological studies and one prospective study in populations with high rates of ginseng use (70% users) suggested that oral ingestion of ginseng may decrease the incidence of some human cancers.[108] It has been hypothesized that the possible anticancer effects of ginseng may be due to its stimulating effects on the immune system.[69]

HISTORICAL EVIDENCE

This review is limited to the scientific/clinical evidence available within the biomedical model. However, it would be a disservice to this herb to discount its historical use within the Traditional Chinese Medical paradigm. In using this herb it is important to remember that extensive empirical evidence exists. This is reviewed extensively in several texts.[15, 109]

ADVERSE EFFECTS

The most common adverse effect noted is insomnia.[64] Other reported effects included diarrhea, skin eruptions, vaginal bleeding[52] and breast tenderness.[100, 101] One case each of Stevens-Johnson syndrome,[110] mania,[111] and cerebral arteritis[112] possibly associated with ingestion of ginseng have been reported; however, the ginseng products were not tested for purity, thus these reactions may have been caused by adulterated products.[113] In addition, given the widespread use of ginseng products worldwide, such reactions are very rare indeed.

The term "Ginseng Abuse Syndrome" has been used to describe symptoms of overstimulation, including: hypertension, diarrhea, restlessness, nervousness, euphoria, insomnia and skin eruptions, which may occur in the overuse of the product.[114, 115] However, this description has been criticized due to the fact that the majority of the individuals in this study were also ingesting high levels of caffeine.

CAUTIONS/CONTRAINDICATIONS

Ginseng should be used with caution in: hypertension, acute illness, premenopausal women with unstable hormonal cycles, controlled diabetics and concomitant use of stimulants.[52] As well, given that ginseng is considered a tonic, its use may not be appropriate in young, robust individuals.[3] The safety of *Panax ginseng* and *Panax quinquefolius* has not been established in children, pregnant and/or lactating women. Ginseng should not be ingested in the evening due to its ability to induce insomnia.

DRUG INTERACTIONS

Ginseng is generally considered to have an additive effect when used concomitantly with MAOIs.[116] This caution is derived from a case study describing symptoms of headache and tremulousness in a 64-year-old woman who was taking phenelzine and added ginseng to her regimen.[117] Three years later a re-challenge with ginseng in the same woman resulted in the same symptoms.[118] A second possible case of an interaction between ginseng (contained in an ingredient in a herbal tea) and phenelzine has also been reported.[119]

One study found that ginseng augmented the hypnotic effect of pentobarbital,[16] while others have found no effect.[81, 82] However, potentiation of amphetamine-induced increase in motility and stereotypy as well as potentiation of haloperidol induced catalepsy have been reported in animal studies.[82] Caution with concomitant use of centrally-acting medications is recommended.

DOSAGE REGIMENS

The typical dose (taken from one to three times daily) ranges from 100 mg to 500 mg of standardized extract (4% to 8% ginsenosides).[11] The raw root may be taken by decoction (boiling in water or broth) in a dose of 0.6 to 4 g and is usually taken in the morning.[11] In cases of long term administration, ginseng is usually taken for a period of 15 to 20 days, followed by a 2 week resting period.[11, 35]

Premium ginseng root is extremely expensive, often costing thousands of dollars per kilogram, which leads one to question the quality of cheaper brands of the product. Commercially, ginseng is available in a wide range of forms including: teas, capsules, extracts, tablets, roots, chewing gum, cigarettes, and candies.[12] It is extremely difficult to determine the quality and quantity of ginseng present in some of these dosage forms. A study done in the late 1970s (and currently being repeated by the American Botanical Council) reported that 60% of the 54 North American ginseng products tested did not contain enough ginsenosides to be considered pharmacologically active and that 25% contained no ginsenosides at all.[120] Another study of 17 commercial ginseng products available in Sweden found that only one out of the 5 brands which listed their ginsenoside content on the label met the label claim.[121] In a follow up study of 50 ginseng products from eleven countries, the same team of researchers reported a range of 1.9% to 9.0% ginsenoside content, with 6 products (gathered from Sweden, the USA and the UK) which did not contain any ginsenosides.[122, 123] Several cases of athletes consuming adulterated ginseng products (e.g., with ephedrine, psuedophedrine) which have resulted in doping charges have been reported.[122, 124]

REFERENCES

1. Wren RC. *Potter's New Encyclopaedia of Botanical Drugs and Preparations.* Saffron Waldon, UK: C.W. Daniel Company; 1988:362.
2. Bradley P. *British Herbal Compendium*. Bournemouth, UK: The British Herbal Medical Association; 1992:239.
3. Mills S. *Essential Book of Herbal Medicine.* London: Penguin; 1991:677.
4. Foster S. American Ginseng: *Panax quinquefolium*. Austin, TX: American Botanical Association; 1991:7.
5. Foster S. Asian Ginseng: *Panax ginseng*. Austin, TX: American Botanical Council; 1991:7.
6. Leung A, Foster S. *Encyclopedia of Common Natural Ingredients Used in Food, Drugs and Cosmetics* 2nd ed. New York, NY: John Wiley and Sons; 1996:649.
7. Shibata S, Tanaka O, Shoji J, Saito H. Chemistry and Pharmacology of Panax. *Economic and Medicinal Plant Research*. 1985;1:217-84.
8. Bahrke MS, Morgan WP. Evaluation of the ergogenic properties of ginseng. *Sports Medicine*. 1994;18(4):229-48.
9. Baek NI, Kim DS, Lee YH, Park JD, Lee CB, Kim SI. Ginsenoside Rh4, a genuine dammarane glycoside from Korean

red ginseng. *Planta Medica*. 1996;62(1):86-7.
10. Baranov AI. Medicinal uses of ginseng and related plants in the Soviet Union: recent trends in Soviet literature. *Journal of Ethnopharmacology*. 1982;6(3):339-53.
11. Murray MT. *The Healing Power of Herbs*. Rocklin, CA: Prima Publishing; 1992:246.
12. Tyler VE. *Herbs of Choice. The Therapeutic Use of Phytomedicinals.* Binghamton, NY: Pharmaceutical Products Press; 1994:209.
13. Lewis WH. Chapter 15. In: Etkin NL, ed *Plants in Indigenous Medicine and Diet: Biobehavioral Approaches* Bedford Hills, N.Y: Regrave Publishing; 1986:290-305.
14. Chang H, But P. *Pharmacology and Applications of Chinese Materia Medica.* Philadelphia, PA: World Scientific; 1986:773.
15. Teegarden R. *Chinese Tonic Herbs.* New York: Japan Publishing Inc; 1985:197.
16. Bensky D, Gamble A. *Chinese Herbal Medicine Materia Medica.* Seattle, WA: Eastland Press; 1986:556.
17. Kumar R, Grover SK, Divekar HM, *et al*. Enhanced thermogenesis in rats by *Panax ginseng*, multivitamins and minerals. *International Journal of Biometeorology*. 1996;39(4):187-91.
18. Caso Marasco A, Vargas Ruiz R, Salas Villagomez A, Begona Infante C. Double-blind study of a multivitamin complex supplemented with ginseng extract. *Drugs Under Experimental and Clinical Research*. 1996;22(6):323-9.
19. Avakia EV, Evonuk E. Effects of *Panax ginseng* extract on tissue glycogen and adrenal cholesterol depletion during prolonged exercise. *Planta Medica*. 1979;36:43-8.
20. Fulder SJ. Ginseng and the hypothalamic-pituitary control of stress. *American Journal of Chinese Medicine*. 1981;9:112-8.
21. Wagner H, Norr H, Winterhoff H. Plant adaptogens. *Phytomedicine*. 1994;1:63-76.
22. Hiai S, Yokoyama H, Oura H. Features of ginseng saponin-induced corticosterone secretion. *Endocrinologia Japonica*. 1979;26:737-40.
23. Hiai S, Yokoyama H, Oura H, Kawashima Y. Evaluation of corticosterone secretion-inducing effects of ginsenosides and their prosapogenins and sapogenins. *Chemical and Pharmaceutical Bulletin*. 1983;31:168-74.
24. Popov IM, Goldwag WJ. A review of the properties and clinical effects of ginseng. *American Journal of Chinese Medicine*. 1973;1(2):263-70.
25. Brekhman II, Dardymov IV. Pharmacological investigation of glycosides from Ginseng and Eleutherococcus. *Lloydia*. 1969;32(1):46-51.
26. Filaretov AA, Bogdanova TS, Podvigina TT, *et al.* Role of pituitary-adrenocortical system in body adtation abilities. *Experimental and Clinical Endocrinology*. 1988;92:129-36.
27. Martinez B, Staba EJ. The physiological effects of *Aralia*, *Panax* and *Eleutherococcus* on excised rats. *Japanese Journal of Pharmacology*. 1984;35(2):79-85.
28. Lewis WH, Zenger VE, Lynch RG. No adaptogen response of mice to ginseng and Eleutherococcus infusions. *Journal of Ethnopharmacology*. 1983;8(2):209-14.
29. Hallstrom C, Fulder S, Carruthers M. Effect of ginseng on the performance of nurses on night duty. *Comparat Med East West*. 1982;6(4):277-82.
30. Knapik JJ, Wright JE, Welch MJ, *et al.* The influence of *Panax ginseng* on indices of substrate utilization during repeated exhaustive exercise in man. [Abstract]. *Federation Proceedings*. 1983;42:336.
31. Pieralisi G, Ripari P, Vecchiet L. Effects of a standardized ginseng extract combined with dimethylaminoethanol bitartrate, vitamins, minerals and trace elements on physical performance during exercise. *Clinical Therapeutics*. 1991;13(3):373-82.
32. Van Schepdael P. Les effects dy ginseng G115 sur la capacite physique de sportifs d'endurance. *Acta Therapeutica*. 1993;19:337-47.
33. Brekman II, Dardymov IV. New substances of plant origin which increase nonspecific resistance. *Ann Rev Pharmacol*. 1969;9: 419-30.
34. Avakian EV, Sugimoto RB, Taguchi S, *et al.* Effect of *Panax ginseng* extract on energy metabolism during exercise in rats. *Planta Medica*. 1984;50:151-4.
35. Brown D. *Herbal Prescriptions for Better Health*. Rocklin, CA: Prima Publishing; 1996:349.
36. D'Angelo L, Grimwaldi R, Caravaggi M, *et al.* A double-blind, placebo-controlled clinical study on the effect of a standardized ginseng extract on psychomotor performance in healthy volunteers. *Journal of Ethnopharmacology*. 1986;16:15-22.
37. Petkov W. The mechanism of action of *P. ginseng*. *Arzneimittelforschung*. 1961;11:288-95.
38. Samira MMH, Attia MA, Allam M, Elwan O. Effect of standardized ginseng extract G115 on the metabolism and electrical activity of the rabbit's brain. *Journal of International Medical Research*. 1985;13:342-8.
39. Petkov VD, Kehayov R, Belcheva S, *et al.* Memory effects of standardized extracts of *Panax ginseng* (G115), *Ginkgo biloba* (GK 501) and their combination Gincosan (PHL-00701). *Planta Medica*. 1993;59(2):106-14.
40. Xiao PG, Xing ST, Wang LW. Immunological aspects of Chinese medicinal plants as antiageing drugs. [Review]. *Journal of Ethnopharmacology.* 1993;38(2-3):167-75.
41. Jeong TC, Kim HJ, Park JI, *et al.* Protective effects of red ginseng saponins against carbon tetrachloride-induced

hepatotoxicity in Sprague Dawley rats. *Planta Medica*. 1997;63(2):136-40.
42. Park HJ, Park KM, Rhee MH, *et al.* Effect of ginsenoside Rb1 on rat liver phosphoproteins induced by carbon tetra chloride. *Biological and Pharmaceutical Bulletin*. 1996;19(6):834-8.
43. Kim MY, Lee KY, Lee SK. Inductive effect of ginsenoside-Rg1 on tyrosine aminotransferase gene expression in rat primary hepatocyte cultures. *Biochem Mol Biol Int*. 1994;34(4):845-51.
44. Lin JH, Wu LS, Tsai KT, *et al*. Effects of ginseng on the blood chemistry profile of dexamethasone-treated male rats. *American Journal of Chinese Medicine*. 1995;23(2):167-72.
45. Oura H, Hiai S, Nabetani S. Effect of ginseng on endoplastic reticulum and ribosome. *Planta Medica*. 1975;28:76-88.
46. Oura H, Nakashima S, Tsukada K. Effect of radix ginseng on serum protein synthesis. *Chemical and Pharmaceutical Bulletin*. 1972;20:980-6.
47. Hikino H, Kiso Y, Sanada S, Shoji J. Antihepatotoxic actions of ginsenosides from *Panax ginseng* roots. *Planta Medica*. 1985;52: 62-4.
48. Oh JS, *et al.* The effect of ginseng on experimental hypertension. *Korean Journal of Pharmacology*. 1968;4:27-31.
49. Siegel RK. Ginseng and high blood pressure [letter]. *Journal of the American Medical Association*. 1980;243:32.
50. Wood WB, Roh BL, White RP. Cardiovascular actions of *Panax ginseng* in dogs. *Japanese Journal of Pharmacology*. 1964;14:284-94.
51. Lee DC, Lee MO, Kim CY, *et al.* Effect of ether, ethanol and aqueous extracts of ginseng on cardiovascular functions in dogs. *Can J Comparat Med*. 1981;45:182-7.
52. Baldwin CA, Anderson LA, Phillipson JD. What pharmacists should know about ginseng. *The Pharmaceutical Journal*. 1986;November 8:583-6.
53. Matsuda H, Namba K, Fukuda S, *et al.* Pharmacological study on *Panax ginseng* C.A. Meyer. III. Effects of red ginseng on experimental disseminated intrvascular coagulation. (2) Effects of ginsenosides on blood coagulation and fibrinolytic systems. *Chemical and Pharmaceutical Bulletin*. 1986;34(3):1153-7.
54. Kimura Y, Okuda H, Arichi S. Effects of various ginseng saponins on 5-hydroxytryptamine release and aggregation in human platelets. *Journal of Pharmacy and Pharmacology*. 1988;40:838-43.
55. Matsuda H, Namba K, Fukuda S, *et al.* Pharmacological study on *Panax ginseng* C.A. Meyer. IV. Effects of red ginseng on experimental disseminated intravascular coagulation. (3) Effect of ginsenoside-R_O on the blood coagulative and fibrinolytic system. *Chemical and Pharmaceutical Bulletin.* 1986;34(5):2100-4.
56. Kuo SC, Tenagg CM, Lee JC, *et al*. Antiplatelet components of *Panax ginseng*. *Planta Medica*. 1990;56:164-7.
57. Park HJ, Lee JH, Song YB, Park KH. Effects of dietary supplementation of lipophilic fraction from *Panax ginseng* on cGMP and cAMP in rat platelets and on blood coagulation. *Biological and Pharmaceutical Bulletin*. 1996;19(11):1434-9.
58. Park HJ, Rhee MH, Park KM, *et al*. Effect of non-saponin fraction from *Panax ginseng* on cGMP and thromboxane A_2 in human platelet aggregation. *Journal of Ethnopharmacology*. 1995;49(3):157-62.
59. Toh HT. Improved isolated heart contractility and mitochondrial oxidation after chronic treatment with *Panax ginseng* in rats. *American Journal of Chinese Medicine.* 1994;22(3-4):275-84.
60. Yamamoto M, Vemura T, Nakama S., *et al.* Serum HDL-cholesterol-increasing and fatty liver-improving action of *Panax ginseng* in High cholesterol diet-fed rats with clinical effect on hyperlipidemia in man. *American Journal of Chinese Medicine*. 1983;11:96-101.
61. Chen X. Cardiovascular protection by ginsenosides and their nitric oxide releasing action. [Review]. *Clinical and Experimental Pharmacology and Physiology*. 1996;23(8):728-32.
62. Choi SR, Saji H, Iida Y, *et al*. Ginseng pretreatment protects against transient global cerebral ischemia in the rat: measurement of local cerebral glucose utilization by [14C] deoxyglucose autoradiography. *Biological and Pharmaceutical Bulletin*. 1996;19(4):644-6.
63. Wen TC, Yoshimura H, Matsuda S, *et al*. Ginseng root prevents learning disability and neuronal l oss in gerbils with 5-minute forebrain ischemia. *Acta Neuropathologica*. 1996;91(1):15-22.
64. Scaglione F, Cattaneo G, Alessandria M, Cogo R. Efficacy and safety of the standardised Ginseng extract G115 for potentiating vaccination against the influenza syndrome and protection against the common cold. [Published erratum appears in *Drugs Exp Clin Res* 1996;22(6):338]. *Drugs Under Experimental and Clinical Research*. 1996;22(2):65-72.
65. See DM, Broumand N, Sahl L, Tilles JG. *In vitro* effects of echinacea and ginseng on natural killer and antibody-dependent cell cytotoxicity in healthy subjects and chronic fatigue syndrome or acquired immunodeficiency syndrome patients. *Immunopharmacology*. 1997;35(3):229-35.
66. Jin R, Wan LL, Mitsuishi T, *et al.* Effect of shi-ka-ron and Chinese herbs on cytokine production of macrophage in immunocompromised mice. *American Journal of Chinese Medicine*. 1994;22(3-4):255-66.
67. Akagawa G, Abe S, Tansho S, *et al*. Protection of C3H/HE J mice from development of *Candida albicans* infection by oral administration of Juzen-taiho-to and its component, Ginseng radix: possible roles of macrophages in the host defense mechanisms. *Immunopharmacology and Immunotoxicology*. 1996;18(1):73-89.
68. Liu J, Wang S, Liu H, *et al.* Stimulatory effect of saponin from *Panax ginseng* on immune function of lymphocytes in the elderly. *Mechanisms of Ageing and Development*. 1995;83(1):43-53.

69. Lee YS, Chung IS, Lee IR, *et al*. Activation of multiple effector pathways of immune system by the antineoplastic immunostimulator acidic polysaccharide ginsan isolated from *Panax ginseng*. *Anticancer Research*. 1997;17(1A):323-31.
70. Tomoda M, Takeda K, Shimizu N, *et al.* Characterization of two acidic polysaccharides having immunological activities from the root of *Panax ginseng*. *Biological and Pharmaceutical Bulletin*. 1993;16(1):22-5.
71. Tomoda M, Hirabayashi K, Shimizu N, *et al*. Characterization of two novel polysaccharides having immunological activities from the root of *Panax ginseng*. *Biological and Pharmaceutical Bulletin*. 1993;16(11):1087-90.
72. Gupta S, *et al.* Panax: a new mitogen and interferon producer. *Clinical Research*. 1980;28:504A.
73. Jie YH, Cammisuli S, Baggiolini M. Immunomodulatory effects of *Panax ginseng* C.A. Meyer in the mouse. *Agents and Actions*. 1984;15:386-91.
74. Singh VK, Agarwal S, Gupta B. Immunomodulatory activity of *Panax ginseng* extract. *Planta Medica*. 1984;51:462-5.
75. Yun TK, Yun YS, Han IW. Anti-carcinogenic effect of long-term oral administration of newborn mice exposed to various chemical carcinogens. *Cancer Detection and Prevention*. 1983;6:515-25.
76. Yeung HW, Cheung K, Leung KN, *et al.* Immunopharmacology of Chinese medicine. I. Ginseng-induced immuno suppression in virus infected mice. *American Journal of Chinese Medicine*. 1982;10:44-54.
77. Kang M, Yoshimatsu H, Oohara A, *et al*. Ginsenoside Rg1 modulates ingestive behavior and thermal response induced by interleukin-1 beta in rats. *Physiology and Behaviour*. 1995;57(2):393-6.
78. Yoshimura H, Watanabe K, Ogawa N. Psychotropic effects of ginseng saponins on agonistic behaviour between resident and intruder mice. *European Journal of Pharmacology*. 1988;146:291-7.
79. Yoshimura H, Watanabe K, Ogawa N. Acute and chronic effects of ginseng saponins on maternal aggression in mice. *European Journal of Pharmacology*. 1988;150:319-24.
80. Bhattacharya SK, Mitra SK. Anxiolytic activity of *Panax ginseng* roots: An experimental study. *Journal of Ethnopharmacology*. 1991;34:87-92.
81. Nguyen TT, Matsumoto K, Yamasaki K, *et al*. Effects of majonoside-R2 on pentobarbital sleep and gastric lesion in psychologically stressed mice. *Pharmacology Biochemistry and Behaviour*. 1996;53(4):957-63.
82. Mitra SK, Chakraborti A, Bhattacharya SK. Neuropharmacological studies on *Panax ginseng*. *Indian Journal of Experimental Biology*. 1996;34(1):41-7.
83. Kim H-S, Jang CG, Lee MK. Antinarcotic effects of the standardized ginseng extract G115 on morphine. *Planta Medica*. 1990;56:158-63.
84. Kim H-S, Oh K, Park WK, *et al*. Effects of *Panax ginseng* on the development of morphine tolerance and dependence. *Korean Journal of Ginseng Science*. 1987;11:182-90.
85. Tokuyama S, Takahashi M, Kaneto H. The effect of ginseng extract on locomotor sensitization and conditioned place preference induced by methamphetamine and cocaine in mice. *Pharmacology Biochemistry and Behaviour*. 1996;54(4):671-6.
86. Kim HS, Kang JG, Seong YH, *et al*. Blockade by ginseng total saponin of the development of cocaine induced reverse tolerance and dopamine receptor supersensitivity in mice. .*Pharmacology Biochemistry and Behaviour*. 1995;50(1):23-7.
87. Kim HS, Kang JG, Rheu HM, Cho DH, Oh KW. Blockade by ginseng total saponin of the development of methamphetamine reverse tolerance and dopamine receptor supersensitivity in mice. *Planta Medica*. 1995;61(1):22-5.
88. Nishiyama N, Cho SI, Kitagawa I, Saito H. Malonylginsenoside Rb1 potentiates nerve growth factor (NGF)-induced neurite outgrowth of cultured chick embryonic dorsal root ganglia. *Biological and Pharmaceutical Bulletin*. 1994;17(4):509-13.
89. Okamura N, Kobayashi K, Akaike A, Yagi A. Protective effect of ginseng saponins against impaired brain growth in neonatal rats exposed to ethanol. *Biological and Pharmaceutical Bulletin*. 1994;17(2):270-4.
90. Abe K, Cho SI, Kitagaw I, Nishiyama N, Saito H. Differential effects of ginsenoside Rb1 and malonylginsenoside Rb1 on long-term potentiation in the dentate gyrus of rats. *Brain Research*. 1994;649(1-2):7-11.
91. Ng TB, Yeung HW. Hypoglycemic constituents of *Panax ginseng*. *General Pharmacology*. 1985;6:549-52.
92. Sotaniemi EA, Haapakoski E, Rautio A. Ginseng therapy in non-insulin-dependent diabetic patients. *Diabetes Care*. 1995;18(10):1373-5.
93. Konno C, Sugiyama, K, Kano M *et al.* Isolation and hypoglycemic activity of panaxans A,B,C,D, and E, glycans of *Panax ginseng* roots. *Planta Medica*. 1984;51:434-6.
94. Waki I, Tamura T, Kimura M. Effects of a hypoglycemic component of ginseng radix on insulin biosynthesis in normal and diabetic animals. *Journal of Pharmacobiodynamics.* 1982;5:547-4.
95. Oshima Y, Sato K, Hikino H. Isolation and hypoglycemic activity of quinquefolans A, B, C, glycans of *Panax quinquefolium* roots. *Journal of Natural Products*. 1987;50(2):188-90.
96. Kim C. Influence of ginseng on mating behaviour of male rats. *American Journal of Chinese Medicine*. 1976;4(2):163-8.

97. Salvati G, Genovesi G, Marcellini L, *et al.* Effects of *Panax Ginseng* C.A. Meyer saponins on male fertility. *Panminerva Med*. 1996;38(4):249-54.
98. Chen X, Lee TJ. Ginsenosides-induced nitric oxide-mediated relaxation of the rabbit corpus cavernosum. *British Journal of Pharmacology*. 1995;115(1):15-8.
99. Punnonen R, Lukola A. Oestrogen-like effects of ginseng. *British Medical Journal*. 1980;281:1110.
100. Palmer BV, Montgomery ACV, Monteiro JC. Ginseng and mastalgia. [Letter]. *British Medical Journal*. 1978;1:1284.
101. Koriech OM. Ginseng and mastaglia. *British Medical Journal*. 1978;1:1556.
102. Ben-Hur E, Fulder S. Effect of *P. ginseng* saponins and *Eletherococcus senticosus* on survival of cultured mammalian cells after ionizing radiation. *American Journal of Chinese Medicine*. 1981;9:48-56.
103. Yun TK, Shoi SY. A Case controlled study of ginseng intake in cancer. *International Journal of Epidemiology*. 1990;19(4):871-6.
104. Mochizuki M, Yoo YC, Matsuzawa K, *et al.* Inhibitory effect of tumor metastasis in mice by saponins, ginsenoside-Rb2, 20(R)- and 20(S)-ginsenoside-Rg3, of red ginseng. *Biological and Pharmaceutical Bulletin*. 1995;18(9):1197-202.
105. Sato K, Mochizuki M, Saiki I, *et al.* Inhibition of tumor angiogenesis and metastasis by a saponin of *Panax ginseng*, ginsenoside-Rb2. *Biological and Pharmaceutical Bulletin*. 1994;17(5):635-9.
106. Tode T, Kikuchi Y, Kita T, *et al.* Inhibitory effects by oral administration of ginsenoside Rh_2 on the growth of human ovarian cancer cells in nude mice. *Journal of Cancer Research and Clinical Oncology*. 1993;120(1-2):24-6.
107 Lee YN, Lee HY, Chung HY, *et al. In vitro* induction of differentiation by ginsenoides in F9 teratocarcinoma cells. *European Journal of Cancer*. 1996;8:1420-8.
108. Yun TK. Experimental and epidemiological evidence of the cancer-preventive effects of *Panax ginseng* C.A. Meyer [Review]. *Nutrition Reviews*. 1996;54(11 Pt 2):S71-81.
109. Foster S, Chongxi Y. *Herbal Emissaries. Bringing Chinese Herbs to the West.* Rochester, Vermont: Healing Arts Press; 1992:356.
110. Dega H, Laporte JL, Frances C, *et al.* Ginseng as a cause for Stevens-Johnson syndrome? [Letter; see comments]. *Lancet*. 1996;347(9011):1344.
111. Gonzalez-Seijo JC, Ramos YM, Lastra I. Manic episode and ginseng: report of a possible case. [Letter]. *Journal of Clinical Psychopharmacology*. 1995;15(6):447-8.
112. Ryu SJ, Chien YY. Ginseng-associated cerebral arteritis. *Neurology*. 1995;45(4):829-30.
113. Faleni R, Soldati F. Ginseng as cause of Stevens-Johnson syndrome? [Letter; comment]. *Lancet*. 1996;348(9022):267.
114. Sonnenborn U, Hansel R, De Smit. *Adverse Effects of Herbal Drugs.* Berlin: Springer; 1992:296
115. Siegel RK. Ginseng Abuse Syndrome. *Journal of the American Medical Association*. 1979;241:1644-5.
116. Stockley I. *Drug Interactions. A Sourcebook of Adverse Interactions, Their Mechanisms, Clinical Importance, and Management.* 3rd ed. Cambridge, UK: Blackwell Scientific Press; 1994.
117. Shader RI, Greenblat DJ. Phenelzine and the dream machine-ramblings and reflections. *Journal of Clinical Psychopharmacology*. 1985;5(2):65.
118. Shader RI, Greenblatt DJ. Bees, ginseng and MAOIs revisited. *Journal of Clinical Psychopharmacology.* 1988;8(4):235.
119. Jones BD, Runikis AM. Interaction of ginseng with phenelzine. *Journal of Psychopharmacology*. 1987;7(3):201-2.
120. Liberti LE, der Marderosian A. Evaluation of commercial ginseng products. *Journal of Pharmaceutical Sciences*. 1978;67:1487-9.
121. Cui JF, Garle M, Bjorkhem I, Eneroth P. Determination of aglycones of ginsenosides in ginseng preparations sold in Sweden and in urine samples from Swedish athletes consuming ginseng. *Scandinavian Journal of Clinical and Laboratory Investigation.* 1996;56(2):151-60.
122. Cui J, Garle M, Eneroth P, Bjorkhem I. What do commercial ginseng preparations contain? [Letter]. *Lancet*. 1994;344(8915):134.
123. Walker AF. What is in ginseng? [Letter; comment]. *Lancet*. 1994;344(8922):619.
124. Watt J, Bottomley MB, Read MTF. Olympic athletics medical experience, Seoul — personal views. *British Journal of Sports Medicine*. 1989;23(2):76-9.

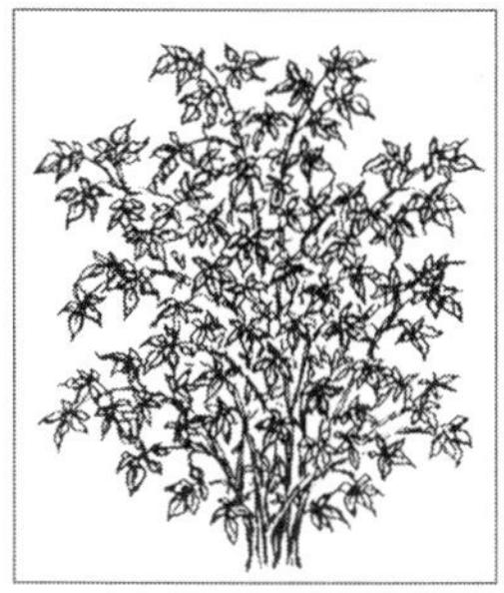

GINSENG, SIBERIAN

Eleutherococcus senticosus (Rupr. & Maxim.) Maxim.

THUMBNAIL SKETCH

Active Constituents

- Eleutherosides

Common Uses

- Stress, fatigue and general debility
- To increase endurance/performance in work/sports
- General tonic (e.g., for long-term immune stimulation)

Adverse Effects

- Rare; most occur because of adulterated products

Cautions/Contraindications

- Not for use in pregnancy, lactation or children
- Some sources list other cautions, but these are largely unsubstantiated

Drug Interactions

- May increase the duration of action of some sedatives

Doses

- Solid extract (20:1): 100-200 mg (in 1-3 divided doses)

INTRODUCTION

Family: Araliaceae

Synonyms: Eleuthero, Touch-me-not, Devil's shrub, Eleuthero ginseng, Wild pepper[1]

Eleutherococcus senticosus is native to the Russian far east, as well as the parts of Korea, China and Japan north of the 38th latitude. This shrub grows to approximately 2 m in height. The root, which is the part used medicinally, is normally harvested in the fall when the medicinally-active constituents are the most concentrated. The leaves can also be used medicinally.[2]

Although historical documentation of the medicinal use of plants in the Araliaceae family (which also includes *Panax ginseng* C.A. Meyer and *Panax quinquefolium* L.) can be confusing (this is reviewed well by Halstead and Hood 1984)[3], it appears that *Eleutherococcus senticosus* was used within Traditional Chinese Medicine for over 4000 years to increase longevity, improve general health, improve appetite and aid memory.[2, 4] Traditional Chinese Medicine indications for Siberian ginseng also include: benefiting qi (chi) or the vital energy and treating 'yang' deficiency, especially of the spleen and kidney, as well as normalizing body functions.[1] Although documentation of *Eleutherococcus senticosus* in Russia dates back to 1855 when two Russian scientists began studying the plant,[2] interest in its medicinal use began only in the 1960s when researchers in that country became interested in its potential as a substitute for the more expensive and difficult to obtain *Panax* sp. (e.g., *Panax ginseng* and *Panax quinquefolium*) which are reviewed in the previous monograph. Although some of the adaptogenic properties of Siberian ginseng are thought to be similar to those of *Panax ginseng*, it is not the same botanical species, nor are the main active constituents the same. Marketing in North America under the common name Siberian ginseng only compounds the confusion surrounding these species.[1] Today, this species is becoming more commonly known by its abbreviated scientific name, Eleuthero, in an attempt to reduce this confusion.[5, 6]

Constituents [2, 7, 8]

The main active chemical constituents are a group of chemically-dissimilar compounds which have been called eleutherosides. Tyler argues that this was done to make Eleuthro appear more similar to the true ginsengs from the *Panax* sp., whose active constituents are the ginsenosides – a group of triterpenoid saponins.[5] Eleuthero does not contain any of the ginsenosides found in *Panax* spp.

Roots:

- Coumarins: eleutheroside B1 (isofraxidin-7-0-alpha- L-glucoside, also known as beta-caly canthoside), isofraxidin, coumarin X
- Lignans: eleutheroside B4 ((-)-sesamin), eleutheroside D ((-)-syringarsinol di-0- beta-D-glucoside), eleutheroside E (different crystal form of D, also known as acanthoside D)
- Phenylpropanoid: eleutheroside B (syringin), caffeic acid and caffeic acid ethyl ester
- Polysaccharides: eleutheroside C (methyl-alpha-D-galactoside), eleutherans A-G
- Sterols: eleutheroside A (daucosterol)
- Triterpene: oleanolic acid
- Miscellaneous eleutherosides: eleutheroside B2, eleutheroside B3, eleutheroside F, eleutheroside G

Leaves:

- Triterpenes: eleutheroside I (also known as mussenin B), eleutheroside K, eleutheroside L, eleutheroside M (also known as hederasaponin B), senticosides A to D (may be identical to eleutherosides I, K, L and M)

THERAPEUTIC USES & RELEVANT PHARMACOLOGY

Numerous *in vivo*, *in vitro*, and human clinical trials have been conducted on this species in Russia. Unfortunately, few have been translated into the English language. This monograph includes information from review articles (the review by Farnsworth is the most extensive encountered)[2] as well as any original articles available in English.

ADAPTOGENTIC ACTIVITY

Historically, Siberian ginseng has been used as a general tonic, relying on its adaptogenic action. An adaptogen is thought to work in a non-specific manner, drawing the patient toward normal function, irrespective of the direction of the pathologic state.[9, 10] Fulder reports that eleuthero is widely used in Russia by such diverse populations as deep sea divers, mine and mountain rescue workers, soldiers, factory workers, cosmonauts, and athletes largely for its perceived ability to increase endurance and promote the body's ability to tolerate stressful conditions.[11]

Anti-stress Activity

An early study suggested that eleuthero increases non-specific development of resistance to stress, as well as inhibiting the alarm-reaction to stress including decreasing the activation of the adrenal cortex.[12]

Anti-fatigue – Physical

Perhaps the most common use of eleuthero in North America is its use to increase physical endurance and stamina. However, most of the Russian studies of this indication were neither double-blinded nor controlled adequately, making it difficult to assess its true clinical effect. Several animal studies found no significant difference between the length of time that mice ingesting eleuthero could swim in comparison with placebo.[13, 14] One animal study also found no difference in plasma lactic acid, glucagon, insulin or liver glycogen levels in exercised rats who had ingested eleuthero.[14] Yet, in one single-blind, placebo-controlled study in healthy males (n=6), all four parameters of physical capacity (oxygen uptake, oxygen pulse, maximal work capacity and exhaustion time) were significantly increased in the group taking the eleuthero as compared to those taking placebo.[15] In a more recent double-blind, placebo controlled study of 20 highly trained long distance runners, no significant differences were noted between the group who took the eleuthero extract daily for 6 weeks and the placebo group.[16] The authors caution that while eleuthero may not enhance the physical ability of highly-trained athletes, it may still provide some benefit to the average individual.

IMMUNOSTIMULATING EFFECTS

A placebo-controlled, double blind study of healthy volunteers who were given 3- to 40 mL of an eleuthero extract (0.2% w/v eleutheroside B) reported that those ingesting eleuthero experienced a significant increase in total lymphocyte count with the most pronounced effect noticed with the T-lymphocytes. Granulocyte and monocyte levels were unchanged in these individuals.[17]

NEUROLOGICAL EFFECTS

Eleuthero has been reported to have both a sedative action and a stimulant effect in animal experiments.[2] One study found that mice given eleuthero exhibited significantly more aggressive behavior than those given distilled water.[13]

MISCELLANEOUS EFFECTS

Diabetes

Hypoglycemic activity has been reported in animal studies with some forms of induced-hyperglycemia;[18] however, another study found no effect of eleuthero on alloxan-induced hyperglycemia in rats.[2, 19] Positive effects appear to be due to the polysaccharide components also known as eleutherans A-G.[18]

Platelet Aggregation

An anti-aggregatory compound, 3,4-dihydroxybenzoic acid (DBA) has been identified in eleuthero, which is reported to be as potent as ASA in inhibiting collagen- and adenosine-induced platelet aggregation, but less potent at inhibiting arachidonic acid-induced platelet aggregation.[20]

Anti-cancer Properties

Several Russian *in vitro* and *in vivo* studies suggest that eleuthero may have direct cytostatic activity as well as metastasis-preventing effects. These studies are briefly reviewed by Hacker and Medon,[21] who reported that aqueous extracts of eleuthero in combination with cytarabine provided additive antiproliferative effects against L1210 murine leukemia.[21] No human clinical trials could be found for this indication.

Protection from Radiation

Siberian ginseng is noted for its ability to provide protection in animals subjected to both single exposure and long-term X-ray radiation. In one study rats given *Eleutherococcus senticosis* survived twice as long as control rats when exposed to long term radiation (total dose 1620 to 7000 rads). When the rats were given both Eleutherococcus and antibiotics and exposed to radiation (total dose 3000 rads over 60 days), they survived three times as long.[2] An *in vitro* study noted only slight radio protective effects of eleuthro on the survival of cultured mammalian cells, while *Panax ginseng* was found to have significant effects in the same test system.[22] Although no human trials were available for review, Siberian ginseng is thought to be useful as an adjunctive treatment for those undergoing radiation treatment for a variety of cancerous conditions.

ADVERSE EFFECTS

Two reviews of clinical trials in which over 6000 individuals ingested eleuthero for up to 60 days reported no incidences of serious toxicity.[2, 7] In addition, no long-term toxicity was reported in mice at a dose of 5.0 mL/kg of fluid extract.[2] Another comprehensive review of the literature concluded that unlike *Panax ginseng*, eleuthero never produces excitation or a stress-like syndrome in patients.[23] However, the Farnsworth review cites one study in which an unspecified proportion of 64 atherosclerotic patients (taking 4.5 to 6.0 mL of an ethanolic root extract daily for 25 to 30 days, repeated 6-8 times with 3-4 month intervals) experienced hypertension, cardiac problems (e.g., extrasystole, shifts in cardiac rhythm, tachycardia) and insomnia.[2] This review cites a second study in which 2 of 55 patients with rheumatic heart lesions reported headaches, hypertension, pericardial pain and palpitations.[2]

Eleuthero products have been commonly misidentified or adulterated in the past, most commonly with a plant known as *Periploca sepium* Bunge, Asclepiadaceae (the bark of silk vine). The Chinese name for eleuthero is "Ci-wu-jia", while the Chinese name for *Periploca sepium* is "Wu-jia", which may explain the original source of confusion.[1] *Periplocia sepium* is known to contain cardiac glycosides and chemicals with steroidal bases which may explain many of the side effects which have previously been attributed to eleuthero products. The most famous Canadian case is one of maternal-neonatal androgenization attributed to "Siberian ginseng."[24] The "Siberian ginseng" product, was later determined to contain no *Eleuthercoccus senticocus*, but almost certainly *Periploca sepium* instead.[25] However, oral administration of the original adulterated material to rats in a bioassay for androgenization failed to produce positive results. Thus, either the androgenizing effects noted in mother and infant were not due to the implicated herbal product, or the effects were specific to humans or idiosyncratic to the individuals involved.[26]

Tyler reports another Canadian incident in which an eleuthero product was adulterated with 0.5% caffeine, providing a stimulant effect to the user.[5]

Clinically, ingestion of true eleuthero products is associated with very few adverse effects.

CAUTIONS/CONTRAINDICATIONS

Some authors suggest that eleuthero should not be given to individuals with: hypertension (greater than 180/90 mmHg); asthma or emphysema, diabetes, cardiac disorders or those receiving anxiolytic or sedative treatment.[2] Baldwin also suggests caution when treating individuals with acute illness or fever; suffering from mania, schizophrenia or in premenopausal women.[7] Safety has not been established for use in children, and pregnant or lactating women.[8]

Clinically, eleuthero appears significantly less likely to cause problems in most individuals than *Panax* spp. (e.g., *Panax ginseng* and *Panax quinquefolium*).

DRUG INTERACTIONS

Some authors suggest caution with concomitant use of eleuthero and a variety of other therapies including: cardiac, anticoagulant, hypoglycemic, and hypo/hypertensive agents.[2] Eleuthero has been reported to both increase and decrease barbiturate sleeping time in *in vitro* and *in vivo* experiments.[2, 27, 28] In addition, a recent Canadian case study reported that eleuthero may be responsible for elevated serum digoxin levels in a 74-year-old man who presented with elevated serum digoxin levels at a routine check up with no signs of toxic effects. The authors suggested that there were three possible explanations for this finding: 1) some chemical constituent of eleuthero was converted to digoxin *in vivo*; 2) some component of eleuthero interfered with digoxin elimination; or 3) the eleuthero caused a false serum assay result.[29] Dennis Awang, a Canadian expert on herbal products, argues that the eleutherosides are in no way chemically similar to cardiac glycosides such as digoxin and have not been observed to have any cardiotonic effects. He argues that the case reported by McRae is most likely another case in which *Periploca sepium* is substituted for *Eleutherococcus senticosus* because the former contains several cardiac glycosides which provide a more rational explanation for the rise in serum digoxin noted in the patient.[30] It should be noted that the "Siberian ginseng" product in this case has never been tested for eleutheroside content.

DOSAGE REGIMENS[2]

- Dried root: 2-4 grams (in 1-3 divided doses) daily
- Tincture (1:5): 10-20 mL (in 1-3 divided doses) daily
- Fluid extract (1:1): 2-4 mL (in 1-3 divided doses) daily
- Solid extract (20:1): 100-200 mg (in 1-3 divided doses) daily

Most human studies involving long-term administration of eleuthero have involved eleuthero-free periods of 2 to 3 weeks every 30 to 60 days.[27]

REFERENCES

1. Foster S. *Siberian Ginseng: Eleuthercoccus senticosus*. Austin, TX: American Botanical Council; 1991:7
2. Farnsworth NR, Kinghorn AD, Soejarto D, Waller DP. Siberian ginseng (*Eleuthrococcus senticosus*): Current status as an adaptogen. In: Wagner H, Hikino H, Farnsworth NR, eds. *Economic and Medicinal Plant Research*. Orlando, Florida: Academic Press; 1985:155-215.
3. Halstead BW, Hood LL. *Eleutherococcus senticosus Siberian Ginseng: An Introduction to the Concept of Adaptogenic Medicine*. Long Beach, CA: Oriental Healing Arts Institute; 1984:240
4. Leung A, Foster S. Encyclopedia of Common Natural Ingredients Used in Food, Drugs and Cosmetics. 2nd edition. New York, NY: John Wiley and Sons; 1996:649.
5. Tyler VE. *Herbs of Choice. The Therapeutic Use of Phytomedicinals*. Binghamton, NY: Pharmaceutical Products Press; 1994:209.
6. Brown D. *Herbal Prescriptions for Better Health*. Rocklin, CA: Prima Publishing; 1996:349.
7. Baldwin CA, Anderson LA, Phillipson JD. What pharmacists should know about ginseng. *The Pharmaceutical Journal*. 1986;November 8:583-6.
8. Newall CA, Anderson LA, Phillipson JD. *Herbal Medicines: A Guide for Health Care Professionals*. London: The Pharmaceutical Press; 1996:296.
9. Shibata S, Tanaka O, Shoji J, Saito H. Chemistry and Pharmacology of Panax. *Economic and Medicinal Plant Research*. 1985;1:217-84.
10. Bahrke MS, Morgan WP. Evaluation of the ergogenic properties of ginseng. *Sports Medicine*. 1994;18(4):229-48.
11. Fulder S. The drug the builds Russians. *New Science*. 1980;21:576-9.
12. Brekhman II, Kirillov OI. Effect of eleutherococcus on alarm-phase of stress. *Life Sciences*. 1969;8(3):113-21.
13. Lewis WH, Zenger VE, Lynch RG. No adaptogen response of mice to ginseng and Eleutherococcus infusions. *Journal of Ethnopharmacology*. 1983;8(2):209-14.
14. Martinez B, Staba EJ. The physiological effects of *Aralia*, *Panax* and *Eleutherococcus* on excised rats. *Japanese Journal of Pharmacology*. 1984;35(2):79-85.
15. Asano K, Takahashi T, Miyashita M, *et al.* Effect of *Eleutherococcus senticosus* extract on human physical working capacity. *Planta Medica*. 1986;3:175-7.
16. Dowling EA, Redondo DR, Branch JD, *et al*. Effect of *Eleutherococcus senticosus* on submaximal and maximal exercise performance. *Medicine and Sciences in Sports and Exercise*. 1996;28(4):482-9.
17. Bohn B, Nebe CT, Birr C. Flow-cytometric studies with *Eleutherococcus senticosus* extract as an immunomodulatory agent. *Arzneimittelforschung*. 1987;37(10):1193-6.
18. Hikino H, Takahashi M, Otake K, Konno C. Isolation and hypoglycemic activity of eleutherans A, B, C, D, E, F, and G: Gycans of *Eleutherococcus senticosus* roots. *Journal of Natural Products*. 1986;49(2):293-7.
19. Medon PJ, Thompson EB, Farnsworth NR. Hypoglycemic effect and toxicity of *Eleutherococcus senticosus* following acute and chronic administration in mice. *Chung Kuo Yao Li Hsueh Pao*. 1981;2(4):281-5.

20. Yun-Choi HS, Kim J, Lee J. Potential inhibitors of platelet aggregation from plant sources III. *Journal of Natural Products*. 1987;50:1059-64.
21. Hacker B, Medon PJ. Cytotoxic effects of *Eleutherococcus senticosus* aqueous extracts in combination with N6-(delta 2-isopentenyl)-adenosine and 1-beta-D-arabinofuranosylcytosine against L1210 leukemia cells. *Journal of Pharmaceutical Sciences.* 1984;73(2):270-2.
22. Ben-Hur E, Fulder S. Effect of P. ginseng saponins and *Eletherococcus senticosus* on survival of cultured mammalian cells after ionizing radiation. *American Journal of Chinese Medicine*. 1981;9:48-56.
23. Barnanov AI. Medicinal uses of ginseng and related plants in the Soviet Union: recent trends in the Soviet literature. *Journal of Ethnopharmacology*. 1982;6:339-53.
24. Koren G, Randor S, Martin S, Danneman D. Maternal ginseng use associated with neonatal androgenization. *Journal of the American Medical Association*. 1990;264(22):2866.
25. Awang DVC. Maternal use of ginseng and neonatal androgenization [Comment]. *Journal of the American Medical Association*. 1991;265:1839.
26. Waller DP, Martin AM, Farnsworth NR, Awang DVC. Lack of androgenticity of siberian ginseng. [Letter] *Journal of the American Medical Association*. 1992;267(17):2329.
27. Bradley P. *British Herbal Compendium.* Bournemouth, UK: The British Herbal Medical Association; 1992:239.
28. Medon PJ, Ferguson PW, Watson CF. Effects of *Eleutherococcus senticosus* extracts on hexobarbital metabolism *in vivo* and *in vitro*. *Journal of Ethnopharmacology.* 1984;10(2):235-41.
29. McRae S. Elevated serum digoxin levels in a patient taking digoxin and Siberian ginseng. [See comments] *Canadian Medical Association Journal.* 1996;155(3):293-5.
30. Awang DV. Siberian ginseng toxicity may be case of mistaken identity. [Comment] *Canadian Medical Association Journal.* 1996;155(9):1237.

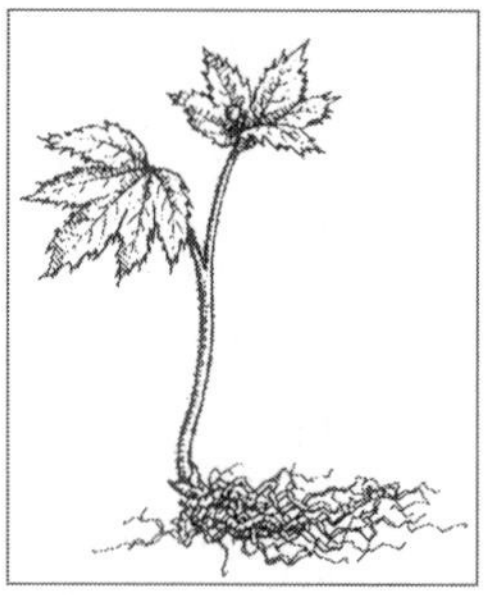

GOLDENSEAL

Hydrastis canadensis L.

THUMBNAIL SKETCH

Active Constituents

- Isoquinoline alkaloids (incl. hydrastine and berberine)

Common Uses

- Infections and inflammation of mucous membranes of the digestive tract, upper respiratory tract and genitourinary tract.

Adverse Effects

- Few at therapeutic doses, but there is a potential of poisoning

Cautions/Contraindications

- Pregnancy, hypertension

Drug Interactions

- None noted in clinical practice

Doses

- 0.5-1g of dried root three times daily
- 2-4mL of hydroalcoholic tincture (1:10, 60% ethanol) three times daily
- 0.3-1mL of liquid extract (1:1, 60% ethanol) three times daily

INTRODUCTION

Family: Ranunculaceae

Synonyms: Hydrastis, Yellow root, Orange root, Indian turmeric, Eye root, Jaundice root, Indian dye, Yellow puccoon, Ground raspberry, Turmeric root[1-3]

Goldenseal is a perennial member of the buttercup family that stands up to 30cm in height and produces a single white/green flower. The knotty distinctively yellow rhizome is the part that is used medicinally.[4] While it was once found commonly throughout Central and Eastern United States and Southern Ontario, over-collection has now seriously diminished its numbers.[1, 4] It is now considered an endangered species. Goldenseal has enjoyed a long medicinal history, originally used by the peoples of the First Nations for a variety of conditions, including skin diseases, ulcers, liver conditions, digestive conditions and infections.[1, 5] Given its bright yellow color, it was also used commonly as a dye.[1, 2] The early eclectic physicians continued to use goldenseal into the beginning of the 20th century. Goldenseal is now mentioned in most of the world's herbal pharmacopoeias.

Constituents [1, 3, 4, 6-10]

- Alkaloids: isoquinoline alkaloids (berberine, hydrastine, canadine), canadaline, hydrastidine, isohydrastidine, berberastine.
- Miscellaneous: meconin, saturated and unsaturated fatty acids, chlorogenic acid, carbohydrates (D-fructose, D-galactose, sucrose)

THERAPEUTIC USES & RELEVANT PHARMACOLOGY

COMMON USES

While herbalists use goldenseal for many conditions, it is considered especially useful in the management of infections and conditions of mucous membranes. It is often referred to by herbalists as the 'king of the tonics of the mucous membranes'.[11] Indications include inflammatory and infectious conditions of the gastrointestinal tract (gastritis, digestive problems, infectious diarrhea),[1] upper respiratory tract, eyes and genitourinary system. As a bitter and a cholagogue, it is used to aid digestion and treat dyspepsia.[12, 13]

Given its astringent action, goldenseal is also used to treat menorrhagia and post-partum hemorrhage (see cautions/contraindications).[12, 13] Externally it has been suggested useful in the treatment of various skin conditions such as eczema, ringworm, athlete's foot, impetigo and pruritis.[12, 14]

Goldenseal is often used to treat the common cold, either alone or in combination with echinacea. Bergner has recently questioned its effectiveness in the management of this condition. Firstly, the active antimicrobial agent (berberine) is poorly absorbed following oral administration and secondly because of the lack of historical data to support this indication. Its popularity in this situation is more likely due to an inappropriate transposition of modern antibiotic protocols.[15] It has been suggested that goldenseal acts in these cases not as an 'antibiotic-like' agent but rather as an alterative, aiding the body's inherent defensive processes.[15]

Goldenseal has often been used to mask detection of illegal substances, such as marijuana and heroin, by urinalysis.[16] However, there is no data to support this use. It has been shown that even large doses of goldenseal have no influence on the excretion of narcotics.[17, 18] In a review article, Foster concludes that this myth originated from a fictional novel written by a prominent 19th-century eclectic physician.[19]

ANTIMICROBIAL

Most of the evidence used to support the antimicrobial action of goldenseal is actually taken from information relating to the use of berberine salts (especially sulfate). *In vitro* studies have shown berberine to be effective against a large number of bacteria including members of *Bacillus* sp., *Streptococcus* sp., *Staphylococcus* sp., *Klebsiella* sp., *Proteus* sp., *Corynebacterium diptheria, Enterobacter aerogenes, Salmonella typhi, Vibrio cholerae, Shigella boydii, Pseudomonas aeruginosa, Mycobacterium tuberculosis, Escherichia coli* and *Xanthomonas citri.*[5, 6, 15, 20] In addition it is active against a wide variety of fungi (including *Candida albicans, Cryptococcus neoformans, Saccharomyces cerevisiae, Trichophyton mentagrophytes, Sporothrix schenkii*) and parasites (including *Giardia lamblia, Entamoeba histolytica, Leishmania donovani).*[5, 6, 20-23] Using chick embryos, berberine at a dose of 0.5mg per egg offered protection from *Chlamydia trachomatis*. This action was comparable to that afforded by a dose of 1mg of sulphadiazine per egg.[24]

Berberine sulfate has been shown to prevent the adherence of streptococci to host cells and this could in part explain its 'antibiotic' properties.[25] *In vitro* experiments have shown that the pH of the medium influences the antimicrobial action of berberine salts[20], with the action increasing with the basic nature of the medium used (e.g., when pH=8 antimicrobial activity is 2-4x greater than when the medium has a pH of 7).[5] Both berberine sulfate and berberine hydrochloride appear to have similar antimicrobial properties.[20]

In a randomized controlled trial, a single dose of berberine sulfate (400 mg) was shown to decrease the mean stool volume and duration of diarrhea when given to adult individuals (n=165) suffering from acute diarrhea due to *Escherichia coli.* In patients with diarrhea caused by *Vibrio cholerae*, the decrease in stool volume was slight and was not additive to the effects of tetracycline.[26] In another randomized, placebo controlled, double blind clinical trial of adults (n=400) presenting with acute watery diarrhea, the effects of berberine hydrochloride (HCl) (100 mg 4x daily), berberine HCl (100 mg 4x daily) plus tetracycline (500 mg 4x daily) and tetracycline (500 mg 4x daily) alone were studied. In the subgroup suffering from cholera (n=186), a significant reduction in duration, frequency and need for rehydration fluid was noted in the tetracycline and tetracycline/berberine group. Berberine HCl by itself was shown to have no antisecretory action (a reduction of stool volume by 1L which was not clinically significant) but did decrease the number of excreted vibrios in the stool. The authors suggest that an antisecretory action may not have been demonstrated because the dose given was too low. Both berberine HCl and tetracycline were shown to be ineffective in patients (n=215) suffering from non-cholera diarrhea.[27]

An uncontrolled study showed that berberine administered orally in children (n=137, aged 5 months to 14 yrs) was comparable to other medications in the management of giardiasis. The author suggested that it could be of use in this situation especially due to the ease of administration and lack of unpleasant adverse effects. It should be noted that there was an increased rate of relapse after one month when compared to conventional treatments such as metronidazole.[28]

In determining the use of goldenseal for its reputed antimicrobial properties it must be remembered that the above information comes from the use and applications of berberine salts. Some authors have suggested that the claims made for this botanical medicine are exaggerated.[16]

CARDIAC ACTION

In vitro studies have produced contradictory results. While hydrastine has been shown to have a vasoconstrictive and thus hypertensive action[9], it has also been noted that berberine and hydrastine have a hypotensive action.[6, 9] In addition, berberine has been shown to: have anticoagulant properties in human blood;[6] have a dose dependant action on cardiac function;[6] increase coronary blood flow;[6] and to exert a protective effect in dogs following ventricular failure.[1]

ANTI-CANCER

Berberine sulfate has been shown to inhibit the tumor promoting action of 12-0-tetradecanoylphorbol-13-acetate and telecodin *in vitro*.[29] In addition, berberine was shown to have antineoplastic activity *in vivo* against malignant human and rat brain tumors cell lines.[30]

HEPATIC ACTIVITY

The historical choleretic action of berberine has been demonstrated in a number of clinical trials.[5] Berberine has been shown to decrease elevated tyramine levels commonly associated with liver cirrhosis by inhibiting tyrosine decarboxylase produced by gut flora.[5]

MISCELLANEOUS

While not exhibiting a hypoglycemic effect, goldenseal has been shown to decrease polydipsia in streptozotocin-induced diabetic mice.[31]

ADVERSE EFFECTS

As for the therapeutic action, possible adverse effects are due to the isoquinoline alkaloids, notably hydrastine and berberine. In high doses (details not given), goldenseal has been noted to cause: oral and pharyngeal irritation, nausea, vomiting, diarrhea, parasthesia, convulsions, weak pulse, hypotension and death from respiratory or cardiac paralysis.[32] Given the lack of cases of adverse reactions, some authors suggest the dangers posed by the use of this herb medicinally have been exaggerated.[15] Some authors argue that the trials mentioned above support this position;[26, 28] however, most were conducted using berberine alone, and not whole goldenseal products (which are those normally seen in clinical practice).

Contact ulceration has been noted when goldenseal root is applied externally to mucous membranes, such as in the form of vaginal douches.[6] In addition, drying of the mucous membranes has been noted after the oral administration of goldenseal, even at doses within the therapeutic range.[15] High doses of plants rich in berberine may cause functional vitamin B problems due to altered metabolism.[33]

The administration of a plant rich in berberine (*Coptis chinensis* Franch., Ranunculaceae) to neonates suffering from glucose 6 phosphate dehydrogense deficiency has resulted in jaundice and hemolytic anemia. While the exact mode of action is yet unknown, berberine appears to exert a bilirubin displacing action. These reported adverse effects have, in part, led to a restriction of sale of berberine rich herbs in general.[34] The applicability of these cautions to the use of goldenseal has been questioned.[15]

The risk of complications due to the destruction of gut flora commonly seen with conventional antibiotics has yet to be completely determined. Many authors suggest this to be unlikely,[5, 15] a possible explanation being that berberine salts are also active against opportunistic fungi such as *Candida albicans.*[5]

CAUTIONS/CONTRAINDICATIONS

Due to the fact that the isoquinoline alkaloids are reputed to have a stimulant action on the uterus, goldenseal is contraindicated in pregnancy.[35] Goldenseal should also be used with caution in cases of hypertension.[11]

DRUG INTERACTIONS

While no specific drug interactions could be found for goldenseal, berberine has been noted to increase the sleeping time induced by barbiturates in rats.[6]

DOSAGE REGIMENS

- 0.5-1 g of dried root and rhizome, dry or as decoction, three times a day[3]
- 2-4 mL of hydroalcoholic tincture (1:10, 60% ethanol) three times a day[3]
- 0.3-1 mL of liquid extract (1:1, 60% ethanol) three times daily[3]
- 250 mg of solid extract (4:1) three times daily[5].
- 250-500 mg of an extract standardized to 5% hydrastine three times daily[36]

Bergner cautions that the myth that goldenseal is a 'natural antibiotic' has led to the herb being used inappropriately in a large number of cases. [15]

Liquid products containing goldenseal are bright yellow in color and will stain clothing if spilled accidentally.

RELATED PLANTS

Other plants containing berberine used medicinally include Bayberry (*Berberis vulgaris* L., Berberidaceae) and Oregon Grape/Trailing Mahonia (*Mahonia aquifolium* (Pursh) Nutt., Berberidaceae).

REFERENCES

1. Marie Snow J. Hydrastis Canadensis. *The Protocol Journal of Botanical Medicine*. 1997;2(2):25-28.
2. Hutchens A. *Indian Herbology of North America*. Boston, MA: Shambhala Press; 1991:382.
3. Bradley P. *British Herbal Compendium.* Bournemouth, UK: BHMA; 1992:239.
4. Leung A, Foster S. *Encylcopedia of Common Natural Ingredients Used in Food, Drugs and Cosmetics.* 2nd ed. New York, NY: John Wiley and Sons; 1996:649.
5. Murray M, J P. *Hydrastis Canadensis, Berberis Vulgaris, Berberis Aquifolium*, and other Berberine-containing Plants. In: Murray M, Pizzorno J, eds. *The Textbook of Natural Medicine.* Seattle, WA: Bastyr University; 1992.

6. Newall C, Anderson L, Philipson JD. *Herbal Medicines: A Guide for Health Care Professionals.* London: The Pharmaceutical Press; 1996:296.
7. Gleye J, *et al.* La canadaline:nouvel alcaloide *d'Hydrastis canadensis. Phytochemistry.* 1974;13:675-6.
8. El-Masry S, *et al.* Colorimetric and spectrophotometric determination of *Hydrastsis* alkaloids in pharmaceutical preparations. *Journal of Pharmaceutical Sciences.* 1980;69:597-8.
9. Genest K, Hughes DW. Natural products in Canadian pharmaceuticals iv. *Hydrastis canadensis. Canadian Journal of Pharmaceutical Science.* 1969;4:41-5.
10. Wisniewski W, Furmanczyk Z, Zapasnik M. Determination of hydrastine, hydrastinine and berberine in the liquid extract of hydrastis. *Acta Poloniae Pharmaceutica.* 1970;27(5):487-91.
11. Mills S. *The Essential Book of Herbal Medicine.* 2nd ed. London: Penguin Publ; 1991:677.
12. Hoffmann D. *Holistic Herbal.* Rockport, CA: Element Books; 1996:256.
13. Chevallier A. *The Encyclopedia of Medicinal Plants.* London: Reader's Digest; 1996:336.
14. Bove M. *An Encylopedia of Natural Healing For Children and Infants.* New Canaan, CT: Keats; 1996:303.
15. Bergner P. Goldenseal and the common cold: The antibiotic myth. *Medical Herbalism.* 1996-97;8(4):1-10.
16. Tyler V. *The Honest Herbal.* 3rd ed. Binghamton, NY: Pharmaceutical Products Press; 1993:375.
17. Nebelkopf E. Herbal therapy in the treatment of drug abuse. *International Journal of the Addictions.* 1987;22(8):695-717.
18. Crombie J, Nugent T, Tobin T. Inability of goldenseal to interfere with the detection of morphine in urine. *Equine Veterinary Science.* 1982;Jan/Feb:16-21.
19. Foster S. Goldenseal masking of drug tests. *Herbalgram.* 1989;21:7.
20. Amin A, Subbaiah T, Abbasi K. Berberine sulphate: Antimicrobial activity, bioassay, and mode of action. *Canadian Journal of Microbiology.* 1969;15(9):1067-76.
21. Kaneda Y, Torii M, Tanaka T, Aikawa M, *et al. In vitro* effects of berberine sulphate on the growth of *Entamoeba histolytica*, *Giardia lamblia* and *Trichomonas vaginalis*. *Annals of Tropical Medicine and Parasitology.* 1991;85:417-25.
22. Mahajan V, Sharma A, Rattan A. Antimycotic activity of berberine sulphate: An alkaloid from an Indian medicinal herb. *Sabouraudia.* 1982;20:79-81.
23. Subbaiah T, Amin A. Effect of berberine sulphate on *Entamoeba histolytica*. *Nature.* 1967;215(100):527-8.
24. Sabir M, Mahajan V, Mohapatra L, Bhide N. Experimental study of the antitrachoma action of berberine. *Indian Journal of Medical Research.* 1976;64(8):1160-7.
25. Sun D, Courtney H, Beachey E. Berberine sulfate blocks adherence of *Streptococcus pyogenes* to epithelial cells, fibronectin, and hexadecane. *Antimicrobial Agents and Chemotherapy.* 1988;32(9):1370-1374.
26. Rabbani GH, Butler T, Knight J, *et al.* Randomised controlled trial of berberine sulphate therapy for diarrhoea due to enterotoxigenic *Escherichia coli* and *Vibrio cholerae*. *Journal of Infectious Diseases.* 1987;155:979-84.
27. Khin-Maung U, Myo-Kin, Nyunt-Nyaunt-Wai, Aye-Kyaw, Tin-U. Clinical trial of berberine in acute watery diarrhoea. *British Medical Journal.* 1985;291:1601-5.
28. Gupte S. Use of berberine in the treatment of giardiasis. *American Journal of Diseases of Children.* 1975;129:866.
29. Nishino H, Kitagawa K, Fujiki H, Iwashima A. Berberine sulphate inhibits tumour-promoting activity of teleocidin in two stage carcinogenesis on mouse skin. *Oncology.* 1986;43:131-4.
30. Zhang R, Dougherty D, Rosenblum M. Laboratory studies of berberine used alone and in combination with 1,3-Bis (2-chloroethyl-1-nitrosurea) to treat malignant brain tumours. *Chinese Medicine Journal.* 1990;103(8):658-65.
31. Swanston-Flatt S, Day C, Bailey C, Flatt P. Evaluation of traditional plant treatments for diabetes: Studies in streptozotocin diabetic mice. *Acta Diabetologica Latina.* 1989;26(1):51-5.
32. Brinker F. *Toxicology of Botanical Medicine.* 2nd ed. Portland, OR: National College of Naturopathic Medicine; 1983:141.
33. Murray M. *The Healing Power of Herbs.* Rocklin, CA: Prima Publishing; 1992:410.
34. De Smet P.A.G.M, Keller K, Hansel R, Chandler R. *Adverse Effects of Herbal Drugs.* Berlin: Springer-Verlag; 1997:250.
35. Farnsworth N, Bingel A, Cordell G, *et al.* Potential Value of Plants as Sources of New Antifertility Agents I. *Journal of Pharmaceutical Sciences.* 1975;64(4):535-598.
36. Murray M, Werbach M. *Botanical Influences on Illness.* Tarzana, CA: Third Line Press; 1994:344.

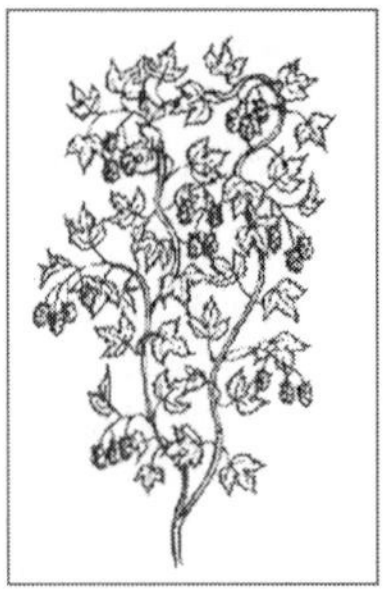

HOPS

Humulus lupulus L.

THUMBNAIL SKETCH

Active Constituents
- Volatile oil
- Resinous components
- Flavonoid glycosides

Common Uses
- Insomnia, agitation, ailments arising from nervous tension such as irritable bowel syndrome, poor digestion.

Adverse Effects
- Contact dermatitis and respiratory difficulties following exposure to the herb itself, disruption of menstrual cycle.

Cautions/Contraindications
- Depression
- Pregnancy

Drug Interactions
- May potentiate the action of hypnotics and alcohol

Doses
- 0.5-1g of dried strobiles three times daily and before bed
- 0.5-1mL liquid extract (1:1, 45% ethanol) three times daily and before bed
- 1-2mL of tincture (1:5, 60% ethanol) three times daily and before bed

INTRODUCTION

Family: Cannabaceae

Synonyms: Humulus, Lupulus, Common hops, European hops.[1-3]

Hops is a climbing perennial herb standing up to 6 m in height found in marshy areas throughout North America, Europe and Asia.[2, 4] It produces a yellowish-green male flower and a 'catkin-like' female flower.[5] The female flowers or strobiles have glandular hairs, which are rich in volatile oils producing a characteristic heavy aroma. These strobiles are the parts used medicinally.[5] Hops is an essential part of the brewing industry, making it arguably one of the most commonly used herbs. It has a long medicinal history, primarily as a mild sedative. In addition to being taken orally, 'hops pillows' are also often used to aid sleep with the aroma allegedly having a calming action.[5] Hops is also said to influence both male and female sexual function. In female hop-pickers it was noted that menarche often occurred early and in men a decrease in 'sexual excess' was seen.[4]

Constituents [1-3, 5-8]

- Volatile oils including: humulene, myrcene and beta-caryophyllene
- Chalcones including: xanthohumol and xanthohumol
- Resinous component: alpha-bitter acids including humulone, cohumulone and adhumulone; beta-bitter acids including lupulone, colupulone, adlupulone; 2-methyl-3-buten-2-ol*
- Flavonoid glycosides: including astargalin, quercetin and rutin
- Miscellaneous: condensed tannins, 'estrogenic substances'

While 2-methyl-3-buten-2-ol exists in small amounts in the plant, the amount is thought to increase on storage from the auto-oxidation of other resinous components.[7] This component is thought to be one of the active sedative constituents.[7, 9, 10]

THERAPEUTIC USES & RELEVANT PHARMACOLOGY

Hops is considered to be a mild sedative and is indicated in the management of insomnia and agitation/restlessness.[1, 2, 5, 11-13] It has also been used in the treatment of conditions related to nervous tension such as irritable bowel syndrome, palpitations and nervous coughs.[4, 5, 11] Given the bitter nature of the resinous material, it is used as a digestive aid and to help stimulate appetite.[1, 2, 4, 5, 12, 13]

ANTIMICROBIAL

Components of hops have been shown to exert antibacterial action primarily against Gram-positive bacteria.[2, 3, 14, 15] Humulone and lupulone appear to be particularly responsible for this action.[2, 15] The activity against Gram-negative bacteria is low due to the presence of a phospholipid rich membrane leading to an increased inactivation of the active principles.[15]

Clinically, aqueous extracts of hops have been used to treat various infections, including acute bacterial dysentery and pulmonary tuberculosis.[2] However, no clinical trial investigating these uses could be found.

Activity against a number of fungi and yeasts, including *Trichophyton*, *Candida, Fusarium* and *Mucor* spp, has been demonstrated.[3, 14, 16] The action of one component, 3-isopentenylphlorisovalerophenone, was compared favorably to griseofulvin in potency against *Trichophyton* spp.[16] A more recent evaluation noted no action against the yeast *Candida albicans.*[14]

SEDATIVE ACTION

A sedative/hypnotic action has been attributed to 2-methyl-3-butene-2-ol *in vivo.*[7, 10, 17, 18] The sedative action of commercial products containing hops could be due to the *in vivo* formation of 2-methyl-3-butene-2-ol.[7, 17] This volatile product can induce an hypnotic effect when inhaled[9] and exists in relatively high concentrations in bath products,[7] giving possible credence to the use of items such as 'hops pillows'. However, Tyler questions whether enough 2-methy-3-buten-2-ol exists in most commercial products to support its use as a sedative.[9]

Oral administration of a commercial product (Seda-Kneipp®), which contains valerian in addition to hops, has been shown to decrease the impact of noise on sleep patterns (both slow-wave and REM).[19] Combination products containing both valerian and hops have been shown not to cause morning 'hangover' effects but may impair performance a few hours after ingestion.[20] In both the above scenarios it should be noted that valerian (*Valeriana officinalis* L. Valerianaceae) has been shown to possess hypnotic characteristics of its own.[21, 22]

MISCELLANEOUS

Metabolism

Both colupulone and 2-methyl-3-buten-2-ol have been shown to induce cytochrome P4503A in mice and rats[23-26] and cytochrome P4502B in rats.[26]

Anti-inflammatory

Humulone has been shown to possess anti-inflammatory properties, reducing 12-O-tetradecanoylphorbol-13-acetate induced inflammatory ear edema in mice.[27] The mechanism of action suggested is an inhibition of arachidonic acid metabolism.[28]

Oncology

Hops has been used historically in the treatment of cancer.[2] Humulone has been shown to inhibit the tumor-promoting effect of 12-O-tetradecanoylphorbol-13-acetate on skin tumor formation in mice.[28]

Endocrine

Using the uterine-weight assay of immature female mice as a determinant, no estrogenic properties could be shown for various components of hops, including the essential-oil fraction and bitter acids.[8] This finding contradicts others which have stated that hops has 'appreciable estrogenic activity'[5] and could aid in the treatment of hot flushing resulting from hormonal imbalance.[29] A disruption of menstrual cycle in female-hop pickers and decrease in male libido has been documented.[5]

ADVERSE EFFECTS

Components of hops are known to have allergenic potential resulting in instances of contact dermatitis as well as respiratory allergy and distress following frequent contact with hops.[3, 30, 31] The parenteral administration of large doses of hops has proved fatal *in vivo*.[3] The implication for clinical practice is unknown.

CAUTIONS/CONTRAINDICATIONS

Products containing hops should not be taken by individuals diagnosed with depression.[1, 3, 5, 11]

Given its possible 'estrogenic' action, hops may disrupt menstrual cycles[5] and the documentation of *in vitro* uterine anti-spasmodic activity suggests that hops should be avoided during pregnancy.[3, 5]

DRUG INTERACTIONS

While no clinical instances were found, caution is prudent when herbal products containing hops are used with hypnotic medications and alcohol.[3] The implication of induction of components of the cytochrome P450 system on concurrent drug therapy has yet to be evaluated.

DOSAGE REGIMENS[1]

- 0.5-1g of dried strobiles three times daily and before bed
- 0.5-1ml liquid extract (1:1, 45% ethanol) three times daily and before bed
- 1-2mL of tincture (1:5, 60% ethanol) three times daily and before bed

REFERENCES

1. Bradley P. *British Herbal Compendium.* Bournemouth, UK: BHMA; 1992:239.
2. Leung A, Foster S. *Encylcopedia of Common Natural Ingredients Used in Food, Drugs and Cosmetics.* 2nd ed. New York, NY: John Wiley and Sons; 1996:649.
3. Newall C, Anderson L, Philipson JD. *Herbal Medicines: A Guide for Health Care Professionals.* London: The Pharmaceutical Press; 1996:296.
4. Weiss R. *Herbal Medicine*. 6th ed. Gothenburg, Sweden: AB Arcanum; 1988:362.
5. Mills S. *The Essential Book of Herbal Medicine.* 2nd ed. London: Penguin; 1991:677.
6. Wren R. *Potter's New Encyclopaedia of Botanical Drugs and Preparations.* Saffron Walden: C.W Daniel Company; 1988:362.
7. Hansel R, *et al.* The sedative-hypnotic principle of hops. 3. Communication: Contents of 2-methyl-3-butene-2-ol in hops and hop preparations. *Planta Medica*. 1982;45:224-8.
8. Fenselau C, Talalay P. Is oestrogenic activity present in hops? *Food Cosmetics and Toxicology.* 1973;11:597-603.
9. Tyler V. *Herbs of Choice.The Therapeutic Use of Phytomedicinals.* Binghampton, NY: Pharmaceutical Products Press; 1994:208.
10. Wohlfart R, Wurm R, Hansel R, Schmidt H. Detection of sedative-hypnotic active ingredients in hops.5. Degradation of bitter acids to 2-methy-3-buten-2-ol, a hop constituent with sedative-hypnotic activity. *Archiv der Pharmazie*. 1983;316(2):132-7.
11. Hoffmann D. *Holistic Herbal*. Rockport: Element Books; 1996:256.
12. Chevallier A. *The Encyclopedia of Medicinal Plants.* London: Reader's Digest; 1996:336.
13. Bove M. *An Encylopedia of Natural Healing for Children and Infants.* New Canaan, CT: Keats; 1996:303.
14. Langezaal CR, Chandra A, Scheffer JJ. Antimicrobial screening of essential oils and extracts of some *Humulus lupulus* L. cultivars. *Pharmaceutisch Weekblad*. 1992;14(6):353-6.
15. Schmalreck AF, Teuber M. Structural features determining the antibiotic potencies of natural and synthetic hop bitter resins, their precursors and derivatives. *Canadian Journal of Microbiology.* 1975;21:205-12.

16. Mizobuchi S, Sato Y. Antifungal activities of hop bitter resins and related compounds. *Agric Biol Chem*. 1985;49:399-405.
17. Hansel R, Wohlfart R. Narcotic action of 2-methyl-3-butene-2-ol contained in the exhalation of hops. *Zeitschrift fur Naturforschung*. 1980;35(11-12):1096-7.
18. Wohlfart R, Hansel R, Schmidt H. The sedative-hypnotoc principle of hops. 4. Communication: Pharmacology of 2-methyl-3-buten-2-ol. *Planta Medica*. 1983;48:120-3.
19. Muller-Limmroth W, Ehrenstein W. Experimental studies of the effects of Seda-Kneipp on the sleep of sleep disturbed subjects; implications for the treatment of different sleep disturbances. *Medizinische Klinik*. 1977;72(25):1119-25.
20. Gerhard U, Linnenbrink N, Georghaidou C, Hobi V. Vigilance-decreasing effects of 2 plant-derived sedatives. *Schweizerische Rundschau fur Medizin Praxis*. 1996;85(15):473-81.
21. Houghton P. Valerian. *Pharmaceutical Journal*. 1994;253:95-6.
22. Hobbs C. Valerian. *Herbalgram*. 1989;21:19-34.
23. Mannering GJ, Shoeman JA, Deloria LB. Identification of the antibiotic hops component, colupulone, as an inducer of hepatic cytochrome P-4503A in the mouse. *Drug Metabolism and Disposition*. 1992;20(2):142-7.
24. Mannering GJ, Shoeman JA, Shoeman DW. Effects of colupulone, a component of hops and brewer's yeast, and chromium on glucose tolerance and hepatic cytochrome P450 in ondiabetic and spontaneously diabetic mice. *Biochemical and Biophysical Research Communications*. 1994;200(3):1455-62.
25. Mannering GJ, Shoeman JA. Murine cytochrome P4503A is induced by 2-methyl-3-buten-2-ol, 3-methyl-1-penyn-3-ol (meparfynol, and tert-amyl alcohol). *Xenobiotica*. 1996;26(5):487-93.
26. Shipp E, Mehigh C, Helferich W. The effect of colupulone (a HOPS beta-acid) on hepatic cytochrome P-450 enzymatic activity in the rat. *Food and Chemical Toxicology*. 1994;32(11):1007-14.
27. Yasukawa K, Yamaguchi A, Arita J, *et al.* Inhibitory effect of edible plant extracts on 12-O-tetradecanoylphorbol-13-acetate-induced ear oedema in mice. *Phytotherapy Research*. 1993;7:185-189.
28. Yasukawa K, Takeuchi M, Takido M. Humulon, a bitter in the hop, inhibits tumor promotion by 12-O-tetradecanoylphorbol-13-acetate in two stage carcinogenesis in mouse skin. *Oncology*. 1995;52(2):156-8.
29. Goetz P. Traitement des bouffees de chaleur par insuffisance ovarienne par l'extrait de houblon (*Humulus lupulus*). *Rev. Phytother Prat*. 1990;December(4):13-15.
30. O'Donovan W. Hops dermatitis. *Lancet*. 1924;2:597.
31. Newmark FM. Hops allergy and terepene sensitivity: An occupational disease. *Annals of Allergy*. 1978;41:311-12.

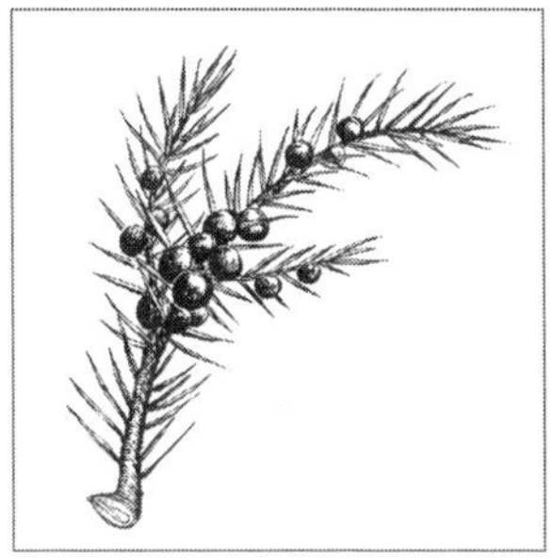

JUNIPER

Juniperus communis L.

THUMBNAIL SKETCH

Active Constituents
- Volatile oils (monoterpenes and sesquiterpenes)

Common Uses

Minor genitourinary tract infections including:
- Cystitis
- Chronic arthritic conditions
- Digestive upset

Adverse Effects

Internal:
- 'Kidney pain', urination, hematuria, albuminuria, tachycardia, hypertension

External:
- burning, blistering, erythema and inflammation

Cautions/Contraindications
- Pregnancy
- Chronic or acute kidney disease (disputed)

Drug Interactions
- Avoid with conventional hypoglycemic and diuretic therapy

Doses
- 1-2g of fruit three times daily
- 2-4mL of liquid extract (1:1 in 25% alcohol) three times daily
- 1-2mL of tincture (1:5 in 45% alcohol) three times daily

INTRODUCTION

Family: Cupressaceae

Synonyms: Buccae juniperi, Genievre, Wacholderbeeren, Juniper bush.[1, 2]

Juniperus communis is an evergreen shrub native to Northern and Central Europe.[3, 4] The tree itself can stand up to 6m and produces distinctive fruit,[3, 4] which while they are often referred to as berries, are in fact fleshy cone scales.[3-5] These 'berries' are rich in essential oils and have been used for centuries for both culinary and medicinal purposes.[6] For best effect, the berries should be harvested in the second year when they are dark blue/purple in color.[5] Most adults will be familiar with its distinctive odor and taste since juniper berries are the principal flavoring agent in gin. Unfortunately, gin contains insufficient amounts of the essential oil to afford it any medicinal properties.[6]

Constituents [2-4, 7-10]

- Volatile oil: monoterpenes (including 1,4-cineole, terpin-4-ol, sabinene, limonene, myrcene), sesquiterpenes (including caryophyllene, cadinene and elemene)
- Tannins: proanthocyanins and gallotannins
- Flavonoid glycosides: including rutin, isoquercitin and quercetin
- Miscellaneous: sugars, junionone, resin, vitamin C, diterpene acids, glucuronic acid

THERAPEUTIC USES & RELEVANT PHARMACOLOGY

COMMON USES

While Juniper has many medicinal uses, it is primarily considered to be useful in the treatment of conditions of the genitourinary tract and musculoskeletal system.[5, 11-14] It is also considered a 'urinary antiseptic' and diuretic and is used in conditions such as cystitis.[5, 11] Weiss considers it useful both internally and externally in chronic arthritis, chronic gout, neuralgia and other rheumatic conditions.[5, 12]

Given its aromatic quality, it is also classified as a bitter and carminative and used for digestive upset and colic as well as to stimulate appetite.[5, 12]

PHARMACOLOGY

Most of the evidence supporting the therapeutic usefulness of juniper is empirical, and what little research there is, is often not available in English. The diuretic action of juniper is attributed to the terpinen-4-ol portion which is purported to stimulate glomerular filtration.[6] Juniper has also been demonstrated to have a hypoglycemic action in both rats and mice.[15, 16] This action appears to be primarily extrapancreatic in origin.[15] In a variety of *in vitro* and *in vivo* models, juniper has been shown to have antifungal, antiviral (against herpes simplex virus 1) and anti-inflammatory properties.[2] Finally, oral administration of an extract of juniper berries was seen to decrease experimentally-induced foot edema in rats.[17]

ADVERSE EFFECTS

Adverse effects have been reported following consumption or topical application of the oil. External application has been seen to result in burning, erythema, inflammation, blistering and edema. Internally, lower back pain in the kidney area, urination, discolored urine, hematuria, albuminuria, tachycardia and hypertension have been reported.[2] Positive patch test reactions following the topical application of an extract of juniper resulting in a dermatitis have also been noted.[18]

CAUTIONS/CONTRAINDICATIONS

Juniper berries are generally considered to be contraindicated in cases of chronic and/or acute kidney disease[2, 6, 12] because of the high concentration of the irritant terpene hydrocarbons such as alpha and beta pinenes relative to the diuretic terpenin-4-ol.[19] A recent review article has challenged this opinion, suggesting that this warning arises from the administration of high doses of juniper and terpentine oil in veterinary medicine. In addition, the author argues that the clouding of urine seen following administration of high doses of the oil probably results from the excretion of juniper oil metabolites and is not an indication of kidney irritation.[20] Oil distilled from the needles, branches and unripe fruit may be particularly high in the irritant components and should still be of concern to the practitioner.[21] Given the present situation, the oil should be administered only under medical supervision.[2]

Juniper has been shown to have uterostimulant, anti-implantation and possible antifertility properties and should not be used in pregnancy.[2, 22].

DRUG INTERACTIONS

Juniper should be used with caution in cases of concomitant conventional hypoglycemic and diuretic therapy.[2]

DOSAGE REGIMENS [2]

- 1-2 g of fruit three times daily.
- 1-2 mL of tincture (1:5 in 45% alcohol) three times daily
- 0.03-0.2 mL of essential oil (1:5 in 45% alcohol) three times daily

REFERENCES

1. Hutchens A. *Indian Herbology of North America*. Boston, MA: Shambhala Press; 1991:382.
2. Newall C, Anderson L, Philipson JD. *Herbal Medicines: A Guide for Health Care Professionals*. London: The Pharmaceutical Press; 1996:296.
3. Leung A, Foster S. *Encyclopedia of Common Natural Ingredients Used in Food, Drugs and Cosmetics*. 2nd ed. New York, NY: John Wiley and Sons; 1996:649.
4. Evans W. *Trease and Evan's Pharmacognosy*. 13th ed. London: Bailliere Tindall; 1989:832.
5. Bergner P. Juniper berries. *Medical Herbalism*. 1994;6(2):13.
6. Tyler V. *The Honest Herbal*. 3rd ed. Binghamton, NY: Pharmaceutical Products Press; 1993:375.
7. Thomas AF, Ozainne M. 'Junionone' {1-(2,2-Dimethylcyclobutyl)but-1-2en-3-one], the first vegetable monocyclic cyclobutane monoterpenoid. *J C S Chem Comm*. 1973:746.
8. Chandler RF. An inconspicuous but insidious drug. *Rev Pharm Can*. 1986:563-6.
9. Friedrich H, Engelshowe R. Tannin producing monomeric substances in Juniperus communis. *Planta Medica*. 1978;33:251-7.

10. Wren R. *Potter's New Encyclopaedia of Botanical Drugs and Preparations.* Saffron Walden: C.W Daniel Company; 1988:362.
11. Hoffmann D. *Holistic Herbal*. Rockport, CA: Element Books; 1996:256.
12. Weiss R. *Herbal Medicine.* 6th ed. Gothenburg, Sweden: AB Arcanum; 1988:362.
13. Mills S. *The Essential Book of Herbal Medicine*. 2nd ed. London: Penguin; 1991:677.
14. Chevallier A. *The Encyclopedia of Medicinal Plants*. London: Reader's Digest; 1996:336.
15. Sanchez de Medina F, Gamez M, Jimenez I, *et al*. Hypoglycemic activity of juniper "berries". *Planta Medica*. 1994;60(3):197-200.
16. Swanston-Flatt S, Day C, Bailey C, Flatt P. Traditional plant treatments for diabetes. Studies in normal and streptozotocin mice. *Diabetologia*. 1990;33(8):462-4.
17. Mascolo N, *et al.* Biological screening of Italian medicinal plants for anti-inflammatory activity. *Phytotherapy Research*. 1987;1:28-31.
18. Mathias CG, Maibach HI, Mitchell JC. Plant dermatitis-patch test results (1975-78). Note on *Juniperus* extract. *Contact Dermatitis*. 1979;5:336-7.
19. Tyler V. *Herb's of Choice.The Therapeutic Use of Phytomedicinals*. Binghampton, NY: Pharmaceutical Products Press; 1994:208.
20. Schilcher H, Heil BM. Nephrotoxicity of juniper berry preparations: A critical review of the literature from 1844 to 1993. *Zeitschrift fur Phytother*. 1994;15:203-13.
21. Bone K. Juniper berry is not a kidney irritant. *Medical Herbalism*. 1994;6(2):12.
22. Farnsworth N, Bingel A, Cordell G, *et al*. Potential value of plants as sources of new antifertility agents I. *Journal of Pharmaceutical Sciences*. 1975;64(4):535-598.

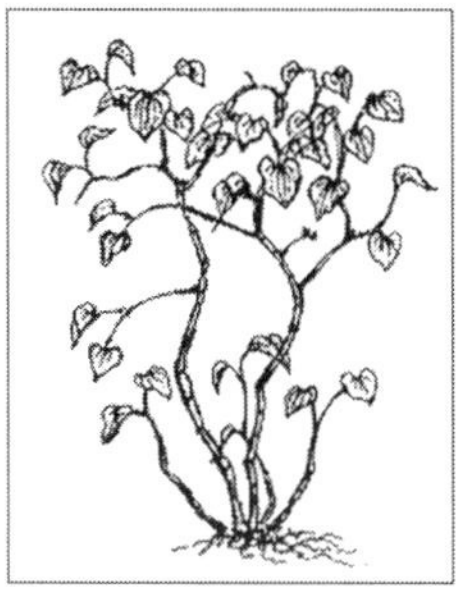

KAVA

Piper methysticum G.Forst

THUMBNAIL SKETCH

Active Constituents

- Kavalactones (kavapyrones)

Common Uses

- Anxiety, states of tension and restlessness, conditions associated with muscle tension/spasm and pain

Adverse Effects

- Disturbances of vision (photophobia, diplopia and oculomotor paralysis), yellowing of the skin, problems with equilibrium, pruritic skin condition (allergy), dizziness and stupor, gastrointestinal discomfort

Cautions/Contraindications

- Pregnancy, lactation, Parkinson's Disease; not recommended for prolonged use (> 3 months)

Drug Interactions

- May potentiate the action of other centrally acting drugs

Doses

- 100mg of kava extract standardized to 70% kavalactone 2-3 times daily.
- 1.5-3g of dried rhizome daily in divided doses
- 3-6mL of alcoholic extract (1:2) daily in divided doses

INTRODUCTION

Family: Piperaceae

Synonyms: Kawa, Kava-Kava[1, 2]

Kava is a perennial shrub standing up to 3 m in height and found throughout Polynesia and the Pacific islands.[1, 3] The substantial, juicy rootstock (rhizome) is the part used medicinally.[1, 3, 4] It was first described in the West by the British explorer, Captain James Cook, in the 18th century during his exploration of the South Pacific.[4]

In addition to its importance as a medicinal agent, kava plays an important role in many social and religious customs of the Polynesian indigenous peoples. Consumption of a beverage made from kava occurred during funeral and marriage ceremonies as well as to honor visiting guests and dignitaries. The preparation of the beverage made from kava was a deeply orchestrated procedure, which often included chewing the root to aid extraction.[3] Kava beverage (kava-kava) is considered to a be a social beverage which causes numbness of the mouth followed by a pleasant mellow and relaxed state when consumed.[4, 5] Fortunately, hangovers do not seem to be a common occurrence.[4]

Constituents[1, 3, 4, 6, 7]

- Kavalactones including the pyrones: kavain (kawain), dihydrokavain, methysticin, dihydromethysticin, and yangonin.
- Alkaloids: cepharadione A (an isoquinoline), pipmethystine (a pyridone, in the leaf only)
- Miscellaneous: flavonoids and benzyl-ketones.

THERAPEUTIC USES & RELEVANT PHARMACOLOGY

COMMON USES

Kava is considered by many to be one of the most effective herbal medicines for the treatment of anxiety.[4, 5, 8] As a muscle relaxant it is used in conditions associated with muscle tension such as headaches.[4, 8] It is also reputed to be effective in the management of mild insomnia and pain,[4, 8] stress and restlessness[9], the treatment of urinary tract infections[10] and arthritic conditions.[8] Application of the raw herb has been reported to ease dental pain and canker sores.[8, 11]

PHARMACOLOGY

Most interest, and investigation, has been focused on the resinous pyrones or kavalactones. Their affinity for various GABA and benzodiazepine binding sites is debatable with conflicting evidence being found on investigation.[12, 13] Kavalactones are very poorly soluble in water, so for medicinal use they must be placed in colloidal solution or at least converted to a finely divided form to promote absorption of the suspension from the gastrointestinal tract.[14, 15] Kava, or its constituents, have been reported to exhibit neuroprotective effects against ischemia,[16] produce EEG changes similar to those exhibited by diazepam,[17] block the voltage dependent sodium ion channel,[18] exert an anticonvulsive action,[4, 19-21] possess antifibrillatory properties,[6] exert an analgesic effect,[4] relax skeletal smooth muscle,[6] inhibit conditioned reflexes in a number of animal models,[22] have local anaesthetic properties[4, 6] and possess antispasmodic and tranquilizing characteristics.[4, 6]

A number of clinical trials, published primarily in German, have shown that kava extracts may prove beneficial in the management of anxiety and tension of non-psychotic origin.[4, 5] In a recent double-blind placebo controlled trial, administration of 100 mg of kava extract (standardized to 70% kavalactone) to patients diagnosed with anxiety (n=58) three times daily for four weeks resulted in significant improvement as measured by the Hamilton anxiety scale. Improvement was noted within the first week and no significant adverse effects were noted.[23] In contrast to benzodiazepines, experience with the therapeutic use of kava preparations has shown no evidence that there is any potential for physical or psychological dependency.[15] Nine double-blind studies have been completed with the isolated compound DL-kawain, comparing it to reference drugs and placebo, with results similar to kava extract.[15]

Anti-fungal activity [4] and antimycobacterial activities[7] have been noted *in vitro*.

A number of excellent English reviews of this plant's medicinal action and historical/cultural importance exist.[3, 4, 6, 24]

ADVERSE EFFECTS

Excessive consumption of kava beverage can result in disturbances of vision (photophobia, diplopia and oculomotor paralysis), yellowing of the skin, problems with equilibrium, dizziness and stupor.[1, 4, 5] These effects have only been reported following consumption of the beverage and it is unlikely that they are of any particular concern in practice.[4] Kava does not appear to adversely affect cognitive function, mental acuity or coordination in comparison to oxazepam, as measured by event-related potentials during cognitive testing.[25]

Chronic administration of kava has resulted in a characteristic scaling of the skin on the extremities associated with intense itching.[1, 3, 4] It was originally hypothesized that this was due to a deficiency in vitamin B3 but the patients symptoms were not improved following administration of nicotinamide (100mg daily for 3 weeks).[4] It is now considered to be an allergic skin reaction.[15]

CAUTIONS/CONTRAINDICATIONS

Due to its dopaminergic properties, kava should be used with caution in cases of Parkinsons disease.[26]

Use is currently considered to be contraindicated in pregnancy, lactation and depression.[1]

DRUG INTERACTIONS

Concomitant administration of kava with barbiturates and centrally acting conventional medication may result in a potentiation of their action.[1, 4] Administration of dihydromethysticin is known to potentiate the action of hexobarbital in animal models.[6] While large doses of alcohol are known to potentiate the action of kava in mice, similar effects have not been confirmed in humans. Excessive alcohol consumption is still best to be avoided in people taking kava because of the perceived potential for interaction.[27]

A possible interaction between kava and a benzodiazepine (alprazolam) has been reported in a 54-year-old man. The individual was admitted to hospital in a "lethargic and disorientated" state after recently introducing kava to his supplement regimen. The patient was also taking cimetidine and terazosin.[28]

DOSAGE REGIMEN

- 100mg of kava extract standardized to 70% kavalactones two or three times daily.[5]
- 1.5-3g of dried rhizome daily in divided doses[4]
- 3-6mL of alcoholic extract (1:2) daily in divided doses[4]
- Generally the duration of use should not exceed 3 months.[15]

REFERENCES

1. Leung A, Foster S. *Encyclopedia of Common Natural Ingredient Used in Food, Drugs and Cosmetics.* 2nd ed. New York, NY: John Wiley and Sons; 1996:649.
2. Wren R. *Potter's New Encyclopedia of Botanical Drugs and Preparations*. Saffron Walden: C.W. Daniel Company; 1988:362.
3. Singh Y, Blumenthal M. Kava: An overview. *Herbalgram*. 1997;39:34-54.
4. Bone K. Kava — A safe herbal treatment for anxiety. *British Journal of Phytotherpy*. 1993/94;3(4):147-153.
5. Brown D. *Herbal Prescriptions for Better Health*. Rocklin,CA: Prima Publishing; 1995:349.
6. Hansel R, (translated by A. Clay and R. Reichert). Kava-kava in modern drug research: Portrait of a medicinal plant. *Quarterly Review of Natural Medicine*. 1996;4(4):259-274.
7. Farnsworth N. NAPRALERT natural products computer database. *University of Illinois at Chicago program for Collaborative Research in the Pharmaceutical Sciences*. Chicago; 1998.
8. Chevallier A. *The Encyclopedia of Medicinal Plants*. London: Reader's Digest; 1996:336.
9. Blumenthal M, Busse WR, Goldberg A, *et al. The Complete German Commission E Monographs: Therapeutic Guide to Herbal Medicine.* Austin, TX: American Botanical Council; 1998:685.
10. Mills S. *The Essential Book of Herbal Medicine*. 2nd ed. London: Penguin Publ; 1991:677.
11. Duke J. *The Green Pharmacy.* New York: Rodale Press Inc.; 1997:617.
12. Jussogie A, Semiz A, Heimke C. Kavapyrone extract enriched from *Piper methysticum* as modulator of the GABA binding site in different regions of the rat brain. *Psychopharmacology (Berlin)*. 1994;116:469-74.
13. Davies L, Drew C, Duffield P, *et al.* Kava pyrones and resin: Studies on GABA(A), GABA (B), and benzodiazepine binding sites in the rodent brain. *Pharmacology and Toxicology*. 1992;71(2):120-6.
14. Reichling J, Saller R. Quality control in the manufacturing of modern herbal remedies. *Quarterly Review of Natural Medicine*. 1998;6(1):21-28.
15. Schulz V, Hansel R, Tyler V. *Rational Phytotherapy: A Physicians' Guide to Herbal Medicine*. Berlin: Springer-Verlag; 1998:306.
16. Backhauss C, Krieglstein J. Extract of kava and its methysticin constituents protect brain tissues against ischemic damage in rodents. *European Journal of Pharmacology.* 1992;215:265-9.
17. Gebner B, Cnota P. Extract of Kava-kava rhizome in comparison with diazepam and placebo. *Zeitschrift fur Phytother*. 1994;15:30-37.
18. Glietz J, Beile A, Peters T. Kawain inhibits vetradine-activated voltage-dependent Na+ channels in syunaptosomes prepared from rat cerebral cortes. *Neutopharmacology*. 1995;24:1133-8.
19. Kretzschmar R, Meyer H. Comparative experiments on the anticonvulsant efficacy of *Piper methysticum* pyrone bonds [German]. *Arch. Int. Pharmacodyn*. 1969;177:261-77.
20. Kretzschmar R, Meyer H, Teschendorf H, Zollner B. Antagonistic effect of natural 5,6-hydrated kava pyrones on strychnine poisoning and experimental local tetanus. [German]. *Ach Int. Pharmacodyn*. 1969;182:251-68.
21. Meyer H, Kretzschmar R. Research on the relationship between molecular structure and pharmacological effect if aryl-substituted 4-methoxy pyrones of the Kava pyrone type. [German]. *Arzneimittelforschg*. 1969;19:617-23.
22. Duffield P, Jamieson D, Duffield A. Effect of aqueous and lipid-soluble extracts of Kava on the conditioned

avoidance response in rats. *Arch Int Pharmacodyn*. 1989;301(81-90).
23. Lehmann E, Kinzler E, Friedemann J. Efficacy of a special kava extract (*Piper methysticum*) in a patients with states of anxiety, tension and excitedness of non-mental origin-a double-blind placebo-controlled study of four weeks treatment. *Phytomedicine*. 1996;3(2):113-9.
24. Schulz V, Hubner W, Ploch M. Clinical trials with phyto-psychopharmacological agents. *Phytomedicine*. 1997;4(4):379-387.
25. Munte T, Heinze H, Matzke M, Steitz J. Effects of oxazepam and an extract of Kava roots (*Piper methysticum*) on event-related potentials in a word recognition task. *Neuropsychobiology*. 1993;27:46-53.
26. Schelosky L, Raffauf C, Jendroska K, *et al.* Kava and dopamine antagonism. *Journal of Neurology, Neurosurgery and Psychiatry*. 1995;58:639-40.
27. Herberg K. Effect of special extract WS 1490 combined with ethyl alcohol on safety-relevant performance para meters. *Blutalkohol*. 1993;30:96-105.
28. Almeida J, Grimsley E. Coma from the health food store: Interaction between kava and alprazolam. *Annals of Internal Medicine*. 1996;125:940-41.

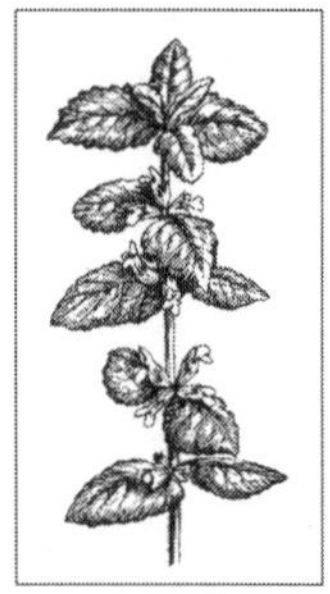

LEMON BALM

Melissa officinalis L.

THUMBNAIL SKETCH

Active Constituents

- Volatile oils, tannins, flavonoids (rosmarinic acid)

Common Uses

Internal:

- Insomnia, anxiety, and situations resulting from nervous tension including digestive and cardiac conditions, pediatric conditions

Topical:

- Cold sores

Adverse Effects

- None reported

Cautions/Contraindications

- Existing thyroid conditions

Drug Interactions

- The potential exists for interactions with concomitant thyroid medications.

Doses

- Oral: 1-4g of dried herb three times daily
- Topical: 70:1 concentrate of dried herb applied to affected area 2 to 4 times daily

INTRODUCTION

Family: Lamiaceae (also known as Labiatae)

Synonyms: Melissa, Common balm, Bee balm, Balm, Honeyplant, Sweet balm, Cure-all[1-3]

Lemon balm is a perennial herb standing up to 1 m in height native to Mediterranean Europe, North Africa and Western Asia.[2] Like most members of the mint family, it is aromatic, producing a characteristic lemony scent.[1, 2] Lemon balm has enjoyed a long medicinal history. The aerial parts have many reputed actions. As one of the primary nervines, it is commonly used for conditions arising from situations of nervous tension.[1, 4] Given its reputation as a gentle herbal product, it is considered particularly well-suited to pediatric conditions.

Constituents [1-3, 5]

- Volatile oils (0.1-0.2%): citral a and b, caryophyllene oxide, citronellal, geraniol, linalool, nerol
- Flavonoids including: isoquercetrin, apigenin-7-O-glucoside, rhamnocitrin, luteolin-7-O-glucoside
- Henylpropanoids including: triterpenoids, rosmarinic acid
- Miscellaneous: tannins, ursolic acid, caffeic acid, and polyphenolic agents

THERAPEUTIC USES & RELEVANT PHARMACOLOGY

COMMON USES

Lemon balm is reputed to have sedative,[1, 6, 7] antispasmodic,[1, 2, 6-8] carminative,[1, 6-8] antiemetic,[4, 7] antimicrobial,[4] antihormonal and diaphoretic properties.[1, 4, 7]

Oral consumption is considered useful in the treatment of anxiety, insomnia, colds/fevers and digestive upset (bloating). It is considered by many to be especially useful as a children's remedy.[1, 4] Topically lemon balm is effective in the treatment of cold sores. Inhalation of the essential oil is reputed to have a direct influence on the nervous system, instilling calmness and improving mood.[4, 7] It is particularly well-suited to the management of conditions, often cardiac or digestive, where the etiology has a psychological component.[1, 6]

NERVOUS SYSTEM

A lyophilized hydroalcoholic extract of *Melissa officinalis* has been shown to exert hypnotic and peripheral analgesic activity in mice.[9] A German trial demonstrated that a combination herbal product containing valerian (160mg/tablet) and lemon balm (80mg/tablet) promoted sleep (1 tablet at bedtime) as effectively as triazolam 0.125mg (Halcion®) at a similar regimen.[10] It should be noted that valerian has a long established hypnotic action of its own. This combination product did not influence concentration or induce daytime sedation[10, 11] and did not potentiate the effects of alcohol.[11]

ANTIMICROBIAL

The essential oil fraction of *Melissa officinalis* exerts an antimicrobial action *in vitro* against a variety of bacteria and fungi.[2, 12] In addition, antiviral properties of *Melissa officinalis* have been demonstrated on many occasions.[13-16] The active constituents appear to be primarily the polyphenols and tannins.[16, 17] Most interest has been focused on the action of *Melissa officinalis* in the management of herpes simplex infections. In a recent multi-center clinical study (n=115) and subsequent placebo controlled double-blind study (n=116), the topical application of 1% dried extract of lemon balm appeared effective in the management of herpes simplex. Improvement of symptoms was noted by day 2 of the treatment and the test agent was considered superior to placebo by both physicians and patients. For optimum results the authors suggest that treatment be started at the onset of the infection.[15]

ENDOCRINE

Extracts of *Melissa officinalis* have long been documented to possess antithyrotropic activities.[2, 18, 19] Aqueous extracts contain components, notably certain phenolic agents, that inhibit the extrathyroidal metabolism of both T3 and T4 in a dose related manner.[18] *In vitro* studies have demonstrated that a freeze-dried extract of *Melissa officinalis* inhibits the binding, in a dose dependent manner, of thyroid stimulating hormone (TSH) to thyroid membrane. It was hypothesized that components present in the freeze-dried extract interacted with TSH preventing its binding to the membrane bound TSH receptor.[20] In addition, components of the freeze-dried extract of *Melissa officinalis* inhibited the binding of immunoglobulin G found in Grave's disease to TSH receptors.[21] This may in part support the historical use of lemon balm in the management of some thyroid conditions.[21]

Freeze dried extracts of *Melissa officinalis* that demonstrate the above antithyrotropic properties also possess antigonadotropic characteristics preventing the binding of human chorionic gonadotrophin (HCG) to rat testis *in vitro.*[20]

MISCELLANEOUS

Antioxidant

Hydroalcoholic extracts of *Melissa officinalis* have been shown to possess antioxidant properties, thought in part to be due to the presence of rosmarinic acid.[22]

Anti-inflammatory

Rosmarinic acid isolated from *Melissa officinalis* has been shown to influence complement activity. This may be explained in part by its ability to inhibit the action of C3-convertase[23] and C5 convertase.[24] Studies in animal models suggest that rosmarinic acid also exerts an anti-inflammatory action in complement-dependent inflammatory processes.[23]

ADVERSE EFFECTS

No examples of unpleasant adverse effects could be found for this phytomedicine.

CAUTIONS/CONTRAINDICATIONS

While no specific examples could be found, lemon balm should be used cautiously in patients with thyroid conditions. Safety in pregnancy has not been established. Lemon balm appears to have no mutagenic properties.[25]

DRUG INTERACTIONS

While no clinical examples could be found, products containing lemon balm may interact with conventional thyroid medications.

A lyophilized hydroalcoholic extract of *Melissa officinalis* has been noted to promote the hypnotic action of pentobarbital in mice.[9]

DOSAGE REGIMEN

Oral:

- 1-4g taken three times daily, as an infusion or in a comparable dosage for a tincture or fluid extract.[1]

Topical:

- Concentrated extract (70:1) applied 2 to 4 times daily in the management of cold sores.[15]

Since Lemon Balm is rich in volatile oils, infusions should be made in a closed container.[6]

REFERENCES

1. Mills S. *The Essential Book of Herbal Medicine.* 2nd ed. London: Penguin; 1991:677.
2. Leung A, Foster S. *Encyclopedia of Common Natural Ingredients Used in Food, Drugs and Cosmetics.* 2nd ed. New York, NY: John Wiley and Sons; 1996:649.
3. Wren R. *Potter's New Encyclopaedia of Botanical Drugs and Preparations.* Saffron Walden: C.W Daniel Company; 1988:362.
4. Bove M. *An Encyclopedia of Natural Healing for Children and Infants.* New Canaan, CT: Keats; 1996:303.
5. Mulkens A. Flavonoids of the leaves of *Melissa officinalis* L. *Pharmaceutica Acta Helvetiae*. 1987;62(1):19-22.
6. Weiss R. *Herbal Medicine.* 6th ed. Gothenburg, Sweden: AB Arcanum; 1988:362.
7. Hoffmann D. *Holistic Herbal.* Rockport, CA: Element Books; 1996:256.
8. Chevallier A. *The Encyclopedia of Medicinal Plants.* London: Reader's Digest; 1996:336.
9. Soulimani R, Fleurentin J, Mortier F, *et al.* Neurotropic action of the hydroalcoholic extract of *Melissa officinalis* in the mouse. *Planta Medica*. 1991;57(2):105-9.
10. Dressing H, Riemann D, *et al.* Insomnia: Are valerian/balm combination of equal value to benzodiazepine? *Therapiewoche*. 1992;42:726-36.
11. Albrect M, Berger W. Psychopharmaceuticals and safety in traffic. *Zeits Allegmeinmed*. 1995;71:1215-221.
12. Larrondo JV, Agut M *et al.* Antimicrobial activity of essences from labiates. *Microbios*. 1995;82(332):171-2.
13. Kucera L, Cohen R, Herrmann E. Antiviral activites of extracts of the Lemon balm plant. *Annals of the New York Academy of Sciences*. 1965;130(1):474-82.
14. Kucera L, E H. Antiviral substances in plants of the mint family (labiatae).I. Tannin of *Melissa officinalis*. *Proceedings of the Society for Experimental Biology and Medicine*. 1967;124(3):865-9.
15. Wobling R, Leonhardt K. Local therapy of herpes simplex with dried extract from *Melissa officinalis*. *Phytomedicine*. 1994;1(1):25-31.
16. Dimitrova Z, Dimov B, Manolova N, *et al.* Antiherpes effect of *Melissa officinalis* L. extracts. *Acta Microbiologica Bulgarica*. 1993;29:65-72.
17. Foster S. Clinical assessment of *Melissa officinalis* (lemon balm) in herpes treatment. *Quarterly Review of Natural Medicine*. 1995;3(2):3-5.
18. Auf'molk M, Köhrle J, Gumbinger H, *et al.* Antihormonal effects of plant extracts: Iodothyronine deiodinase of rat liver is inhibited by extracts and secondary metabolites of plants. *Hormone and Metabolic Research*. 1984;16(4):188-92.
19. Brinker F. Inhibition of endocrine function by botanical agents. *Journal of Naturopathic Medicine*. 1990;1(1):10-18.

20. Auf'mkolk M, Ingbar JC, Amir SM, *et al.* Inhibition by certain plant extracts of the binding and adenylate cyclase stimulatory effect of bovine thyrotropin in human thyroid membranes. *Endocrinology*. 1984;115(2):527-34.
21. Auf'mkolk M, Ingbar J, Kubota K, *et al.* Extracts and auto-oxidized constituents of certain plants inhibit the receptor-binding and the biological activity of Graves' immunoglobulin. *Endocrinology*. 1985;116(5):1687-93.
22. Lamaison J, Petitjean-Freytet C, Carnat A. Medicinal Laminaceae with antioxidant properties, a potential source of rosmarinic acid. *Pharmaceutica Acta Helvetiae*. 1991;66(7):185-8.
23. Englberger W, Hadding V, Etschenberg E, *et al.* Rosmarinic acid: A new inihibitor of complement C3-convertase with anti-inflammatory activity. *International Journal of Immunopharmacology*. 1988;10(6):729-37.
24. Peake P, Pussell BA, Martyn D, *et al.* The inhibitory effect of rosmarinic acid on complement involves the C5 convertase. *International Journal of Immunology*. 1991;13(7):853-7.
25. Ramos Ruiz A, De la Toree R, Alonso N, A V, *et al.* Screening of medicinal plants for induction of somatic segregation activity in *Aspergillus nidulans*. *Journal of Ethnopharmacology*. 1996;52(3):123-127.

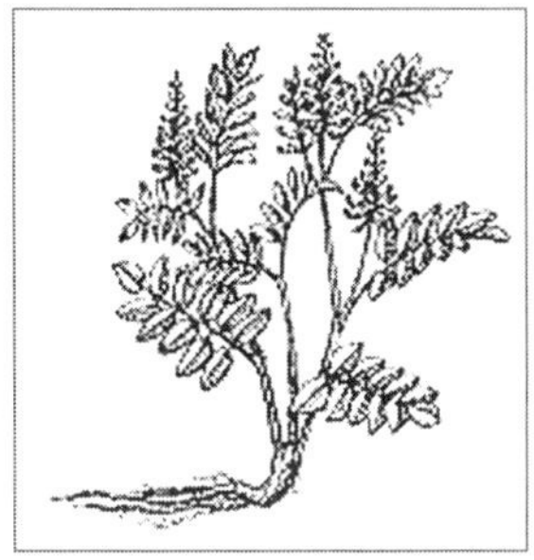

LICORICE

Glycyrrhiza glabra L.

THUMBNAIL SKETCH

Active Constituents

- Glycyrrhizin, glycyrrhetinic acid

Common Uses

- Inflammation of the GI tract (e.g., peptic and duodenal ulcers, gastritis)
- Inflammation of the skin (e.g., oral herpes lesions, canker sores)
- Productive coughs/bronchitis
- Adrenocorticoid insufficiency (e.g., due to stress and overwork)
- Sweetening and flavouring agent

Adverse Effects

- Pseudoaldosteronism which presents as hypernatremia, hypokalemia, hypertension, headache, edema, lethargy, and can lead to congestive heart failure

Cautions/Contraindications

- Caution recommended in patients with pre-existing cardiovascular disease, and liver or kidney dysfunction; safety in pregnancy has not been established.

Drug Interactions

- Increases the half-life of hydrocortisone and prednisolone; possible interactions with medications whose action is closely linked to potassium levels including cardiac glycosides, and both loop and potassium-sparing diuretics

Doses

- Powdered root: 1-4 g daily in three divided doses
- Solid (dry powdered) extract (4:1): 250-500 mg daily in three divided doses
- Deglycyrrhizinated licorice tablets: 380-1,140 mg (1-3 chewable tablets) three times daily

INTRODUCTION

Family: Fabaceae (also known as Leguminosae)

Synonyms:[1-4] Liquorice, Glycyrrhiza, Sweet wood, Liquiritiae, Glycyrrhizae radix

Licorice is a small (1-2 m in height) perennial shrub which grows in temperate regions. The roots and underground horizontal stems called rhizomes or stolons are the parts used medicinally.[3, 5] Licorice has been used medicinally for over 4000 years.[1] Historically it was used as an expectorant, an antitussive and a mild laxative.[5] It is also a very important herb within Traditional Chinese Medicine where its uses include treating peptic ulcers, asthma, and malaria.[6] Within Traditional Chinese Medicine, licorice (*Glycyrrhiza uralensis* Fisch. In DC.[7]) is considered to be a sweet, neutral herb which clears phlegm and tonifies the spleen.

Although licorice has significant pharmacological actions, it is often added to botanical formulations because of its distinctive flavor and its sweetening action: glycyrrhizin is 50 to 100 times sweeter than sucrose.[5, 6, 8] The amount of licorice in products varies dramatically.[9, 10] Most of the licorice candy available in North America is flavored not with licorice, but with anise oil.[11] One study found that authentic licorice candy contained between 0.26 mg/g and 7.9 mg/g of glycyrrhizin; while medicinal products ranged from 0.30 mg/g to 47.1 mg/g of glycyrrhizin.[9] In addition, licorice flavoured chewing tobacco contained between 1.5 mg/g to 4.1 mg/g of glycyrrhizin.[9]

Constituents[1, 3, 5, 12, 13]

- Terpenoids: glycyrrhizin (also called glycyrrhizic or glycyrrhizinic acid) which yields glycyrrhetinic acid (also called glycyrrhetic or glycyrretic acid) and glucuronic acid after hydrolysis; glycyrrhetol, glabrolide, licoric acid, liquiritic acid
- Flavonoids and isoflavonoids including: isoflavonol, kumatakenin, licoricone, glabrol, formononetin, chalcone and chalcone derivatives including isoliquiritigenin, licochalcone A and B
- Coumarins: umbelliferone, herniarin, glycyrin, liqcoumarin
- Volatile oils including: anethole, benzaldehyde, cumic alcohol, eugenol, fenchone
- Miscellaneous: acetylsalicylic acid, salicylic acid, methylsalicylate

THERAPEUTIC USES & RELEVANT PHARMACOLOGY

PHARMACOLOGY

The pharmacology of licorice has been extensively studied and several good reviews discuss this in detail.[1, 4, 14-18] In summary, glycyrrhizin inhibits three enzymes: two (15-hydroxyprostaglandin dehydrogenase and delta13 - prostaglandin reductase) are involved in the metabolism of two prostaglandins (E and F2a) and the third, which is found primarily in the kidneys and liver (11 beta-hydroxysteroid dehydrogenase) catalyzes the production of cortisone (inactive) from cortisol (active).[2, 19, 20] Thus, corticosteroid receptors become increasingly activated by cortisol, which may result in hypertension. In addition, glycyrrhizin and glycyrrhetinic acid bind weakly to mineralocorticoid and glucocorticoid receptors;[14, 20, 21] influences aldosterone secretion and elimination;[14, 22] suppress plasma renin activity;[17, 23] and decrease angiotensin levels.[16] Licorice has also been shown to increase atrial natriuretic peptide (ANP) and decrease vasopressin levels.[24]

Licorice is considered a "phytoestrogen," that is the steroid-like configuration of several of the components of licorice including the isoflavones and glycyrrhetinic acid, have the ability to influence estrogen metabolism. Generally, if estrogen levels are high, these constituents inhibit estrogen action by binding to the estrogen receptors and blocking the binding of endogenous estrogen. However, if estrogen levels are low, they appear to potentiate the action of estrogen. For this reason it is often referred to as being "amphoteric" (partial agonist) in nature. Phytoestrogens have between 1/20 and 1/100 the action of estrogen.[5, 12]

Pharmacokinetics

Peak serum concentration of glycyrrhizin occurs approximately 4 hours after ingestion, but varies widely among individuals ingesting the same amount of glycyrrhizin. In contrast, glycyrrhetinic acid levels peak at approximately 24 hours. Glycyrrhizin serum concentration decreases quickly and is no longer detectable by 96 hours. Glycyrrhetinic acid levels decrease more slowly.[3, 25] Consumption of 100 to 200 g licorice daily will result in plasma concentrations of glycyrrhetinic acid of 80 to 480 ng/mL.[19] It appears that the bioavailability (i.e. intestinal absorption) of glycyrrhizin is higher when it is consumed alone than when it is consumed as a constituent of licorice root or licorice root extract,[26-28] but it does not appear to be influenced by the presence of food.[3, 29] Glycyrrhizin is excreted mainly (80%) by the liver into the bile by a process which can become saturated.[30]

GASTROINTESTINAL EFFECTS

Perhaps one of the most well-known uses for licorice is its use in gastrointestinal conditions. Licorice has been used to treat dyspepsia for centuries. In fact, two pharmaceutical products, deglycyrrhizinated licorice and carbenoxolone, have been available since the mid-1960s, both of which enhance the body's ability to protect the gastrointestinal lining in a variety of ways including: "increasing the number of mucous-secreting cells (thereby increasing the amount of protective mucosubstances secreted); improving the protective nature mucous produced; increasing the life span of the surface intestinal cells; and enhancing the microcirculation of the gastrointestinal tract lining." This mechanism of action is described in detail elsewhere.[31]

Carbenoxolone

This derivative of glycyrrhetinic acid has been marketed for the treatment of both duodenal and gastric ulcers. Although its exact mechanism of action has not yet been elucidated, it appears to increase synthesis and secretion of mucus. Although efficacy studies have reported conflicting results, one study showed that maintenance therapy of carbenoxolone decreased the recurrence rate of gastric ulcers significantly more than either antacids or a placebo.[1] Several randomized, double-blind, controlled trials have demonstrated that carbenoxolone is also more effective than placebo in the treatment of duodenal ulcers.[1] No information could be found comparing the effects of carbenoxolone with standard combination antibiotic therapy used in the management of peptic ulcer disease. Carbenoxolone is rarely used today because its adverse effects include water retention, as well as increased blood pressure. This will be discussed in detail in the Adverse Effects section of this monograph.

Deglycyrrhizinated Licorice (DGL)

Deglycyrrhicinated licorice or DGL was developed in an attempt to reduce the adverse effects, which are largely caused by the glycyrrhizin content of licorice products. DGL has a glycyrrhizin content of < 3% [1] and no known adverse effects.[5] Although the active constituent of DGL has not been identified, it is believed to be a spasmolytic agent.[1] The majority of randomized, placebo-controlled trials of DGL tested a specific product currently only available in Europe called Caved-S®, which is a chewable tablet. Another European brand, Ulcedal®, which was available in capsule form (it has since been removed from the market) appeared to be ineffective, leading some researchers to hypothesize that DGL must mix with saliva to be effective.[5] One study (n=100) reported that DGL (760 mg three times daily between meals) had comparable efficacy to cimetidine (200 mg three times daily and 400 mg at bedtime) in its ability to increase the healing rate of gastric ulcers.[32] This study also found no significant difference in ulcer recurrence after one year when they compared maintenance therapy of DGL (760 mg twice daily) and cimetidine (400 mg at bedtime).[32] In addition, DGL has been shown to be equivalent to ranitidine in treatment of gastric ulcers.[33]

Several studies also report the effectiveness of DGL in the treatment of duodenal ulcers.[34, 35] One (n=40) showed that both 3 g DGL daily for 8 weeks and 4.5 g daily for 16 weeks provided substantial improvement in most patients within 5 to 7 days; however, the higher dose was reported to be significantly more effective.[34] A second study (n=874) reported no significant difference in the rate of healing at 12 weeks between patients treated with DGL (380 mg three times daily), antacids (15 mL suspension of aluminum-magnesium hydroxide equivalent to 3 g/day) or cimetidine (200 mg three times daily and 400 mg at bedtime).[35]

ANTI-INFECTIVE AGENT

Anti-viral

Several studies have found evidence of licorice's antiviral activity.[36, 37] *In vitro* studies document the ability of glycyrrhizin to directly inhibit the growth of several different viruses including: herpes simplex,[36, 38, 39] herpes genitalis and herpes zoster,[40] influenza virus A2,[37] hepatitis A virus[41] and HIV.[38, 42, 43] In addition, both glycyrrhizin and glycyrrhetinic acid have been reported to induce the production of interferon.[44]

A few clinical studies have been conducted which indicate that the topical application of glycyrrhetinic acid or its derivatives decreases the pain and increases the rate of healing of oral and genital herpes lesions.[45-47]

Anti-bacterial/Anti-fungal

Extracts of licorice have been shown *in vitro* to inhibit the growth of a variety of bacteria and fungi including: *Candida albicans*, *Staphylococcus aureus*, *Streptococcus mutans* and *Mycobacterium smegmatis*.[48] The isoflavonoid components appear to be the components responsible for this action. One study found that they had *in vitro* activity comparable to streptomycin against *Staphylococcus aureus*, *Mycobacterium smegmatis* and *Candida albicans*.[1]

Anti-parasitic

Licochalcone A, a component of licorice, has been shown to inhibit both chloroquine-susceptible and chloroquine-resistant strains of *Plasmodium falciparum*[49] and *Leishmania* major and *Leishmanian donovani* promastigotes and amastigotes[50, 51] *in vitro*.

ANTI-INFLAMMATORY AND ANTI-ALLERGIC ACTIVITY

The cortisol-like action of licorice confers an ability to inhibit the formation and secretion of inflammatory compounds. A recent study suggests that glycyrrhetinic acid may also have a direct anti-inflammatory action by selectively inhibiting the classical complement cascade (it has no affect on the alternative pathway).[52] In addition, a recent study reported that glycyrrhizin is a selective inhibitor of thrombin (however it did not effect the clotting activity of thrombin), which may be another mechanism of action for its anti-inflammatory activity.[53] Glycyrrhizin has been shown to inhibit allergenic reactions produced under controlled experimental conditions.[5]

HEPATOPROTECTIVE ACTIVITY

The role of licorice in liver disease is reviewed in detail by Hikino and Kiso.[54] Intravenous administration of glycyrrhizin is used in the treatment of hepatitis in Japan.[55, 56] This indication is supported by several double-blind, controlled studies which have reported that glycyrrhizin is an effective treatment in the management of viral hepatitis.[57] It has been hypothesized that glycyrrhizin may bind to hepatocytes, modifying the expression of hepatitis B virus (HBV) antigens on their surface, thus suppressing their sialylation.[55, 58]

In addition, several *in vitro* studies indicate that glycyrrhizin may protect the liver from damage caused by chemical toxins such as CCl_4 (carbon tetrachloride).[59] The mechanism of action for this is hypothesized to be an inhibition of the cytochrome P-450 system conversion of CCl_4 to CCl_3.

MISCELLANEOUS

Premenstral Syndrome (PMS)

PMS symptoms have been associated with an increased estrogen:progesterone ratio. Phytoestrogens such as licorice are thought to be useful in decreasing the symptoms associated with PMS.[5]

Canker Sores

Licorice has been reported to decrease the pain and speed the healing rate of canker sores in the mouth.[5] One double-blind, cross-over trial (n=24) reported that a mouth wash containing glycyrrhetinic acid reduced the pain associated with mouth ulcers, as well as significantly decreasing the number of new ulcers which developed.[60]

Expectorant/Anti-tussive

Although the mechanism of action has not yet been elucidated, licorice has a long historical use as an expectorant and antitussive.[3, 61] Its use for these indications continues to be widespread in North America today.[2, 6]

Protection from Diabetic Complications

Many diabetic complications improve with the addition of inhibitors of aldose reductase (the first enzyme in the polyol pathway) to the therapeutic regimen.[12, 62, 63] Isoliquiritigenin, a component of licorice has been shown *in vitro* and *in vivo* to inhibit aldose reductase, thus decreasing the conversion of glucose to sorbitol and inhibiting sorbitol accumulation.[12, 62, 63]

Use in Burn Victims

Glycyrrhizin has been shown to decrease the generation of burn-associated suppressor T cells (BTs cells) in thermally injured mice. Other reports have found an increasing incidence of septic infections with an increased number of BTs cells. The authors hypothesize that glycyrrhizin may play a role in the future treatment of burns.[64, 65]

Anti-cancer

A variety of compounds in licorice have been shown to have anti-mutagenic activity and to decrease the growth of some cancer cell lines *in vitro*.[66, 67] The clinical significance of these findings is unknown.

Anti-fatigue

Licorice is considered by some medical herbalists to be an adrenocorticotrophic agent (tonic to the adrenal glands). Consequently, it is used in the management of stress and fatigue.

ADVERSE EFFECTS

Licorice is considered safe in low doses; however, adverse effects are common at doses of more than 20 g of licorice root daily. Adverse symptoms have also been seen in doses significantly lower than this.[3] Because the adverse effects appear at widely differing doses in different individuals,[12, 14, 68] it is important to monitor patients. The adverse effects most commonly experienced are mineralocorticoid-related including: headache, lethargy, sodium and water retention, excessive excretion of potassium, hypokalemic myopathy,[12, 69, 70] and high blood pressure.[2, 12] Because of the low serum potassium, cardiac arrhythmias and ECG abnormalities may also occur.[3] Together these constitute what has been called pseudo(hyper)aldosteronism. Spironolactone will reverse these adverse effects.[3] Amenorrhea and hyperprolactemia (possibly resulting in infertility) have also been reported.[71, 72]

Several deaths have resulted from the ingestion of licorice products.[3, 73] Most often these adverse effects are caused by the consumption of large amounts of licorice candy and/or in those with pre-existing cardiovascular or renal impairment.[3, 74] One much-quoted case of severe congestive heart failure and pulmonary edema occurred when a 53-year-old man ate 700 g of licorice candy over 8 days.[75] Another study reports on the successful treatment of a 63-year-old patient with severe postural hypotension.[76]

Chandler suggests that a maximum of 10 mg of glycyrrhizin (approximately 5 g of authentic licorice candy) can be safely consumed daily over long periods.[3] The Dutch Nutrition Information Bureau suggests that no more than 200 mg of glycyrrhizin should be consumed daily.[3]

Deglycyrrhizinated licorice (DGL) does not appear to cause the adverse effects described above.[3]

CAUTIONS/CONTRAINDICATIONS

Caution should be used in patients with high blood pressure or any other existing cardio-vascular disorders, renal failure, and liver disease.[3-5, 12] Safety in pregnancy has been questioned.[3, 4, 12]

DRUG INTERACTIONS

Licorice may interfere with hormonal therapy or hypoglycemic therapy.[12] For example, Chandler hypothesizes that glycyrrhizin may combine with insulin to cause increased electrolyte disturbances.[3] Newall suggests that potential for interaction exists with any drugs with a narrow therapeutic index or mechanism of action dependent upon potassium levels (e.g., cardiac glycosides, loop diuretics and potassium-sparing diuretics).

Glycyrrhetinic acid increases the half-life of hydrocortisone applied topically,[77] and also potentiates the action of hydrocortisone in lung tissue.[78] There are also several reports that oral administration of glycyrrhizin inhibits the metabolism of prednisolone, thus increasing plasma concentations.[79]

DGL (deglycyrrhizinated licorice) has been reported to increase the bioavailability of nitrofurantoin over 50% if they are administered together; however, it also appears to decrease feelings of nausea associated with nitrofurantoin ingestion.[3]

DOSAGE REGIMENS

- Powdered root: 1-4 g daily in three divided doses[5, 12]
- Fluid extract (1:1): 4-6 mL daily in three divided doses
- Solid (dry powdered) extract (4:1): 250-500 mg daily in three divided doses
- Deglycyrrhizinated licorice tablets: 380-1,140 mg (1-3 chewable tablets) three times daily[5]
- Licorice extract: 0.6-2 g daily[12]

Often prepared as a decoction: add 2-4 g (1 teaspoonful) of herb to 120 mL (1/2 cup) of boiling water and simmer for 5 minutes. Strain and drink this quantity three times daily after meals.[2]

Lozenges/candies as expectorant and cough suppressant (make sure they actually contain real licorice).[2]

Commission E has approved the indication for ulcer treatment (200 to 600 mg of glycyrrhizin daily) for a maximum of 4 to 6 weeks.[80]

REFERENCES

1. Chandler RF. Licorice, more than just a flavour. *Canadian Pharmaceutical Journal*. 1985;September:421-4.
2. Tyler VE. *Herbs of Choice. The Therapeutic Use of Phytomedicinals.* Binghamton, NY: Pharmaceutical Products Press; 1994:209.
3. Chandler RF. *Glycyrrhiza Glabra*. In: De Smet PAGM, Keller K, Hansel R, Chandler RF, eds. *Adverse Effects of Herbal Drugs*. Volume 3 ed. New York: Springer; 1997:67-87.
4. Snow JM. *Glycyrrhiza glabra* L. (Leguminaceae). *The Protocol Journal of Botanical Medicine*. 1996;1(3):9-14.
5. Murray MT. *The Healing Power of Herbs.* Rocklin, CA: Prima Publishing; 1992:246.
6. Leung A, Foster S. *Encyclopedia of Common Natural Ingredients Used in Food, Drugs and Cosmetics.* 2nd ed. New York, NY: John Wiley and Sons; 1996:649.
7. Foster S, Chongxi Y. *Herbal Emissaries. Bringing Chinese Herbs to the West*. Rochester, VT: Healing Arts Press; 1992:356.
8. Mizutani K, Kuramoto T, Tamura Y, *et al.* Sweetness of glycyrrhetic acid 3-O-beta-D-monoglucuronide and the related glycosides. *Bioscience, Biotechnology and Biochemistry.* 1994;58(3):554-5.
9. Spinks EA, Fenwick GR. The determinationof glycyrrhizin in selected UK liquorice products. *Food Additives and Contaminants*. 1990;7:769-78.
10. Stormer FC, Reistad R, Alexander J. Glycyrrhizic acid in liquorice — evaluation of health hazard. *Food and Chemical Toxicology*. 1993;31:303-312.
11. Tyler V. *The Honest Herbal.* 3rd ed. Binghamton, N.Y.: Pharmaceutical Products Press; 1993:375.
12. Newall CA, Anderson LA, Phillipson JD. *Herbal Medicines: A Guide For Health Care Professionals*. London: The Pharmaceutical Press; 1996:296.
13. Kitagawa I, Chen WZ, Hori K, *et al.* Chemical studies of Chinese licorice-roots. I. Elucidation of five new flavonoid

constituents from the roots of *Glycyrrhiza glabra* L. collected in Xinjiang. *Chemical and Pharmaceutical Bulletin (Tokyo)*.1994;42(5):1056-62.
14. Walker BR, Edwards CR. Licorice-induced hypertension and syndromes of apparent mineralocorticoid excess. *Endocrinology and Metabolism Clinics of North America.* 1994;23(2):359-77.
15. Shimojo M, Stewart PM. Apparent mineralocorticoid excess syndromes. *Journal of Endocrinological Investigation.* 1995;18(7):518-32.
16. Schambelan M. Licorice ingestion and blood pressure regulating hormones. *Steroids*. 1994;59(2):127-30.
17. Biglieri EG. My engagement with steroids: A review. *Steroids*. 1995;60(1):52-8.
18. White PC, Mune T, Agarwal AK. 11 beta-Hydroxysteroid dehydrogenase and the syndrome of apparent mineralo corticoid excess. *Endocrine Reveiws.* 1997;18(1):135-56.
19. Stewart PM, Wallace AM, Valentino R, *et al.* Mineralcorticoid activity of liquoirce: 11-Beta- hydroxysteroid dehydrogenase deficiency comes of age. *Lancet*. 1987;II:821-4.
20. Armanini D, Lewicka S, Pratesi C, *et al.* Further studies on the mechanism of the mineralocorticoid action of licorice in humans. *Journal of Endocrinological Investigation*. 1996;19(9):624-9.
21. Armanini D, Karbowiak I, Funder J. Affinity of glycyrrhetinic acid and its derivatives for mineralocorticoid and glucocorticoid receptors. *Clinical Endocrinology*. 1983;19:609-12.
22. Epstein M, Espiner E, Donald R, Hughes H. Effect of eating liquorice on the renin-angiotensin aldosterone axis in normal subjects. *British Medical Journal*. 1977;1:488-90.
23. Conn J, Rovner D, Cohen EL. Licorice-induced pseudoaldosteronism. Hypertension, hypokalaemia, aldosteroneopenia, and suppressed plasma renin activity. *Journal of the American Medical Association*. 1968;205:492-6.
24. Forslund T, Fyhrquist F, Froseth B, Tikkanen I. Effects of licorice on plasma atrial natriuretic peptide in healthy volunteers. *Journal of Internal Medicine*. 1989;225:95-99.
25. Krahenbuhl S, Hasler F, Frey BM, *et al*. Kinetics and dynamics of orally administered 18 beta-glycyrrhetinic acid in humans. *Journal of Clinical Endocrinology and Metabolism*. 1994;78(3):581-5.
26. Cantelli-Forti G, Maffei F, Hrelia P, *et al.* Interaction of licorice on glycyrrhizin pharmacokinetics. *Environmental Health Perspectives*. 1994;102(Suppl 9):65-8.
27. Raggi MA, Maffei F, Bugamelli F, Cantelli Forti G. Bioavailability of glycyrrhizin and licorice extract in rat and human plasma as detected by a HPLC method. *Pharmazie*. 1994;49(4):269-72.
28. Wang Z, Nishioka M, Kurosaki Y, *et al*. Gastrointestinal absorption characteristics of glycyrrhizin from glycyrrhiza extract. *Biological and Pharmaceutical Bulletin*. 1995;18(9):1238-41.
29. Nishioka Y, Kyotani S, Miyamura M, Kusunose M. Influence of time of administration of a Shosaiko-to extract granule on blood concentrations of its active constituents. *Chemical and Pharmaceutical Bulletin*. 1992;40:1335-7.
30. Ichikawa T, Ishida S, Sakiya Y, *et al.* Biliary excretion and enterohepatic cycling of glycyrrhizin in rats. *Journal of Pharmaceutical Science*. 1986;75:672-5.
31. Baker ME. Licorice and enzymes other than 11 beta-hydroxysteroid dehydrogenase: an evolutionary perspective. *Steroids*. 1994;59(2):136-41.
32. Morgan AG, McAdam WAF, Pacsoo C, Darnborough A. Comparison between cimetidine and Caved-S in the treatment of gastric ulceration, and subsequent maintenance therapy. *Gut*. 1982;23:545-51.
33. Glick L. Deglycyrrhizinated liquorice for peptic ulcer. *Lancet*. 1982;2:817.
34. Tewari SN, Wilson AK. Deglycyrrhizinated liquorice in duodenal ulcer. *Practitioner*. 1972;210:820-5.
35. Kassir ZA. Endoscopic controlled trial of four drug regimens in the treatment of chronic duodenal ulceration. *Irish Medical Journal*. 1985;78:153-6.
36. Pompei R, Pani A, Flore O, *et al*. Antiviral activity of glycyrrhizic acid. *Experientia*. 1980;36:304-5.
37. Utsunomiya T, Kobayashi M, Pollard RB, Suzuki F. Glycyrrhizin, an active component of licorice roots, reduces morbidity and mortality of mice infected with lethal doses of influenza virus. *Antimicrobial Agents and Chemotherapy*. 1997;41(3):551-6.
38. Hirabayashi K, Iwata S, Matsumoto H, *et al.* Antiviral activities of glycyrrhizin and its modified compounds against human immunodeficiency virus type 1 (HIV-1) and Herpes simplex virus type 1 (HSV-1) *in vitro*. *Chemical and Pharmaceutical Bulletin*. 1991;39:112-5.
39. Dargan DJ, Subak-Sharpe JH. The effect of triterpenoid compounds on uninfected and herpes simplex virus-infected cells in culture. I. Effect on cell growth, virus particles and virus replication. *Journal of General Virology.* 1985;66:1771-84.
40. Baba M, Shigeta S. Antiviral activity of glycyrrhizin against *varicella zoster* virus *in vitro*. *Antiviral Research*. 1987;7:999-107.
41. Crance JM, Biziagos E, Passagot J, *et al.* Inhibition of hepatitis A virus replication *in vitro* by antiviral com pounds. *Journal of Medical Virology*. 1990;31:155-160.
42. Hattori T, Ikematsu S, Koito A, *et al.* Preliminary evidence for inhibitory effect of glycyrrhizin on HIV replication in patients with AIDS. *Antiviral Research*. 1989;11:255-62.
43. Ito M, Sato A, Hirabayashi K, *et al.* Mechanism of inhibitory effect of glycyrrhizin on replication of human

immunodeficiency virus (HIV). *Antiviral Research*. 1988;10:289-98.
44. Abe N, Ebina T, Ishida N. Interferon induction by glycyrrhizin and glycyrrhetinic acid in mice. *Microbiology and Immunology*. 1982;26:535-9.
45. Partridge M, Poswillo D. Topical carbonoxolone sodium in the management of herpes simplex infection. *British Journal of Oral Maxillofacial Surgery*. 1984;22:138-45.
46. Csonka G, Tyrrell D. Treatment of herpes genitalis with carbonoxolone and cicloxolone creams: A double blind placebo controlled trial. *British Journal of Venereal Disease*. 1984;60:178-81.
47. Poswillo DE, Roberts GL. Topical carbenoxolone for orofacial herpes simplex infections. *Lancet*. 1981;2:142-144.
48. Mitscher L, Park Y, Clark D. Antimicrobial agents from higher plants. Antimicrobial isoflavonoids from glycyrrhiza glabra L. var. typica. *Journal of Natural Products*. 1980;43:259-69.
49. Chen M, Theander TG, Christensen SB, *et al*. Licochalcone A, a new antimalarial agent, inhibits *in vitro* growth of the human malaria parasite *Plasmodium falciparum* and protects mice from *P. yoelii* infection. *Antimicrobial Agents and Chemotherapy*. 1994;38(7):1470-5.
50. Chen M, Christensen SB, Blom J, *et al.* Licochalcone A, a novel antiparasitic agent with potent activity against human pathogenic protozoan species of Leishmania. *Antimicrobial Agents and Chemotherapy*.1993;37(12):2550-6.
51. Christensen SB, Ming C, Andersen L, *et al.* An antileishmanial chalcone from Chinese licorice roots. *Planta Medica*. 1994;60(2):121-3.
52. Kroes BH, Beukelman CJ, van den Berg AJ, *et al*. Inhibition of human complement by beta-glycyrrhetinic acid. *Immunology*. 1997;90(1):115-20.
53. Mauricio I, Francischetti B, Monteiro RQ, Guimaraes JA. Identification of glycyrrhizin as a thrombin inhibitor. *Biochemical and Biophysical Research Communications*. 1997;225:259-63.
54. Hikino H, Kiso Y. Natural products for liver diseases. *Economic and Medicinal Plant Research*. 1988;2:39-72.
55. Sato H, Goto W, Yamamura J, *et al.* Therapeutic basis of glycyrrhizin on chronic hepatitis B. *Antiviral Research*. 1996;30 (2-3):171-7.
56. Yamashiki M, Nishimura A, Suzuki H, *et al*. Effects of the Japanese herbal medicine "Sho-saiko-to" (TJ-9) on *in vitro* interleukin-10 production by peripheral blood mononuclear cells of patients with chronic hepatitis C. *Hepatology*. 1997;25(6):1390-7.
57. Suzuki H, Ohta Y, Takino T, Fugisawa Kea. Effects of glycyrrhizin on biochemical tests in patients with chronic hepatitis — Double blind trial. *Asian Medical Journal*. 1984;26:423-38.
58. Takahara T, Watanabe A, Shiraki K. Effects of glycyrrhizin on hepatitis B surface antigen: a biochemical and morphological study. *Journal of Hepatology*. 1994;21(4):601-9.
59. Kiso Y, Tohkin M, Hikino H, *et al.* Mechanism of antihepatotoxic activity of glycyrrhizin, I. effect on free radical generation and lipid peroxidation. *Planta Medica*. 1984;50:298-302.
60. Poswillo D, Partridge M. Management of recurrent aphthous ulcers. *British Dentistry Journal*. 1984;157:55-7.
61. Anderson DM, Smith WG. The antitussive activity of glycyrrhetinic acid and its derivatives. *Journal of Pharmacy and Pharmacology*. 1961;13:396-404.
62. Aida K, *et al.* Isoliquiritigenin: A new aldose reductase inhibitor from *Glycyrrhizae radix*. *Planta Medica*. 1990;56:254-8.
63. Yun-ping Z, Jia-qing Z. Oral baicalin and liquid extract of licorice reduce sorbital levels in red blood cells of diabetic rats. *Chinese Medical Journal*. 1989;102:203-6.
64. Kobayashi M, Schmitt DA, Utsunomiya T, *et al*. Inhibition of burn-associated suppressor cell generation by glycyrrhizin through the induction of contrasuppressor T cells. *Immunology and Cell Biology*. 1993;71(Pt 3):181-9.
65. Nakajima N, Utsunomiya T, Kobayashi M, *et al*. *In vitro* induction of anti-type 2 T cells by glycyrrhizin. *Burns*. 1996;22(8):612-7.
66. Zani F, Cuzzoni MT, Daglia M, *et al*. Inhibition of mutagenicity in Salmonella typhimurium by *Glycyrrhiza glabra* extract, glycyrrhizinic acid, 18 alpha- and 18 beta-glycyrrhetinic acids. *Planta Medica*. 1993;59(6):502-7.
67. Kitagawa K, Nishino H, Iwashima A. Inhibition of 12-0-tetradecanoylphorbol-13-acetate-stimulated 3-0-methyl-glucose transport in mouse Swiss 3T3 fibroblasts by glycyrrhetic acid. *Cancer Letters*. 1984;24:157-63.
68. Kato H, Kanaoka M, Yano S, Kobayashi M. 3-Monoglucuronyl-glycyrrhetinic acid is a major metabolite that causes licorice-induced pseudoaldosteronism. *Journal of Clinical Endocrinology and Metabolism*. 1995;80(6):1929-33.
69. Cibelli G, *et al.* Hypokalemic myopathy associated with liquorice ingestion. *Italian Journal of Neurological Science*. 1984;5:463-6.
70. Shintani S, Murase H, Tsukagoshi H, Shiigai T. Glycyrrhizin (licorice) — induced hypokalemic myopathy. *European Neurology*. 1992;32:44-51.
71. Corrocher R, *et al.* Pseudoprimary hyperaldosteronism due to liquorice intoxication. *European Review Med Pharmacol Sci*. 1983;5:467-70.
72. Werner S, Brismar K, Olsson S. Hyperprolactinemia and liquorice. *Lancet*. 1979;1:319.
73. Nielsen I, Pedersen RS. Life-threatening hypokalemia caused by liquorice ingestion. *Lancet*. 1984;1:1305.
74. Megia A, Herranz L, Martin-Almendra MA, Martinez I. Angiotensin I-converting enzyme levels and renin-aldosterone axis recovery after cessation of chronic licorice ingestion. [Letter]. *Nephron*. 1993;65(2):329-30.

75. Chamberlain TJ. Licorice poisoning, pseudoaldosteronism, heart failure. *Journal of the American Medical Association*. 1970;213:1343.
76. Basso A, Dalla Paola L, Erle G, *et al*. Licorice ameliorates postural hypotension caused by diabetic autonomic neuropathy. *Diabetes Care*. 1994;17(11):1356.
77. Teelucksingh S, Mackie ADR, Burt D, *et al.* Potentiation of hydrocortisone activity in skin by glycyrrhetinic acid. *Lancet*. 1990;335:1060-63.
78. Schleimer RP. Potential regulation of inflammation in the lung by local metabolism of hydrocortisone. *American Journal of Respiratory Cell and Molecular Biology*. 1991;4:166-73.
79. Chen M-F, Shimada F, Kato H, *et al*. Effect of oral administration of glycyrrhizin on the pharmacokinetics of prednisone. *Endocrinologica Japonica*. 1991;38:167-74.
80. Blumenthal M, Brusse WR, Goldberg A, *et al. The Complete German Commission E Monographs*. Austin, TX: American Botanical Council; 1998:685.

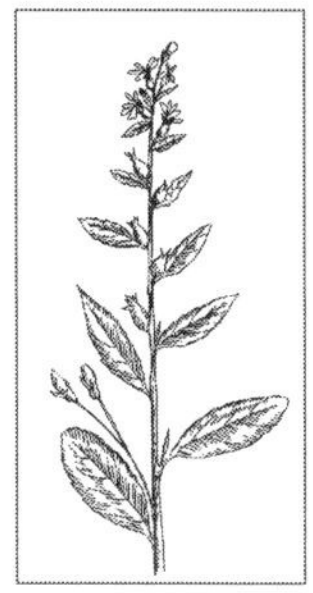

LOBELIA

Lobelia inflata L.

THUMBNAIL SKETCH

Active Constituents

- Piperidine alkaloids notably (-)- lobeline

Common Uses:

- Respiratory conditions such as bronchial asthma and bronchitis
- Tobacco addiction

Adverse Effects

- Nausea, vomiting, diarrhea, coughing and dizziness. Administration of high doses may result in more severe symptoms such as convulsions, hypothermia, coma and even death.

Cautions/Contraindications

- Situations where nicotine is contraindicated, cardiovascular and respiratory disease

Drug Interactions

- None found

Doses

- 0.2-0.6 g of dried herb three times daily
- 0.2-0.6 mL of liquid extract (1:1 in 50% alcohol) three times daily

INTRODUCTION

Family: Campanulaceae

Synonyms: Indian tobacco, Wild tobacco, Asthma weed, Gagroot, Emetic herb, Vomit wort, Puke weed[1-4]

Lobelia is a hairy annual or biennial indigenous to the western parts of North America. It produces pale blue flowers and is often found in acidic soils. While *Lobelia inflata* L.[2, 5] is the plant most common to herbal practice in North America and Western Europe, other members of this genus have a medicinal reputation in many other traditional healing models.[5] For example, in the Chinese Pharmacopoeia, *L. chinensis* Lour. is specified.[6]

Lobelia has a rather infamous medical history. It was used by peoples of the First Nations primarily for respiratory conditions and as an emetic and later became popular amongst the early settlers.[4, 5] Lobelia was also smoked in a similar fashion to tobacco, hence one of the synonyms, Indian tobacco.[5] One New England healer, Samuel Thomson, used it as one of his primary botanical medicines, naming it 'old #1.'[7] When one of his patients died after taking the herb, Thomson was charged (and later acquitted) with murder. Many still consider lobelia to be a poison rather than a medicine.[4]

Constituents[1, 2, 8, 9]

- Alkaloids: ≥14, notably of the piperidine type including (-)- lobeline (main one at 0.36-2.25% dry wt), lobelanine, norlobelanine, lobelanidine, norlobelanidine, lelobanidine, lobinine and isolobinine.
- Miscellaneous: lobelacrin (a bitter glycoside), chelidonic acid, beta- amyrin palmitate, resins and gums.

THERAPEUTIC USES & RELEVANT PHARMACOLOGY

COMMON USES

Lobelia is considered to have expectorant,[5] diaphoretic,[5, 10] emetic,[5, 10] antispasmodic,[5, 10] sedative,[10] and respiratory stimulant properties.[5, 10] It is primarily used for conditions of the respiratory tract, such as bronchial asthma and bronchitis.[5, 10, 11] Expectorant and decongestant drugs containing lobelia are available in Canada.[12] External applications of lobelia have been used to relieve muscle spasm and tension.[5] Indian tobacco is also used in the treatment of tobacco addition.[5] Commercial cigarette smoking deterrents containing lobelia herb are available in Canada[12] and Europe,[6] while the purified alkaloidal salts, lobeline hydrochloride or lobeline sulphate, are marketed for this purpose in several other countries (but not in Canada).[6, 12] Its use as an emetic seems primarily to be an historical one.

PHARMACOLOGY

The medicinal action of lobelia appears to be primarily due to lobeline's nicotinic properties. The exact action of lobeline at the nicotine receptor site appears complex and novel.[13, 14] Lobeline is known to cause stimulation of the central nervous system followed by severe respiratory depression. Administration in a number animal studies has resulted in bronchoconstriction, while bronchodilation was also reported in guinea pigs.[15] A proposed explanation for these differing results is that guinea pigs are particularlly sensitive to adrenergic bronchodilating agents.[15] Bronchodilation resulting from adrenal stimulation has also been reported.[16]

Animal studies suggest that lobeline acts as a cardiovascular stimulant, causing sympathetically mediated hypertension as well as parasympathetically mediated bradycardia.[17] Lobeline has also been shown to inhibit intestinal motility in dogs.[15] Vomiting commonly seen with lobeline use, is centrally mediated.[16] An antidepressant action has been reported in mice following administration of beta-amyrin palmitate extracted from *Lobelia inflata* L.

A number of human clinical trials of lobeline, either alone or combined with other substances, have reported that it is effective in the treatment of tobacco addition.[18-21]

It is important to note that no clinical trials could be found in which the action of the herb lobelia, rather than the alkaloid lobeline, was investigated.

ADVERSE EFFECTS

Adverse effects are similar to those of nicotine and include nausea, vomiting, diarrhea, coughing and dizziness. Administration of high doses may result in more severe symptoms, such as convulsions, hypothermia, coma and even death.[1] Many practitioners comment that the plant's emetic properties limit the potential for serious adverse effects.[22] Tyler does not recommend use of the crude herb due to the lack of standardized products and the relatively high risk to benefit ratio.[23]

A case of death following inhalation of an herbal asthma product containing lobeline (together with stramonium) in a 48-year-old asthmatic female has been documented.[24] It should be noted that stramonium (*Datura stramonium* L., Solanaceae) is a plant rich in alkaloids with a very high potential for toxicity.

CAUTIONS/CONTRAINDICATIONS

Lobelia should be used with caution by patients with cardiovascular disease, respiratory conditions and where nicotine is contraindicated. It should be considered contraindicated in pregnancy and lactation.[1]

DRUG INTERACTIONS

No clinical cases of drug interactions could be found. Given the pharmacological action of lobeline, this herb should be used cautiously with conventional medication in general.

DOSAGE REGIMEN

- 0.2-0.6 g of dried herb three times daily [1]
- 0.2-0.6 mL of liquid extract (1:1 in 50% alcohol) three times daily[1]

Given its potential for adverse effects, it is questionable whether lobelia is appropriate for self-medication

REFERENCES

1. Newall C, Anderson L, Phillipson J. *Herbal Medicines: A Guide for Health Care Professionals*. London: The Pharmaceutical Press; 1996:296.
2. Leung A, Foster S. *Encyclopedia of Common Natural Ingredients Used in Food, Drugs and Cosmetics.* 2nd ed. New York, NY: John Wiley and Sons; 1996:649.
3. Wren R. *Potter's New Encyclopedia of Botanical Drugs and Preparations.* Saffron Walden: CW Daniel Company; 1988:362.
4. Micheletti E, Winterberg A, Humbert G, *et al.*. *North American Folk Healing*. Westmount, QC: Reader's Digest; 1998:408.
5. Chevallier A. *The Encyclopedia of Medicinal Plants*. London: Reader's Digest; 1996:336.
6. Reynolds J. *Martindale: The Extra Pharmacopoeia.* 13th ed. London: The Pharmaceutical Press; 1993:2363.
7. Saunders P. Personal Communication; 1998.
8. Subarnas A, Tadano T, Nakahata N, *et al.* A possible mechanism of antidepressant activity of beta-amyrin palmitate isolated from Lobelia inflata leaves in the forced swimming test. *Life Sciences*. 1993;52(3):289-96.
9. Krochmal A, Wilken L, Chien M. Lobeline content of four Appalachian lobelias. *Lloydia*. 1972;35(3):303-4.
10. Hoffman D. *Holistic Herbal.* Rockport, CA: Element Books; 1996:256.
11. Mills S. *The Essential Book of Herbal Medicine*. London: Penguin; 1991:677.
12. Canada H. Drug Product Database, Ottawa: Health Canada; 1998.
13. Damaj MI, Patrick GS, Creasy KR, Martin BR. Pharmacology of lobeline, a nicotinic receptor ligand. *Journal of Pharmacology & Experimental Therapeutics*. 1997;282(1):410-9.
14. Rao TS, Correa LD, Lloyd GK. Effects of lobeline and dimethylphenylpiperazinium iodide (DMPP) on N-methyl-D-aspartate (NMDA)-evoked acetylcholine release *in vitro*: Evidence for a lack of involvement of classical neuronal nicotinic acetyl choline receptors. *Neuropharmacology*. 1997;36(1):39-50.
15. Cambar P, Shore S, Aviado D. Bronchopulmonary and gastrointestinal effects of lobeline. *Archives Internationoves de Pharmacodynamie et de Therapie*. 1969;177(1):1-27.
16. Murray M. *The Healing Power of Herbs.* 2nd ed. Rocklin, CA: Prima Publishing; 1995:410.
17. Korczyn AD, Bruderman I, Braun K. Cardiovascular effects of lobeline. *Archives Internationales de Pharmacodynamie et de Therapie*. 1969;182(2):370-5.
18. Becker L. Helping patients quit smoking. *Journal of Family Practice*. 1998;46(3):195-6.
19. Plakun A, Ambrus J, Bross I, Graham S, Levin M, Ross C. Clinical factors in smoking withdrawal: Preliminary report. *American Journal of Public Health.* 1966;56(3):434-441.
20. Ross C. Smoking withdrawal research clinics. *American Journal of Public Health*. 1967;57(4):677-681.
21. Ford S, Ederer F. Breaking the cigarette habit. *Journal of the Amerian Medical Association*. 1965;194(2):119-122.
22. Willard T. *Wild Rose Scientific Herbal*. Calgary, AB: Wild Rose College of Natural Healing; 1991:416.
23. Tyler V. *Herbs of Choice. The Therapeutic Use of Phytomedicinals.* Binghamton, NY: Pharmaceutical Products Press; 1994:209.
24. McLaren G. Sudden death in asthma. *British Medical Journal*. 1968;4(628):456.

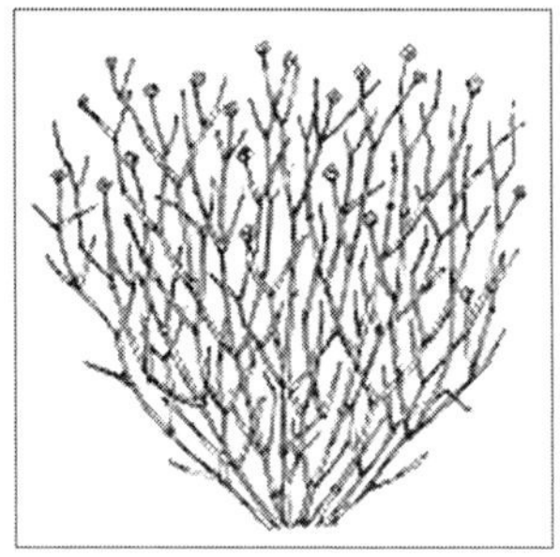

MA HUANG

Ephedra sinica Stapf.

THUMBNAIL SKETCH

Active Constituents

- Alkaloids including ephedrine and pseudoephedrine

Common Uses

- Diseases of the respiratory tract including asthma and bronchitis
- Weight loss

Adverse Effects:

- Dizziness, headache, insomnia, decreased appetite, gastrointestinal distress, tachycardia, sweating, hypertension, psychosis, stroke, seizures and death

Cautions/Contraindications

- Heart disease, hypertension, thyroid disease, diabetes, prostate conditions, anxiety, glaucoma,
- Impaired cerebral circulation, pheochromocytoma, thyrotoxicosis
- Should be avoided in pregnancy and lactation

Drug Interactions

- Similar precautions should be applied as for conventional medicines containing ephedrine and pseudoephedrine, including anti-hypertensives and antidepressants

Doses

- FDA guidelines suggest a maximum dose of 8 mg of ephedrine every six hours up to 24mg per day for no more than 7 days

INTRODUCTION

Family: Ephedraceae

Synonyms: Ephedra, Chinese Ephedra, Herba Ephedrae, Cao mahuang.[1, 2]

Many members of the genus *Ephedra* are reputed to have medicinal properties. This monograph will concentrate primarily on ma huang which is the one most often encountered in North America. Other members of this genus with medicinal applications include: *Ephedra intermedia* Shrenk ex C. A. Mey. (Intermediate ephedra), *Ephedra equisetina* Bunge (Mongolian ephedra), *Ephedra geradiana* Wallich ex Stapf (Pakistani ephedra) and *Ephedra nevadensis* S. Wats (Mormon tea)[1, 3, 4]

Ma huang is a fragrant perennial shrub native to many parts of Asia.[5] It is one of the smallest members of the genus, with greenish herbaceous stems and producing small white flower-like cones.[1, 5] Usually the aerial parts of the plant are used medicinally.[1, 6]

Ma huang has a long medicinal history within Traditional Chinese Medicine where it is used for a number of conditions, most notably of the respiratory system, including asthma, colds and coughs.[3, 7] This herb, or more correctly one of the alkaloids found in it (ephedrine), was probably the first traditional Chinese herbal product to receive acceptance in the West.[3] Ephedra species native to North America such as *Ephedra nevadensis* S. Wats do not contain any alkaloids.[3]

Constituents:[1, 2, 8-10]

- Alkaloids of the protoalkaloid class including (-)- ephedrine (L-ephedrine, major portion), (+)-pseudoephedrine, (+)- norpseudoephedrine, and (-)- norephedrine
- Tannins: catechin, gallic acid, condensed tannins
- Miscellaneous including: ephedrans (glycans), ephedradine, volatile oil and flavonoid glycosides
- Roots: macrocyclic spermine alkaloids (e.g. ephedradine) and L-tyrosine betaine (maokonine)

Note: The alkaloid content may vary from 0.5% to 2.5% (dry wt.), 30% to 90% of which is ephedrine, depending on the species.[10] *E. sinica* contains approximately 1.3% alkaloids with ephedrine making up 60% of this amount.[1]

THERAPEUTIC USES & RELEVANT PHARMACOLOGY

COMMON USES

As has already been mentioned, ma huang is considered an herb of particular importance within many Asian healing models.[1, 7] Ma huang is considered to be particularly useful in the treatment of respiratory conditions associated with fever,[7, 8] asthma,[4, 7, 8, 11] allergic rhinitis[6-8] and bronchitis.[6, 8] It is also considered to be a stimulant and hypertensive agent.[6, 7] Ma huang is often included in weight loss formulas because of its stimulant action.[4]

GENERAL PHARMACOLOGY

The alkaloids, especially ephedrine and pseudoephedrine, are the main constituents responsible for this plant's medicinal action. Ephedrine acts primarily in the periphery as an indirect adrenomimetic agent, causing an increased release of norepinephrine. While it has a longer duration of action than norepinephrine, its peripheral action is limited since tachyphylaxis occurs. It is less potent than norepinephrine but is effective after oral administration.[12]

Ephedrine and pseudoephedrine are known to cross the blood brain barrier resulting in a stimulant action.[1, 12] Administration of ephedrine results in direct bronchodilation.[12] Pseudoephedrine appears to work in a similar manner but is generally considered less potent than ephedrine.[4]

Localized anti-inflammatory properties have been demonstrated for both ephedrine and pseudoephedrine in a number of animal models.[13]

RESPIRATORY SYSTEM

As mentioned above, ephedrine has bronchodilating properties, causing prolonged relaxation of smooth muscles upon oral administration.[12] Constriction of the blood vessels in the mucosa of the respiratory system results in decreased mucous production, providing a decongestant action.[14] Health Canada has published a labelling standard for *Ephedra*-containing products as nasal decongestants,[15] an indication for which approximately 20 ma huang products have been registered as non-prescription drugs. There are also 3 commercial products containing ma huang registered in Canada as vasoconstrictors, 7 as sympathomimetics, and 4 as homeopathic products.[16] The presence of the 'drying' astringent tannins and aromatic volatile oils may also be playing a part in the treatment of bronchial asthma and bronchitis.[1, 8] While ephedrine was once used to treat asthma, the fact that its action is selective to beta-2 adrenoreceptors is a significant disadvantage. It has now been superceded by more selective agents such as salbutamol/albuterol, which have fewer adverse effects.[17]

CARDIOVASCULAR SYSTEM

Administration of ephedrine results in vasoconstriction as well as increased systolic and diastolic blood pressure, force of cardiac contraction and cardiac output.[12, 14] Pseudoephedrine appears to have a weaker hypertensive action than ephedrine.[1] A number of medical herbalists comment that the hypertensive action of plant extracts seem to be less pronounced that those seen with ephedrine alone.[8, 18]

Paradoxically parenteral administration of mahuangen (the roots of Ma huang) has been reported to cause vasodilation in a number of animal models.[1] A variable effect on blood pressure may be observed depending on the relative concentrations of hypotensive ephedradines (ganglionic blocking agents) versus hypertensive maokonine, due to phytochemical differences between the various *Ephedra* species.[10]

OBESITY

A number of clinical studies have shown that supplementation with ephedrine, normally combined with other agents, can result in significant weight loss in both animals[19-21] and humans.[22-29] This action appears to be more pronounced when combined with other methylxanthines, notably caffeine and theophylline. Addition of aspirin to the protocol has been shown to potentiate this effect further.[30, 31]

Ephedrine appears to act as a thermogenic agent, increasing the ability of the body to produce heat from food. It has been suggested that this action is deeply influenced by adrenoreceptor stimulation and that ephedrine can influence all the receptor sub-types. The increased action of ephedrine/methylxanthine and ephedrine/aspirin combinations over ephedrine alone could be due to inhibition of feed-back mechanisms.[32] The thermogenic action appears to be more pronounced with chronic administration.[33] Ephedrine also appears to reduce appetite.[33] The ephedrine/caffeine combination also seems to be protective against reducing HDL-cholesterol during weight loss.[34]

While ma huang may be of use in the treatment of obesity, there is no reason to believe that it will offer any preferential benefits over ephedrine alone. Obesity is not generally considered a traditional indication for ma huang and therefore there is no significant empirical evidence to support its use. Tyler comments that the both the safety and effectiveness of ma huang is open to debate (see adverse effect section).[3] Claims for use of ephedra-containing products as stimulants or diet aids for weight loss are not allowed by Health Canada under the Herbs and Natural Products drug category.[16]

ATHLETIC PERFORMANCE

In a review article, Clarkson and Thompson conclude that there is very little evidence to support the use of ephedrine or pseudoepherine to improve sporting performance. While some athletes may take ephedrine to reduce body fat and promote muscle mass, there is no evidence to support this indication in individuals who are not overweight. It should also be noted that products containing ephedrine or pseudoephedrine are prohibited by a number of sporting authorities.[35]

Most of the evidence purported to support the use of ma huang for the indications described above comes from work carried out using ephedrine or pseudoephedrine alone and not the herb ma huang. While a substantial amount of historical and empirical evidence exists regarding this herb's medicinal usefulness, it is primarily restricted to the treatment of asthma, bronchitis and conditions of the upper respiratory tract.

ADVERSE EFFECTS

Numerous concerns have been voiced regarding the increased popularity of 'natural' commercial products containing ma huang. These products include sports supplements, diet aids and products intended to induce euphoria and increase sensory acuity.[36, 37] While consumption does provide central nervous system stimulation, high amounts can lead to hallucinations, paranoia, and psychosis. A number of fatalities have resulted from consumption of these products in the United States.[38, 39]

In one case, a 23-year-old healthy male died of "patchy myocardial necrosis" after taking a commercial product containing ma huang and caffeine for approximately six weeks. The individual appears to have followed the instructions appearing on the product label.[40]

Products containing ma huang intended for weight loss have been implicated in cases of both mania and psychosis.[41, 42]

Adverse effects seen following consumption of ephedrine products include dizziness, headache, decreased appetite, gastrointestinal distress, irregular heart beat, tachycardia, sweating, insomnia, hypertension, stroke, seizures and death.[36, 43]

In response to these concerns, Health Canada has warned consumers not to use products containing ma huang unless the product label carries a Drug Identification Number and the consumer follows strictly the dosage directions and precautions.[44] The Food and Drug Administration (FDA) of the United States has proposed that products containing ephedrine should: contain no more than 8 mg per unit dose, daily intake should not exceed more than 24 mg, duration of treatment should be limited to a maximum of 7 days, proper contraindications should appear on labels and ephedrine should not be combined with other stimulants such as caffeine.[45]

One case exists of acute hepatitis resulting from administration of ma huang. Given the lack of cases of hepatotoxicity associated with this botanical medicine, the authors conclude that an adulterant in the product was probably responsible rather than the ma huang itself.[46]

Concerns have been expressed that prolonged administration of products containing ma huang may result in a "weakening" of the adrenal gland. Subsequently some practitioners may combine it with 'adrenal tonics' such as licorice.[4]

DRUG INTERACTIONS

Concomitant administration with stimulants or any centrally acting medication such as antidepressants and anti-hypertensives should be avoided. It would seem prudent to apply the restrictions associated with ephedrine to that of ma huang. The action of ephedrine is known to be affected by antacids and agents which alter the pH (acidity) of the urine.[47] Ephedrine is also known to interact with corticosteroids and theophylline.[47] The German Commission E monograph further warns of possible interactions with cardiac glycosides or halothane, resulting in disturbance of heart rhythm: guanetjidine resulting in enhancement of the sympathomimetic effect; monoamine oxidase inhibitors resulting in greatly increased sympathomimetic action of the ephedrine; and secale alkaloid derivatives or oxytocin, resulting in development of hypertension.[48]

CAUTIONS/CONTRAINDICATIONS

Products containing ephedrine should not be taken by people suffering from heart disease, hypertension, thyroid disease, diabetes or conditions associated with enlarged prostate.[4], anxiety,[6] glaucoma, impaired circulation of the cerebrum, pheochromocytoma, or thyrotoxicosis.[48]

Since ephedrine has uterostimulant properties,[1] ma huang should be avoided in pregnancy and lactation.

DOSAGE REGIMENS

Maximum: 8mg of ephedrine every six hours up to a maximum of 24mg per day for no more than 7 days.[45]

Given the above concerns, it is highly questionable whether ma huang products containing appreciable amounts of alkaloids are appropriate for self-medication. Consultation with an appropriately trained health-care provider is advisable.

REFERENCES

1. Leung A, Foster S. *Encyclopedia of Common Natural Ingredients used in Food, Drugs and Cosmetics*. 2nd edition ed. New York, NY: John Wiley and Sons; 1996:649.

2. Wren R. Potter's *New Encyclopedia of Botanical Drugs and Preparations*. Saffron Walden: CW Daniel Company; 1988:362.
3. Tyler V. *Herbs of Choice. The Therapeutic Use of Phytomedicinals.* Binghamton, NY: Pharmaceutical Products Press; 1994:209.
4. Murray M. *The Healing Power of Herbs.* 2nd ed. Rocklin, CA: Prima Publishing; 1995:410.
5. Willard T. *Wild Rose Scientific Herbal.* Calgary, AB: Wild Rose College of Natural healing; 1991.
6. Hoffman D. *Holistic Herbal.* Rockport: Element Books; 1996:256.
7. Chevallier A. *The Encyclopedia of Medicinal Plants*. London: Reader's Digest; 1996:336.
8. Mills S. *The Essential Book of Herbal Medicine*. London: Penguin Publishing; 1991:677.
9. Trease G, Evans W. *Pharmacognosy.* London: Bailliere and Tindall; 1989:832.
10. Olin B. *The Review of Natural products; The Ephedras*. St.Louis: Facts and Comparisons, a Wolters Kluwer Company; 1995.
11. Duke J. *The Green Pharmacy*. Pennsylvania: Rodale Press Inc; 1997:617.
12. Lee T, Stitzel R. Adrenomimetic drugs. In: Craig C, Stitzel R, eds. *Modern Pharmacology*. 4th ed. New York: Little, Brown and Company; 1994:907.
13. Kasahara Y, Hikino H, Tsurufuji S, *et al*. Anti-inflammatory actions of ephedrines in acute inflammations. *Planta Medica.* 1985;51:325-31.
14. Bowman W, Rand M. *Textbook of Pharmacology*. London: Blackwell Scientific Publications; 1980.
15. Health Canada. *Labelling Standard: Ephedra*. Ottawa: Health Canada Drugs Directorate; 1996.
16. Canada H. *Drug Product database.* Ottawa: Health Canada; 1998.
17. King K. The treatment of asthma. *Medical Journal of Australia.* 1985;143:390-394.
18. Hoffmann D. *Therapeutic Herbalism*. s.l.: s.n.; 1992
19. Dulloo AG, Miller DS. The thermogenic properties of ephedrine/methlxanthine mixtures: animal studies. *American Journal of Clinical Nutrition*. 1986;43:388-94.
20. Dulloo AG, Miller DS. Prevention of genetic fa/fa obesity with an ephedrine-methylxanthines thermogenic mixture. *American Journal of Physiology*. 1987;252(3 Pt 2):R507-13.
21. Tulp OL, Buck CL. Caffeine and ephedrine stimulated thermogenesis in LA-corpulent rats. *Comparative Biochemistry & Physiology — C: Comparative Pharmacology & Toxicology*. 1986;85(1):17-9.
22. Breum L, Pedersen JK, Ahlstrom F, *et al*. Comparison of an ephedrine/caffeine combination and dexfenfluramine in the treatment of obesity. A double-blind multi-centre trial in general practice. *International Journal of Obesity & Related Metabolic Disorders.* 1994;18(2):99-103.
23. Daly PA, Krieger DR, Dulloo AG, *et al*. Ephedrine, caffeine and aspirin: safety and efficacy for treatment of human obesity. *International Journal of Obesity & Related Metabolic Disorders.* 1993;17(Suppl 1):S73-8.
24. Astrup A, Breum L, Toubro S, *et al*. The effect and safety of an ephedrine/caffeine compound compared to ephedrine, caffeine and placebo in obese subjects on an energy restricted diet. A double blind trial. *International Journal of Obesity & Related Metabolic Disorders.* 1992;16(4):269-77.
25. Norregaard J, Jorgensen S, Mikkelsen KL, *et al.* The effect of ephedrine plus caffeine on smoking cessation and postcessation weight gain. *Clinical Pharmacology & Therapeutics.* 1996;60(6):679-86.
26. Dulloo AG, Miller DS. The thermogenic properties of ephedrine/methylxanthine mixtures: human studies. *International Journal of Obesity.* 1986;10(6):467-81.
27. Astrup A, Lundsgaard C, Madsen J, Christensen NJ. Enhanced thermogenic responsiveness during chronic ephedrine treatment in man. *American Journal of Clinical Nutrition.* 1985;42(1):83-94.
28. Pasquali R, Cesari MP, Melchionda N, Stefanini C, Raitano A, Labo G. Does ephedrine promote weight loss in low-energy-adapted obese women? *International Journal of Obesity.* 1987;11(2):163-8.
29. Pasquali R, Baraldi G, Cesari MP, *et al.* A controlled trial using ephedrine in the treatment of obesity. *International Journal of Obesity.* 1985;9(2):93-8.
30. Dulloo AG, Miller DS. Aspirin as a promoter of ephedrine-induced thermogenesis: Potential use in the treatment of obesity. *American Journal of Clinical Nutrition.* 1987;45(3):564-9.
31. Horton TJ, Geissler CA. Aspirin potentiates the effect of ephedrine on the thermogenic response to a meal in obese but not lean women. *International Journal of Obesity.* 1991;15(5):359-66.
32. Dulloo A. Ephedrine, xanthines and prostaglandin-inhibitors: action and interactions in the stimulation of thermo genesis. *International Journal of Obesity.* 1993;17((Suppl. 1)):S35-S40.
33. Astrup A. Thermogenesis in human brown adipose tissue and skeletal muscle induced by sympathomimetic stimulation. *Acta Endocrinologica. Supplementum.* 1986;278:1-32.
34. Buemann B, Marckmann P, Christensen NJ, Astrup A. The effect of ephedrine plus caffeine on plasma lipids and

lipoproteins during a 4.2 MJ/day diet. *International Journal of Obesity & Related Metabolic Disorders.* 1994;18(5):329-32.

35. Clarkson PM, Thompson HS. Drugs and sport. Research findings and limitations. *Sports Medicine*. 1997;24(6):366-84.
36. Nightingale SL. From the Food and Drug Administration. *Journal of the American Medical Association*. 1996;275(20):1534.
37. Chase SL. The FDA warns of the dangers of ephedrine. *RN.* 1996;59(12):67.
38. Josefson D. Herbal stimulant causes US deaths. [News]. *British Medical Journal.* 1996;312(7043):1378-9.
39. Maron B, Shirani J, Poliac L, Matherige R, Roberts W, Mueller F. Sudden death in young competitive athletes. *Journal of American Medicine*. 1996;276:199-204.
40. Theoharides TC. Sudden death of a healthy college student related to ephedrine toxicity from a ma huang-containing drink. [Letter]. *Journal of Clinical Psychopharmacology*. 1997;17(5):437-9.
41. Doyle H, Kargin M. Herbal stimulant containing ephedrine has also caused psychosis. [Letter; comment]. British Medical Journal. 1996;313(7059):756.
42. Capwell R. Ephedrine induced mania from a herbal diet supplement. *American Journal of Psychiatry*. 1995;152:647.
43. Kikutani T. Contrary Views on Chinese herbal drugs and side effects. *International Journal of Oriental Medicine.* 1990;15(4):184-188.
44. Canada H. Warning Not to use products containing the herb ephedra, also known as Ma Huang. *Health Canada News Release.* 1997;1997-38.
45. Nightingale SL. From the Food and Drug Administration. *Journal of the American Medical Association*. 1997;278(1):15.
46. Nadir A, Agrawal S, King PD, Marshall JB. Acute hepatitis associated with the use of a Chinese herbal product, ma-huang. [See comments]. *American Journal of Gastroenterology.* 1996;91(7):1436-8.
47. Stockley I. *Drug Interactions, A Source Book of Adverse Interactions, Their Mechanisms, Clinical Importance and Management.* 3rd ed. London: *Blackwell Scientific Publications;* 1994:932.
48. Blumenthal M, Busse WR, Goldberg A, *et al. The Complete German Commission E Monographs: Therapeutic Guide to Herbal Medicine.* Austin, TX: American Botanical Council; 1998:685.

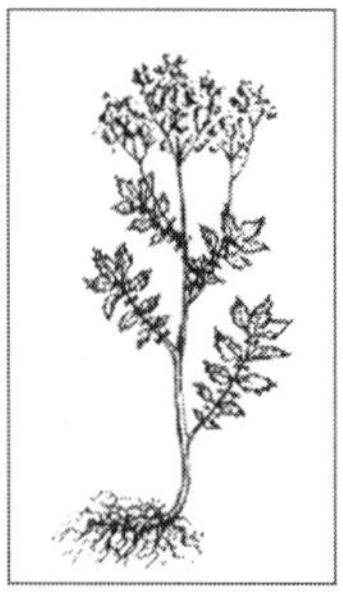

MEADOWSWEET

Filipendula ulmaria (L.) Maxim

THUMBNAIL SKETCH

Active Constituents
- Salicylate-rich volatile oil, flavonoids and tannins

Common Uses
- Digestive upset (including ulceration, dyspepsia and hyperacidity), rheumatic conditions and pain.

Adverse Effects
- None noted

Cautions/Contraindications
- Classic ones applicable to salicylates in general

Drug Interactions
- Classic ones applicable to salicylates in general

Doses
- 4-6 g of dried herb three times daily
- 1.5-6.0 mL fluid extract (1:1 in 25% alcohol) three times daily
- 2-4 mL tincture (1:5 in 45% alcohol) three times daily

INTRODUCTION

Family: Rosaceae

Synonyms: Filipendula, Queen of the meadows, *Spiraea ulmaria* L., Bridewort [1, 2]

Meadowsweet is a stout perennial standing up to 120 cm in height that is native to most parts of Europe and Asia. It produces a thick, pink aromatic root with erect stems and aromatic creamy leaves. The term Spiraea, used in a former binomial name, comes from the fact that the fruits have a twisted appearance.[3] Salicylic acid was first extracted from the flowering buds of this medicinal herb. The term aspirin (acetylsalicylic acid) means "from Spiraea."[3]

Established growths of meadowsweet often completely dominate the marshy areas in which they grow, making another common name, Queen of the meadow, very appropriate.[3] The English herbalist Gerard described the aroma produced by this plant with the following phrase, "for the smell thereof makes the heart merry, delighteth the senses; neither doth it cause headache, or loathsomeness to meat, as some other sweet smelling herbs do."[4] The aerial parts of the plant are used medicinally.

Constituents[1, 2, 5-8]

- Volatile oils: salicylates (including salicylaldehyde, gaultherin, salicin and salicylic acid), vanillin, benzaldehyde
- Flavonoids: rutin, hyperoside, spireoside and kaempferol
- Miscellaneous: hydrolysable tannins, coumarins, mucilage, ascorbic acid.

THERAPEUTIC USES & RELEVANT PHARMACOLOGY

COMMON USES

Meadowsweet is considered by many herbalists to be an important medicinal herb for the management of conditions of the digestive system.[9] It is reputed to have a soothing and healing action and is frequently used to treat such conditions as hyperacidity,[9, 10] indigestion,[9, 10] peptic ulcer disease,[9, 10] nausea,[9, 10] and pediatric diarrhea.[1, 9]

The other primary use of meadowsweet is as an analgesic and anti-inflammatory and it has been suggested that it is useful in the management of pain and rheumatic conditions.[1, 9, 11] It may also act as an antipyretic.[9] While these properties are generally considered to be due to the presence of salicylates in the volatile oil portion, these applications easily predate the identification of these components.

PHARMACOLOGY

Various extracts of meadowsweet have been reported to: lower vascular permeability; increase bronchial tone in cats; increase the bronchospasm induced by histamine in guinea pigs; increase tonus *in vitro* in guinea pig intestine and rabbit uterus; decrease rectal temperature; and potentiate narcotic action.[1,2,6] In addition, an anti-ulcer action has been noted in various animal models, especially with aqueous extracts of the flowers.[1,6,12] In contrast, the ulcerogenic nature of histamine was potentiated by an extract of meadowsweet in the guinea pig.[12]

Extracts of meadowsweet have also been shown to possess bactericidal and bacterostatic properties.[1,2] The flowers and seeds have been shown to exert an anticoagulant and fibrinolytic effect both *in vitro* and *in vivo*.[13] Topical administration of a decoction made from meadowsweet flowers has been shown to decrease the frequency of experimentally induced squamous cell carcinoma of the cervix and vagina in mice. Application of an ointment was shown to increase regression of cervical dysplasia in 32 patients.[14]

ADVERSE EFFECTS

No instances of adverse reactions could be found for this herb.

CAUTIONS/CONTRAINDICATIONS

Given the lack of objective information, the presence of salicylates and the fact that meadowsweet effects uterine smooth muscle *in vitro*, it has been suggested that meadowsweet should be avoided during pregnancy and lactation.[1] While no clinical examples could be found, it has been argued that the classic precautions applicable to salicylates in general are applicable to products containing meadowsweet. Consequently, it should be used with caution in: individuals sensitive to aspirin, asthmatics, gout, diabetes, hemophilia, active peptic ulcer disease, hypoprothrombinemia, kidney and liver disease.[1] Although salicylates are generally considered contraindicated in patients with active peptic ulcer disease, it is important to balance this caution with the empirical uses mentioned previously.

DRUG INTERACTIONS

While no clinical examples could be found, there is every reason to believe that classic drug interactions with salicylates in general (e.g., concomitant oral anticoagulants) are relevant here.[1]

DOSAGE REGIMEN [1,15]

- Dried herb: 4-6 g three times daily
- 1.5-6.0 mL fluid extract (1:1 in 25% alcohol) three times daily
- 2-4 mL tincture (1:5 in 45% alcohol) three times daily

Meadowsweet is often combined with other 'digestive' herbs such as chamomile, licorice, marshmallow and peppermint. Also many herbal painkillers contain meadowsweet often combined with black or white willow bark.

REFERENCES

1. Newall C, Anderson L, Phillipson J. *Herbal Medicines: A Guide for Health Care Professionals*. London: The Pharmaceutical Press; 1996:296.
2. Wren R. *Potter's New Encyclopedia of Botanical Drugs and Preparations.* Saffron Walden: C.W. Daniel Company; 1988:362.

3. Stuart M. *The Encylcopedia of Herbs and Herbalism.* London: Orbis Publishing; 1979:304.
4. Krutch J. *Herbal*. London: Phaidon Press; 1976:255.
5. Scheer T, Wichtl M. On the occurence of Kampferol-4'-O-beta-D-glucopyranoside in *Filipendula ulmaria* and *Allium cepa* [German]. *Planta Medica*. 1987; 53:573-4.
6. Barnaulov OD, *et al.* Chemical composition and primary evaluation of the properties of preparations from *Filipendula ulmaria* (L.) Maxim flowers. *Rastilil'nye Resursy*. 1977; 13:661-9.
7. Valle MG, Nano GM, Tira S. Das atherische ol aus *Filipendula ulmaria*. *Planta Medica*. 1988; 54:181-2.
8. Thieme H. Isolierung eines neuen phenolischen glykosids aus den bluten von *Filipendula ulmaria* (L.) Maxim. *Pharmazie*. 1966; 21:123.
9. Hoffmann D. *Holistic Herbal*. Rockport, CA: Element Books; 1996:256.
10. Mills S. *The Essential Book of Herbal Medicine*. 2nd ed. London: Penguin Publ; 1991:677.
11. Weiss R. *Herbal Medicine.* Beaconsfield: Beaconsfield Publishers Ltd; 1988: 362.
12. Barnaulov OD, Denisenko PP. Antiulcerogenic action of the decoction from flowers of *Filipendula ulmaria* (L.). *Pharmakol-Toxicol* (Moscow). 1980; 43:700-5.
13. Liapina L, Koval'chuk G. A comparative study of the action on the hemostatic system of extracts from the flowers and seeds of the meadowsweet (*Filipendula ulmaria* (L.) Maxim). [Russian]. *Izv Akad Nauk Ser Biol.* 1993; July-Aug(4):625-8.
14. Peresun'ko A, Bespalov V, Limarenko A, Aleksandrov V. Clinico-experimental study using plant preparations from the flowers of *Filipendula ulmaria* (L.) Maxim for the treatment of precancerous changes and preparation of uterine cervical cancer. [Russian]. *Voprosy Onkologii*. 1993; 39(7-12):291-5.
15. Bradley P. *British Herbal Compendium*. Bournemouth: BHMA; 1992.

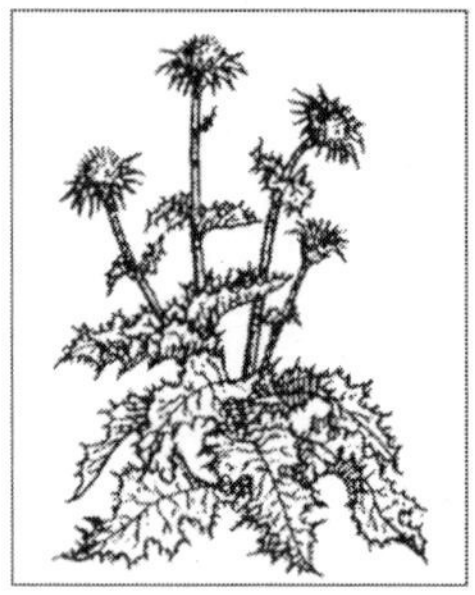

MILK THISTLE

Silybum marianum (L.) Gaertner

THUMBNAIL SKETCH

Active Constituents

- Silymarin

Common Uses

- Liver disorders (including hepatitis and cirrhosis)
- Psoriasis

Adverse Effects

- Very rare; mild diarrhea may occur

Cautions/Contraindications

- Safety in pregnancy and lactation has not yet been established

Drug Interactions

- None known, but may affect the liver metabolism of some medications

Doses

- 200 mg of standardized extract (70% silymarin) three times daily

INTRODUCTION

Family: Asteraceae (also known as Compositae)

Synonyms:[1] Mary thistle, St. Mary thistle, Marian thistle, Lady's thistle, Holy thistle, Silybum, *Carduus marianus* L., *Cnicus marianus*

Although milk thistle originally grew wild throughout much of Europe, it is now naturalized to the east coast of North America, California and South America.[1] This biennial grows up to 1 m in height with spiny leaves which are marked with white along the veins.[2] The specific name *marianum* refers to the legend that the leaves have a white mottling because a drop of the Virgin Mary's milk landed on them. In keeping with this legend, milk thistle has traditionally been used as a galactogogue (i.e., to stimulate milk production in lactating women).[1] Milk thistle is sometimes confused with Blessed thistle (*Cnicus benedictus* L., Asteraceae). Although they are members of the same botanical family, their medicinal actions are quite different.

Milk thistle has been used medicinally for several thousand years. Both the Greeks and the Romans noted its hepatoprotective effects; however, current interest in this product did not begin until the late 1960s when silymarin, a combination of flavonolignans believed to be responsible for the hepatic activity, was first isolated from the ripe seeds.[1] Milk thistle is a clear example in which scientific investigation has confirmed the historical use of an herbal product.

Constituents [1, 3, 4]

- Flavonolignans including: silybin (silibin), silydianin (silidianin), silychristin (silichristin)
- Miscellaneous: apigenin, silbonol, fatty acids

Note that silymarin, the component to which most milk thistle products are standardized, is a mixture of silybin, silydianin, and silychristin.

THERAPEUTIC USES & RELEVANT PHARMACOLOGY

PHARMACOLOGY

Silymarin, the active constituent isolated from the ripe seeds of milk thistle, has been extensively studied. Its actions on the liver are believed to result from three primary mechanisms of action:[1, 5-7]

1. Stimulation of RNA polymerase A (also known as polymerase I) and DNA synthesis:[3, 8, 9] silybin stimulates this enzyme which in turn increases the synthesis of ribosome proteins and thus stimulates cell development, ultimately increasing the regenerative capacity of the liver;
2. Competitive binding with some toxins:[3] silymarin appears to compete with alpha-amanitin and phalloidin (two toxins from the deathcap mushroom) for a receptor on the cell membrane;
3. Antioxidant action via increasing hepatic contents of glutathione (both oxidized and reduced):[3, 10-15] glutathione is a powerful antioxidant which detoxifies a wide variety of substances

in the liver, stomach and intestines; silymarin is reported to be a 10x stronger antioxidant than Vitamin E; it may also increase the enzyme superoxide dismutase (SOD)[16]

Other mechanisms of action which have been hypothesized include: inhibition of lipoxygenase, which catalyses a reaction between polyunsaturated fatty acids and oxygen to produce leukotrienes which may cause liver damage;[17] inhibition of neutrophil function;[18] and inhibition of Kupffer cell functions.[19]

HEPATOPROTECTIVE ACTIVITY

Currently, milk thistle is known primarily for its ability to protect the liver from damage and to restore its function following damage. Tyler feels that animal studies have "shown conclusively that silymarin exerts a liver protective effect against a variety of toxins . . . [and] human trials have also been encouraging for conditions including hepatitis and cirrhosis."[20] In addition, the German Commission E has approved milk thistle as supportive treatment of cirrhosis and chronic inflammatory liver conditions.[21]

Protection from Chemical Toxins

Many animal studies have demonstrated the ability of milk thistle preparations to protect the liver from a variety of toxins including: alpha-amanitin and phalloidin (both from the extremely poisonous Deathcap mushroom),[3, 22-25] carbon tetrachloride, thioacetamide, DL-ethionine,[3] and acetaminophen.[15] In addition, silymarin has been shown to provide significant protection to animals against liver damage typically caused by ethyl alcohol.[3] One double-blind, placebo-controlled trial of "toxic liver damage" (caused by alcohol in most cases) in 33 patients reported that aspartat aminotransferase (AST), and alanine aminotransferase (ALT) values were all significantly improved in the silymarin group in comparison with the control group.[3] This was confirmed in a second double-blind, placebo-controlled study of 106 patients with mild liver disease (most caused by alcohol). AST and ALT serum levels were significantly improved in the group who took 420 mg of silymarin daily when compared with the controls, and there was a positive trend in the concentrations of total and conjugated serum bilirubins in the silymarin group when compared with the control group. Due to the outpatient setting, alcohol consumption was not monitored in this study.[26]

Another double-blind, placebo-controlled trial (n=60) investigated the effect of silymarin in patients who were suffering from hepatotoxicity due to long term treatment with phenothiazines or butyrophenones. All patients taking silymarin (800 mg daily) were reported to have significantly decreased serum levels of malondialdehyde (MDA). Those who stopped taking their psychotropics during the 90 day study experienced the most pronounced decrease; however, those continuing on their psychotropic medication also experienced a decrease which was significant in comparison to the placebo group.[27]

Hepatitis

A variety of studies report the effectiveness of silymarin in treating both acute and chronic hepatitis.[3, 28, 29] One double-blind, placebo-controlled study of patients with acute viral hepatitis (n=28) found that the group taking silymarin had significantly better bilirubin and AST values and a trend toward better ALT values than the control group.[3] Another double-blind, placebo-controlled trial with 20 patients suffering from chronic hepatic diseases showed that silymarin significantly improved seralbumin as well as improving the histopathological outcomes measured including focal necrosis and fibrosis when compared with the placebo group.[3] A more recent double-blind, placebo-controlled study of 20 patients with chronic viral hepatitis reported that those taking silybin-phosphatidylcholine (IdB1016) (two capsules twice daily which was the equivalent of 240 mg of silibinin) experienced a significant decreases in AST, ALT and gamma-glutamyltransferase (GGT) when compared with the levels of the control group.[28] However, two other double-blind, placebo-controlled studies in patients with chronic hepatitis (n=24 and n=12) found no significant difference between the silymarin and placebo groups.[3] To date the majority of clinical trials have tested i.v. silymarin. The applicability of these findings to the ingestion of oral silymarin has been questioned.

Cirrhosis

A double-blind, placebo-controlled trial of 170 individuals with cirrhosis of the liver reported that those taking silymarin (200 mg of milk thistle standardized to 70% silymarin three times daily) had a significantly lower mortality rate over the 2 years of the study period and an additional 2 years of follow-up. Patients with mild alcohol-induced cirrhosis appeared to have received the most benefit from the silymarin treatment. No significant difference in serum concentrations of liver enzymes were noted between the two groups.[30]

PSORIASIS

Some researchers have suggested that milk thistle may also be useful in the management of psoriasis. This may be secondary to its ability to improve liver function or directly due to its ability to decrease leukotriene synthesis by inhibiting lipoxygenase.[2, 31]

ADVERSE EFFECTS

Adverse effects of silymarin appear to be very rare. Because it increases bile flow, it may cause mild diarrhea in some individuals.[2, 5, 20]

CAUTIONS/CONTRAINDICATIONS

Long-term safety and safety in pregnant and lactating women have not yet been established.

DRUG INTERACTIONS

Although no drug interactions could be found in our review of the literature, theoretically the fact that milk thistle increases liver function suggests that it may influence the metabolism of some medications.

DOSAGE REGIMENS

*200 mg of standardized extract three times daily.[5]

*Most products on the Canadian market are standardized to 70% silymarin content. Thus a 200 mg tablet contains 140 mg of silymarin.

Note: silymarin is not very water soluble, thus this herb should not be taken as a 'tea'.[20]

REFERENCES

1. Foster S. *Milk Thistle. Silybum marianum*. Houston, TX: American Botanical Council; 1991:7
2. Murray MT. *The Healing Power of Herbs.* Rocklin, CA: Prima Publishing; 1992:246.
3. Hikino H, Kiso Y. Natural products for liver diseases. *Economic and Medicinal Plant Research*. 1988;2:39-72.
4. Leung A, Foster S. *Encyclopedia of Common Natural Ingredients Used in Food, Drugs and Cosmetics.* 2nd ed. New York, NY: John Wiley and Sons; 1996:649.
5. Brown D. Silymarin educational monograph. *Townsend Newsletter for Doctors*. 1994;136:1282-5.
6. Brown D. Silymarin Education Monograph. *Quarterly Review of Natural Medicine* 1993;Summer:23-36.
7. Leng-Peschlow E. Alcohol-related liver diseases — use of Legalon for therapy. *Quarterly Review of Natural Medicine*. 1996;Summer:103-18.
8. Sonnenbichler J, Goldberg M, Hane L, *et al*. Stimulatory effect of silibinin on the DNA synthesis in partially hepatectomized rat livers: Non-response in hepatoma and other malign cell lines. *Biochemical Pharmacology*. 1986;35(3):538-41.
9. Magliulo P, Carosi G, Minoli L, Gorini S. Studies on the regenerative capacity of the liver in rats subjected to partial hepatectomy and treated with silymarin. *Arzneimittelforschung*. 1973;23:161-7.
10. Valenzuela A, Lagos C, Schmidt K, Videla LA. Silymarin protection against hepatic lipid peroxidation induced by acute ethanol intoxication in the rat. *Biochemical Pharmacology*. 1985;34(12):2209-12.
11. Valenzuela A, Aspillaga M, Vial S, Guerra R. Selectivity of silymarin on the increase of the glutathione content in different tissues of the rat. *Planta Medica*. 1989;55:420-2.
12. Wagner H. Antihepatotoxic flavonoids. In: Cody V, Middleton E, Harbourne JB, eds. *Plant Flavonoids in Biology and Medicine: Biochemical, Pharmacological, and Structure-Activity Relationships.* New York, NY: Alan R Liss; 1986:545-8.
13. Adzet T. Polyphenolic compounds with biological and pharmacological activity. *Herbs Spices Medicinal Plants*. 1986;1:167-84.
14. Hikino H, Kiso Y, Wagner H, Fiebig. Antihepatotoxic actions of flavanolignans from *silybum marianum* fruits. *Planta Medica*. 1984;50:248-50.
15. Campos R, Garrido A, Guerra R, Valenzuela A. Silybin dihemisuccinate protects against glutathione depletion and lipid peroxisation induced by acetaminophen in rat liver. *Planta Medica*. 1989;55:417-9.
16. Muzes G, Deak G, Land I, *et al*. Effect of the bioflavonoid silymarin on the *in vitro* activity and expression of superoxide dismutase (SOD) enzyme. *Acta Physiologica Hungarica*. 1991;78(1):3-9.
17. Fiebrich F, Koch H. Silymarin, an inhibitor of lipoxygenase. *Experentia*. 1979;35:148-50.
18. Alarcon de la Lastra AC, Martin MJ, Motilva V, *et al*. Gastroprotection induced by silymarin, the hepatoprotective principle of *Silybum marianum* in ischemia-reperfusion mucosal injury: Role of neutrophils. *Planta Medica*. 1995;61(2):116-9.
19. Dehmlow C, Erhard J, de Groot H. Inhibition of Kupffer cell functions as an explanation for the hepatoprotective properties of silibinin. *Hepatology*. 1996;23(4):749-54.
20. Tyler VE. *Herbs of Choice. The Therapeutic Use of Phytomedicinals*. Binghamton, NY: Pharmaceutical Products Press; 1994:209.
21. Blumenthal M, Brusse WR, Goldberg A, *et al. The Complete German Commission E Monographs*. Austin, TX: American Botanical Council; 1998:685.
22. Weiss RF. *Herbal Medicine.* Gothenburg, Sweden: Ab Arcanum; 1988:362.
23. Hruby C. Silibinin in the treatment of deathcap fungus poisoning. *Forum*. 1984;6:23-6.
24. Faulstich H, Jahn W, Wieland T. Silybin inhibition of amatoxin uptake in the perfused rat liver. *Arzneimittelforshung*. 1980;30(1):452-4.
25. Tuchweber B, Sieck R, Trost W. Prevention of silybin of phalloidin-induced acute hepatotoxicity. *Toxicology and Applied Pharmacology*. 1979;51:265-75.
26. Salami HA, Sarna S. Effect of silymarin on chemical, functional and morphological alterations of the liver. *Scandinavian Journal of Gastroenterology*. 1982;17:517-21.
27. Palasciano G, Portincasa P, Palmieri V, *et al*. The effect of silymarin on plasma levels of malondialdehyde in patients receiving long-term treatment with psychotropic drugs. *Current Therapeutic Research*. 1994;55(5):537-45.
28. Buzzelli G, Moscarella S, Giusti A, *et al.* A pilot study on the liver protective effect of silybin-phosphatidylcholine complex (IdB1016) in chronic active hepatitis. *International Journal of Clinical Pharmacology Therapy and Toxicology*. 1993;31(9):456-60.
29. Lirussi F, Okolicsanyi L. Cytoprotection in the nineties: Experience with ursodeoxycholic acid and silymarin in chronic liver disease. *Acta Physiologica Hungarica*. 1992;80(1-4):363-7.
30. Ferenci P, Dragosics B, Dittrich H, *et al.* Randomized controlled trial of silymarin treatment in patients with cirrhosis of the liver. *Journal of Hepatology*. 1989;9:105-13.
31. Weber G, Galle K. The liver, a therapeutic target in dermatoses. *Medizinische Welt*. 1983;34:108-11.

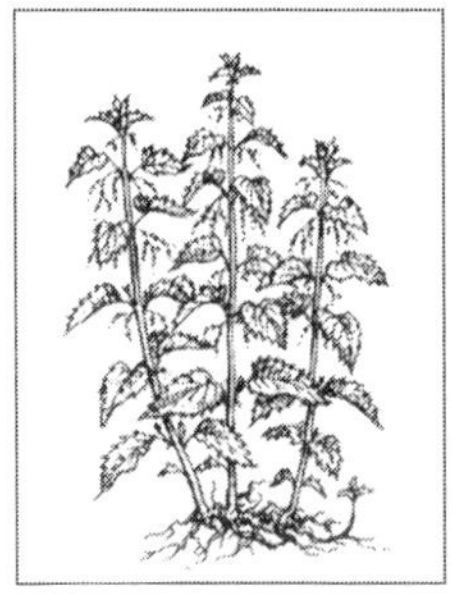

NETTLE

Urtica dioica L., *U. urens* L.

THUMBNAIL SKETCH

Active Constituents

Leaf:

- Flavonoids, amines and carboxylic acids in stinging hairs

Root:

- Sterols, lectins

Common Uses

Leaf:

- Rheumatism, gout, hay fever, as a nutritive supplement

Root:

- Micturition disorders associated with benign prostatic hyperplasia

Adverse Effects

- Skin irritation, gastric distress

Cautions/Contraindications

- Safety not established in pregnancy

Drug Interactions

- Root should be used with caution in cases of concomitant administration with conventional anti-hypertensives, diabetes and diuretic medication.

Doses

Leaf:

- 3-6 g of dried herb three times daily
- 3-4 mL of liquid extract (1:1 in 25% alcohol) three times daily
- 2-6 mL of tincture (1:5 in 45% alcohol) three times daily

Root: ◆4-6 g of root daily

- 1.5-7.5 mL of liquid extract (1:1, 45% ethanol) daily
- 5 mL of tincture (1:5, 40% ethanol) daily

INTRODUCTION

Family: Urticaceae

Synonyms: Stinging nettle, Urtica, Common nettle (*Urtica dioica* L.), Small nettle (*Urtica urens* L.)[1-3]

Nettle is a perennial standing up to 1.5 m in height. Different members of the genus *Urtica* grow naturally throughout most of Europe and North America. While it has enjoyed a long medicinal history in many different models of traditional herbalism, it is considered by many members of the public to be a noxious weed causing a characteristic pruritic rash on contact with the skin. Stinging nettle is also a common homeopathic remedy.[3] The aerial parts and the roots/rhizomes of two species, *U.dioica* L. and *U.urens* L., are used medicinally.[4-6]

Constituents

Leaf [1, 2, 5, 7-9]

- Amines: histamine, choline, acetylcholine, serotonin, etc. (especially in stinging hairs)
- Flavonoids including: isoquercetin, rutin, kaempferol and quercetin
- Minerals including: calcium, potassium, iron and silicon
- Acids including: silicic acid, malic acid, carbonic acid and formic acid
- Miscellaneous: sitosterol, glycoprotein, high levels of chlorophyll, tannins

Roots [2, 4, 10, 11]

- Lectins: Urtica dioica agglutinin (separated into 6 isolectins)
- Sterols (and their glucosides) including 3-beta-sitosterol and sitosterol –3-D-glucoside
- Miscellaneous including lignans, various fatty acids and scopoletin

THERAPEUTIC USES & RELEVANT PHARMACOLOGY

COMMON USES

Within the traditional herbal medicine paradigm, nettle leaves are considered very nutritive and consequently they are often used in situations of convalescence and recuperation.[1] They are also used to aid milk production in nursing mothers.[1] In addition, nettle is used for its astringent properties in the treatment of bleeding conditions such as wounds, hemorrhoids and even uterine hemorrhage.[1, 12]

GENITOURINARY TRACT

Stinging nettle root has become one the major phytomedicines used in the management of benign prostatic hyperplasia (BPH), especially in Europe.[13, 14] It can be taken alone, but is more commonly administered with other phytomedicines used in the management of BPH such as *Serenoa repens* (Bartr.) Small, Arecaceae/Palmae (Saw Palmetto) and *Prunus africana* (Hook. F.) Kalkman,

Rosaceae (African Pygeum).[15, 16] The European Scientific Cooperative on Phytotherapy (ESCOP) lists the 'symptomatic treatment of micturition disorders (nocturia, pollakisuria, dysuria, urine retention) in benign prostatic hyperplasia as one of the indications for stinging nettle root.[4]

Benign Prostatic Hyperplasia (BPH)

Preparations made primarily from the roots of *Urtica dioica* L. have been shown *in vitro* and *in vivo* to affect many aspects of prostate physiology thought to be implicated in BPH. These include: inhibition of sex hormone-binding globulin (SHBG) to human prostatic tissue; possible suppression of prostate cell metabolism and growth; and weak inhibition of aromatase activity.[4, 17] A number of human studies and clinical trials have demonstrated the therapeutic benefit of nettle root in the management of BPH. A more detailed review of these trials, which are primarily published in German, has been published in the ESCOP Urtica radix fascicule. In general the clinical trials had a duration of between 9 weeks and 6 months.[4] It has been suggested that the inclusion of the relatively inexpensive nettle root with more expensive phytomedicines used in the treatment of BPH may form a very cost effective method of treatment.[18]

MUSCULOSKELETAL TRACT

Oral preparations made from nettle leaf have long been used in the management of various arthritic conditions, including rheumatism and gout.[1, 6] It has been suggested that the nettle leaf could have a diuretic effect resulting in an increased elimination of 'toxins' such as uric acid.[1, 6] The localized irritation resulting from topical application of the stinging leaves of this plant is also reputed to be beneficial.[6]

In vitro trials have demonstrated that an hydroalcoholic preparation of the leaves of *Urtica dioica* possesses anti-inflammatory properties. The mechanism of action proposed is that it influences the synthesis of leukotrienes and cyclo-oxygenase derived prostaglandins.[5] It was also reported to decrease the production of a number of inflammatory related cytokines in whole human blood.[19]

A recent open randomized pilot study of patients (n=40) suffering from acute arthritis compared the effectiveness of stewed *Urtica dioica* L. leaves (50 g daily) plus diclofenac (50mg daily) to a larger daily dose of diclofenac (200 mg). Both treatments were administered for 14 days. The drug/herb combination was found to be as effective as the higher dose of NSAID in decreasing elevated acute phase protein concentrations and relieving the clinical arthritic symptoms.

The authors concluded that the action of diclofenac was potentiated by nettle leaves.[20] Although this may seem promising, this was only a pilot study and some criticism has been made regarding the research design.[21]

HAYFEVER

In a double-blind randomized study, the anti-allergic action of a freeze-dried preparation of *Urtica dioica* was compared to placebo. The study was carried out during the peak season for allergic rhinitis. Volunteers (n=98) were assigned to the treatment (300 mg capsules of freeze-dried *Urtica dioica*) or the placebo group and were advised to take two capsules at the onset of the symptoms of allergic rhinitis. Assessment was made by comparing diary symptoms and global response at a follow-up appointment after one week of therapy. Stinging nettle was rated higher than placebo according to the global assessment and slightly higher according to patient diary ratings.[22]

MISCELLANEOUS

In vitro trials have demonstrated that nettle leaves have diuretic, hypotensive, hyperglycemic, central nervous system depressant and analgesic actions.[2, 5] The implication of these findings to clinical practice has not yet been elucidated. In an open study, administration of 15 mL of nettle herb juice was shown to significantly increase the volume of urine excreted by 32 patients suffering from myocardial or chronic venous insufficiency.[5]

ADVERSE EFFECTS

Adverse effects following oral consumption of products containing nettle seem rare. Instances of scanty urination, skin irritation and gastric distress have been noted.[2, 4]

CAUTIONS/CONTRAINDICATIONS

No safety details exist regarding the use of this phytomedicine in pregnancy. Significant contraction of pregnant mouse uterine muscle has been reported *in vitro*.[2, 5]

DRUG INTERACTIONS

No specific cases of drug interactions could be found. Given the information of *in vitro* and *in vivo* studies, caution is advisable in cases of concomitant administration with conventional anti-hypertensive, diabetes and diuretic medications.[2]

DOSAGE REGIMENS

Aerial Parts:[2, 23]

- 3-6 g of dried herb (normally as an infusion) or 3-4 mL of liquid extract (1:1 in 25% alcohol) or 2-6 mL of tincture (1:5 in 45% alcohol) three times daily

Root:[4]

- Daily doses of 4-6 g of root or 1.5-7.5 mL of fluid extract (1:1, 45% ethanol) or 5 mL of tincture (1:5, 40% ethanol)

REFERENCES

1. Mills S. *The Essential Book of Herbal Medicine.* 2nd ed. London: Penguin; 1991:677.
2. Newall C, Anderson L, Phillipson J. *Herbal Medicines: A Guide for Health Care Professionals.* London: The Pharmaceutical Press; 1996:296.
3. Leung A, Foster S. *Encylopedia of Common Natural Ingredients Used in Food, Drugs and Cosmetics.* New York, NY: John Wiley and Sons; 1996:649.
4. ESCOP. *Urticae Radix*/Nettle Root. In: ESCOP Monographs (Fascicule 2)Exeter: ESCOP; 1996:58.
5. ESCOP. *Urticae Folium*/Herba (Nettle Leaf). In: ESCOP Monographs (Fascicule 4). Exeter: ESCOP; 1997:58
6. Weiss RF. *Herbal Medicine*. Beaconsfield, England: Beaconsfield Publishers Ltd.; 1988:362.
7. Chaurasia N, Wichtl M. Flavonolglykoside aus *Urtica dioica*. *Planta Medica*. 1987;53:432-4.
8. Andersen S, Wold JK. Water-soluble glycoprotein from *Urtica dioica* leaves. *Phytochemistry*. 1978;17:1875-7.
9. Barlow RB, Dixon R. Choline acetyltransferase in the nettle *Urtica dioica* L. *Biochemistry Journal*. 1973;132:15-8.
10. Chaurasia N, Wichtl M. Scopolectin, 3-B-sitosterin und 3-B-D-glucosid aus Brennesselwurzel (*Urtica radix*). *Deutsch Apothek Zeitung*. 1986;126:81-3.

11. Chaurasia N, Wichtl M. Sterols and steryl glycosides from *Urtica dioica*. *Journal of Natural Products*. 1987;50:881-5.
12. Hoffmann D. *Holistic Herbal.* Rockport, CA: Element Books; 1996:256.
13. Dreikorn K, Schonhofer P. Status of phytotherapeutic drugs in the treatment of benign prostatic hyperplasia. [German]. *Urologe A.* 1995;34(2):119-29.
14. Buck A. Phytotherapy for the Prostate. *British Journal of Urology*. 1996;78:325-336.
15. Schneider HJ, Honold E, Mashur T. Treatment of benign prostatic hyperplasia. Results of a surveilance study in the practices of urological specialists using a combined plant-based preparation. *Forschritte der Medizin*. 1995;113:37-40.
16. Hartmann R, Mark M, Soldati F. Inhibition of 5 alpha reductase and aromatase by PHL-00801 (Prostatonin), a combination of PY102 (*Pygeum africanum*) and UR102(*Urtica dioica*) extracts. *Phytomedicine.* 1996;3(2):121-128.
17. Hyrb D, Khan M, Romas N, Rosner W. The effect of estracts of the roots of the stinging nettle (*Urtica dioica*) on the interaction of SHBG with its receptor on human prostatic membranes. *Planta Medica*. 1995;61:31-2.
18. McCaleb R. Synergistic action of pygeum and nettle root extracts in prostate disease. *Herbalgram*. 1996;40:18.
19. Obertreis B, Ruttkowski T, Teucher T, *et al*. *Ex-vivo in-vitro* inhibition of lipopolysaccharide stimulated tumor necrosis factor-alpha and interleukin-1 beta secretion in human whole blood by extractum urticae dioicae foliorum. [Published erratum appears in *Arzneimittelforschung* 1996 Sep;46(9):936]. *Arzneimittelforschung*. 1996;46(4):389-94.
20. Chrubasik S, Enderlein W, Bauer R, Grabner W. Evidence for antirheumatic effectivenss of Herba *Urticae dioicae* in acute arthritis: A pilot study. *Phytomedicine*. 1997;4(2):105-108.
21. Rand J. Pilot study indicates that stewed herba urticae dioicae may potentiate the effects of diclofenac in acute arthritis. *Focus on Alternative and Complementary Therapies*. 1997;2(4):156-7.
22. Mittman P. Randomized double-blind study of freeze-dried *Urtica dioca* in the treatment of allergic rhinitis. *Planta Medica*. 1990;56:44-47.
23. Bradley P. *British Herbal Compendium.* Bournemouth: BHMA; 1992:239.

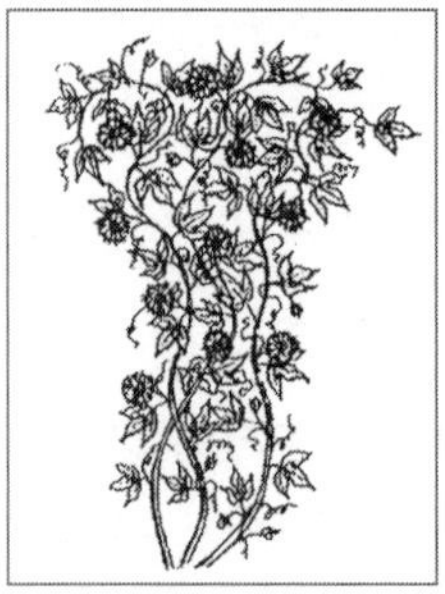

PASSIONFLOWER

Passiflora incarnata L.

THUMBNAIL SKETCH

Active Constituents

∗Multiple including flavonoids

Common Uses

∗Relief of restlessness, tension and insomnia

Adverse Effects

∗Sedation

Cautions/Contraindications

∗Pregnancy and lactation

Drug Interactions

∗The potential exists for interactions with concomitant administration of centrally acting medications

Doses

∗0.25-1.0 g of dried herb
∗0.5 mL-2.0 mL liquid extract (1:1,25% alcohol)
∗2-4 mL (1:8 in 45% alcohol) three times daily

INTRODUCTION

Family: Passifloraceae

Synonyms: Maypop, Maypop passion flower, Passiflora, Apricot vine, Wild passion flower, Passion vine, Grenadille [1, 2]

Passionflower is a perennial vine growing up to 9 m in length which is native to the southern United States. Other members of the genus *Passiflora* are found throughout North, South and Central America.[1] The name arises from the plant's intricate and elaborate flower that blooms only for a maximum of 48 hours.[3] The flower parts are thought to represent the elements of Christ's Passion. For example, the fringe-like crown is said to represent the crown of thorns, while the five anthers represent the five stigmata. 'Passio' means suffering and 'incarnata' means incarnate.[3]

Passionflower was used within many traditional healing models in America. For example, the Aztecs prized it as a sedative.[4] Modern phytotherapy has expanded upon these historical uses. In addition, passionflower is used for similar indications within the homeopathic tradition.[3] While many species of *Passiflora* produce edible fruits, the ones commonly available are not from *P. incarnata* but rather *P. edulis* Sims.[3] The part used medicinally is the leaf.

Constituents [1, 2, 4-11]

- Flavonoids including: vitexin, isovitexin, vitexin-4-O-rhamnoside, rutin, quercetin, kaempferol, apigenin and luteolins (orientin, homoorientin and lucenin)
- Alkaloids including: harman, harmalin, harmalol and harmine (referred to in some texts as harmala alkaloids)
- Miscellaneous: maltol, fatty acids, sugars and gum

THERAPEUTIC USES & RELEVANT PHARMACOLOGY

COMMON USES

Passionflower is reputed to have hypnotic,[4, 12, 13] sedative,[4, 12-14] anodyne (analgesic)[4, 12] and anti-spasmodic properties.[4, 12] The ESCOP monograph lists therapeutic indications of 'tenseness, rest-lessness and irritability with difficulty in falling asleep'.[11] In addition, the French and Swiss herbal pharmacopoeia indicate that it is useful in the management of mild heart conditions.[3] It is thought to be particularly useful in individuals that are weak or exhausted whether from overwork, illness or age.[4] A number of references mention its use in conditions of hysteria and convulsions.[4, 12]

GENERAL PHARMACOLOGY

It was initially thought that the harmala alkaloids were the primary active constituents.[3,13] It has since been shown that they are present only in trace amounts.[3, 4] Another theory is that the medicinal effects may be due at least in part to maltol, which has been shown to have physiological activity in animal models.[15] However, other researchers have argued that maltol may not be present in the original plant, but is formed during the heat extraction processes.[3] While it is likely that no one group of constituents is solely responsible for this plant's medicinal action, it appears that the flavonoid components are the ones of most importance.[3]

CENTRAL NERVOUS SYSTEM

Psychotropic, sedative and anxiolytic properties have been demonstrated following the administration of very large doses of extracts of *P. incarnata* L. in a number of animal models.[3, 11, 16-18] These actions appear to be influenced by the solvent used in the extraction process.[16] Anxiolytic properties are reported to be evident at lower doses with sedation occurring on administration of larger amounts.[17]

Other studies have reported conflicting findings to those mentioned above.[11] Chrysin, a monoflavonoid found in a related species (*P. caerulea* L.), has been shown to exert an anxiolytic action in mice with no subsequent sedation or muscle relaxation. The authors hypothesize that this could be due to its action as a partial antagonist of the central benzodiazepine receptors.[19] An increase in the nociceptive threshold and reduction in locomotor activity have been noted in rats following administration of an hydroalcoholic extract of *P. incarnata* L (160 mg/kg).[18]

A multi-centered, double-blind study (n=182) demonstrated that a commercial product containing passionflower (Euphytose®), was significantly beneficial when compared to placebo in the management of adjustment disorder with anxious mood. The product was given at a dose of two tablets three times daily for 28 days.[20] The impact of passionflower on this outcome is unknown since Euphytose® contains a number of centrally acting phytomedicines, including valerian (*Valeriana officinalis* L., Valerianaceae).

CARDIAC

The evidence supporting the action of passionflower in the treatment of cardiac conditions appears to come from the presence of C-glycosylflavones. These agents (e.g., vitexin, isovitexin) extracted from another plant, hawthorn (*Crataegus monogyna* Jacq., Rosaceae), have been shown to be clinically beneficial in the management of a number of cardiac conditions.[21] Meier makes reference to a randomized, placebo-controlled clinical trial of patients suffering from congestive heart failure (n=40) following administration of a hawthorn/passionflower product (standardized to flavonoid content). While improvement was noted using a number of outcome measures, the importance of the passionflower in the product is not known.[3] Although a hypotensive action from passionflower has been noted *in vivo*,[1] concerns have been raised regarding the lack of clinically relevant information available for this herbal product given its widespread use.[3, 22]

ADVERSE EFFECTS

A case of hypersensitivity vasculitis was noted in a 77-year-old man suffering from rheumatoid arthritis following administration of a herbal product in which '*Passiflora* extract' was the primary ingredient. The patient had been taking conventional medication (diclofenac and cyclopenthiazide) for a period of 5 years and was applying a placebo gel as part of a clinical trial. The authors conclude that the herbal product was the most likely culprit and make reference to another case reported to the CSM (Committee on Safety of Medicines). No reference is made as to whether the authenticity of the product was confirmed.[23] In addition 'altered consciousness' was reported in five people who consumed a commercial product made primarily from the fruit of *P. incarnata* L. (Relaxir ®). Once again, no information is available as to whether attempts were made to authenticate the product.[24]

CAUTIONS/CONTRAINDICATIONS

Excessive use should be avoided during pregnancy and lactation.[2] Passionflower may cause sedation and inhibit the ability to drive or use heavy machinery.[11] No reference could be found regarding the influence of alcohol.

Concerns have been raised because harmala alkaloids found in other plants have been shown to act as monoamine oxidase inhibitors (MAOI). Given the small amounts present in *P. incarnata* L., it is unlikely that this will require the restrictions applied to conventional MAOI therapy.[4]

DRUG INTERACTIONS

Passionflower extracts have been shown to increase the sleeping time induced by pentobarbital or hexabarbital in a number of animal models.[15-18]

Extracts of passionflower also appear to offer protection against convulsions induced by pentylenetetrazole in mice.[15, 18] The clinical relevance of these findings is unknown since the evidence comes solely from animal models and the doses and modes of administration are not generally comparable to those seen in clinical practice. Until more is known, it would be prudent to be cautious when administering products containing this herb concurrently with centrally acting conventional medications.

DOSAGE REGIMENS

- 0.25-1.0 g of dried herb (can be taken as an infusion) or 0.5 -2.0 mL (1:1 in 25% alcohol) or 2-4 mL (1:8 in 45% alcohol) three times daily.[2, 25]
- A number of references note that passionflower is rarely given as a single remedy but rather combined with other phytomedicines determined by the indication.[3, 4]

Since the constituents responsible for the reputed therapeutic action of passionflower have yet to be conclusively determined, Bergner advises against the use of standardized extracts.[4]

REFERENCES

1. Leung A, Foster S. *Encyclopedia of Common Natural Ingredients Used in Food, Drugs and Cosmetics*. New York, NY: John Wiley and Sons; 1996:649.
2. Newall C, Anderson L, Phillipson J. *Herbal Medicines: A Guide for Health Care Professionals*. London: The Pharmaceutical Press; 1996:296.
3. Meier B. *Passiflora incarnata* L. — Passion flower. Portrait of a medicinal plant. *Quarterly Review of Natural Medicine*. 1995;3 (3 Fall):191-202 (Translated from the German *Zeitschrift fur Phytotherapie* 16: 115-26,1995).
4. Bergner P. Passionflower. *Medical Herbalism*. 1995;7(1-2):13-14,26.
5. Congora C, Proliac A, Raynaud J. Isolement et identification de deux glycosyl-luteolines mono-C-substituees et de la diglucosyl-6,8-luteoline di-C-substituee dans les tiges feuillees de *Passiflora incarnata* L. (Isolation and identification of two mono-C-glucosyl-luteolins and of the di-C-subsituted 6,8-diglucosyl-luteolin from the leafy stalks of *Passiflora incarnata* L.). *Helvetica Chimica* Acta. 1986;69:251-3.
6. Quercia V, Turchetto L, Pierini N, *et al*. Identification and determination of vitexin and isovitexin in *Passiflora*

incarnata extracts. *Journal of Chromatography*. 1978;161:396-402.

7. Pietta P, Manera E, Ceva P. Isocratic liquid chromatographic method for the simultaneous determination of *Passiflora incarnata* L. and *Crataegus monogyna* flavonoids in drugs. *Journal of Chromatography*. 1986; 357:233-8.
8. Proliac A, Raynaud J. The presence of C-B-D-6-glucopyranosyl-C-a-L-arabinopyranosyl-8-apigenin in leafy stems of *Passiflora incarnata*. *Pharmazie*. 1986;41:673-4.
9. Geiger H, *et al*. The C-glycosylfavone pattern of *Passiflora incarnata* L. *Zeitung Naturforsch.* 1986;Sept/Oct:949-50.
10. Proliac A, Raynaud J. O-glucosyl-2"-C-glucosyl-6 apegenine de *Passiflora incarnata* L. (Passifloraceae). *Pharmaceutica Acta Helvetiae*. 1988;63(6):174-5.
11. ESCOP. Passiflora Herba/Passiflora. In: *ESCOP Monographs* (Fascicule 4). Exeter: ESCOP; 1997:58.
12. Hoffmann D. *Holistic Herbal*. Rockport, CA: Element Books; 1996:256.
13. Weiss RF. *Herbal Medicine*. Beaconsfield, England: Beaconsfield Publishers; 1988:362.
14. Flynn J. The herbal management of stress. *Australian Journal of Medical Herbalism*. 1996;8(1):15-18.
15. Aoyagi N, Kimura R, Murata T. Studies on *Passiflora incarnata* dry extract. I. Isolation of maltol and pharmacological action of maltol and ethyl maltol. *Chemical and Pharmaceutical Bulletin*. 1974;22:1008-13.
16. Soulimani R, Younos C, Jarmouni S, Bousta D, Misslin R, Mortier F. Behavioural effects of *Passiflora incarnata* L. and its indole alkaloid and flavonoid derivatives and maltol in the mouse. *Journal of Ethnopharmacology*. 1997;57(1):11-20.
17. Della Loggia R, Tubaro A, Redaelli C. Valutazione dell'attivita sul S.N.C del topo di alcuni estratti vegetali e di una loro associazone. [Italian]. *Rivista di Neurologia*. 1981;51:297-310.
18. Speroni E, Minghetti A. Neuropharmacological activity of extracts from *Passiflora incarnata*. *Planta Medica*. 1988;54:488-491.
19. Wolfman C, Viola H, Paladini A, *et al*. Possible anxiolytic effects of chrysin, a central benzodiazepine receptor lig and isolated from *Passiflora coerulea*. *Pharmacology Biochemistry and Behaviour.* 1994;47(1):1-4.
20. Bourin M, Bougerol T, Guitton B, Broutin E. A combination of plant extracts in the treatment of outpatients with adjustment disorder with anxious mood: Controlled study versus placebo. *Fundamental Clinical Pharmacology*. 1997;11(2):127-32.
21. Hobbs C, Foster S. Hawthorn — a literature review. *Herbalgram*. 1990;22:19-33.
22. Tyler V. *Herbs of Choice. The Therapeutic Use of Phytomedicinals*. Binghampton, NY: Pharmaceutical Products Press; 1994:209.
23. Smith GW, Chalmers TM, Nuki G. Vasculitis associated with herbal preparation containing *Passiflora extract.* [Letter]. *British Journal of Rheumatology*. 1993; 32(1):87-8.
24. Solbakken AM, Rorbakken G, Gundersen T. Nature medicine as intoxicant. [Norwegian]. *Tidsskr Nor Laegeforen*. 1997;117(8):1140-1.
25. Bradley P. *British Herbal Compendium*. Bournemouth: BHMA; 1992:239.

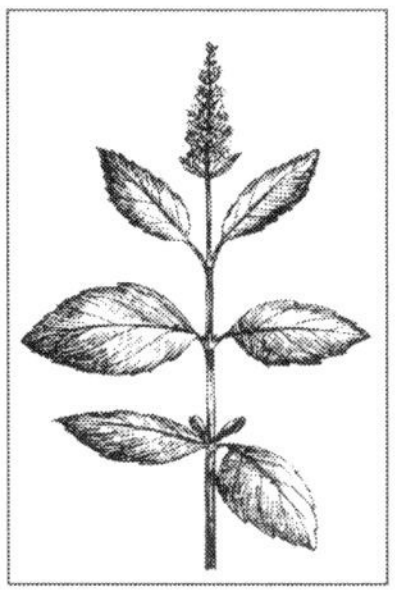

PEPPERMINT

Mentha x piperita L.

THUMBNAIL SKETCH

Active Constituents

- Menthol and its derivatives

Common Uses

- Irritable bowel disease
- Spastic colon
- Adjunctive therapy for colonoscopy and barium enema
- Gastritis

Adverse Effects

- Rare, but include: heartburn and esophageal reflux as well as contact irritation when peppermint is used as a flavoring agent in oral products.

Cautions/Contraindications

- Caution in infants and young children as well as patients with achlorhydria

Drug Interactions

- None known

Doses

- Enteric coated peppermint oil capsules: three times daily away from meals

INTRODUCTION

Family: Laminaceae (also known as Labiatae)

Synonyms: A number of varieties exist, including *M. x piperita* L. var *vulgaris* Sole (Black Mint), and *M. x piperita* L. var *officinalis* Sole (White Mint)[1]

Peppermint (*Mentha x piperita* L.), once thought to be a unique species, is currently thought to be a hybrid of two other members of the mint family: water mint (*Mentha aquatica* L.) and spearmint (*Mentha spicata* L.).[2,3] Although it is native to Europe, peppermint is now an important aromatic/medicinal crop throughout North American temperate zones, especially in the states of Indiana, Wisconsin, Oregon, Washington and Idaho. This perennial grows to a height of approximately 1 m, spreads by surface runners, and has pink to purple flowers.[4] In addition, it has a square stem characteristic of all members of the mint family.[5]

Both the peppermint leaf, often taken as a tea, and the essential oil, which is distilled from the leaves, have a long history of medicinal use. Peppermint is considered a carminitive.[6-8] Peppermint leaf tea has been used for indigestion, nausea, diarrhea, colds, headache and cramps.[4,9] The most common use of peppermint oil today is as a flavouring agent in a variety of oral products, including toothpastes, chewing gum and after-dinner mints.[4,6,10] This review will primarily deal with the use of peppermint when taken orally or applied topically and not on its use as an aromatherapy agent.

Constituents [4,6,9]

- Volatile Oil: (-)-menthol and its esters (acetate and isovalerate), (+)- and (-)-menthone, (+)-isomenthone, (+)-neomethone, (+)-menthofuran, eucalyptol, (-)-limonene
- Miscellaneous: flavonoids, phytol, tocopherols, carotenoids, betain, choline, azulenes, rosmarinic acid, tannins

1-Menthol makes up 29 to 48% of the essential oil, but is considered to be a distinctly different agent, not to be confused with the volatile oil of peppermint.[4] Although menthol can be obtained from peppermint oil, the high price of peppermint oil makes this use very uncommon. Today, menthol is usually produced synthetically by the hydrogenation of thymol. Synthetic menthol differs from that produced from peppermint in that it is racemic.

THERAPEUTIC USES & RELEVANT PHARMACOLOGY

COMMON USES

Peppermint is reputed to have antispasmodic, carminative, antiemetic, diaphoretic, hepatic and antiseptic properties.[1,3,11] As with all carminatives, oral consumption is considered useful in the treatment of many digestive disorders especially nausea, vomiting, bloating, nervous bowel and indigestion.[11,12] It is also commonly used to treat colds and flus.[11]

GASTROINTESTINAL

According to a 1990 study of a variety of over-the-counter (OTC) products conducted by the Food and Drug Administration (FDA) in the United States, there is not sufficient evidence to demonstrate that peppermint oil is effective as a digestive aid. However, this conclusion was based solely on evidence submitted by the manufacturers of the OTC products being reviewed.[13] Tyler heavily criticizes this review.[6] In contrast, the German Commission E's review of the scientific literature has concluded that there is sufficient evidence to demonstrate that peppermint and its volatile oil are effective spasmolytics, and that they promote gastric secretions and the flow of bile.[14]

Several studies have found that in order for peppermint oil to effectively alleviate the symptoms of a variety of bowel conditions, including irritable bowel and spastic colon, the oil must reach the colon in its original state (i.e., unmetabolized state). Thus, most peppermint oil products sold for this purpose in Canada are enteric-coated. Gelatin-coated capsules release the peppermint oil in the stomach where it is metabolized before reaching the colon.[15]

Irritable Bowel Syndrome

Irritable bowel presents with symptoms such as: abdominal pain, feelings of distention, and "variations in bowel habits.[4]" Several clinical trials have demonstrated the clinical effectiveness of enteric-coated peppermint oil (most often the brand Colpermin®) in relieving these symptoms.[16,17] In one double-blind, placebo-controlled, cross-over trial (n=18), enteric-coated peppermint oil capsules (1-2 caps TID depending on severity of symptoms) given between meals significantly decreased patients' symptoms when compared with a placebo (peanut oil).[16]

Antispasmodic

Several *in vitro* studies have demonstrated peppermint oil's ability to relax smooth muscle via blockade of the calcium channel transport mechanism.[18,19] One research team reported that colon spasms during endoscopy were relieved within 30 seconds when diluted suspension of peppermint oil injected along the biopsy channel of the colonoscope in 20 patients. They called for a prospective clinical trial for this indication, but our literature search found none to date.

Several clinical studies have noted that the addition of peppermint to barium enema suspension decreased the incidence of spasm.[21,22] One double-blind study (n=141) found that peppermint oil (added to barium sulphate suspension) was significantly effective at relieving colonic muscle spasm during double contrast barium enema examination. The authors suggest that this simple, safe and inexpensive technique could decrease the need for intravenous spasmolytic agents during barium enema procedures.[22]

Miscellaneous

One double-blind, placebo-controlled, cross-over study (n=6) found that peppermint oil decreases colonic motility in humans.[23] Another double-blind, placebo-controlled, multicentre trial (n=45) found that a peppermint oil (90 mg)/caraway oil (50 mg) combination significantly reduced the symptoms of non-ulcer dyspepsia after four weeks of treatment.[24]

ANTIMICROBIAL ACTIVITY

Antibacterial

In vitro testing indicates that peppermint inhibits the growth of a variety of bacteria, including:

S. aureus, *B. brevis*, *B. circulans*, *Citrobacter sp.*, *E. coli*, *Klebsiella sp.*, *S. Typhi*, *S. Typhimurium*, *S. boydii*, *S. flexneri*, and *V. cholerae*.[25] In addition, peppermint oil was found to be ineffective against *Pseudomonas aeruginosa*.[26] The clinical significance of these findings is unknown.

Antifungal

Peppermint is reported to inhibit the growth *in vitro* of a variety of fungi including: *C. albicans*, *C. neoformans*, *S. schenkii*, *A. citrii*, *A. fumigatus*, *A. oryzae*, *F. oxysporum*, *F. solani*, *H. compactum*, *M. phaseolina*, *S. rolfsii*, and *T. mentagrophytes*.[2] The clinical significance of these findings is unknown.

Antiviral

Peppermint is reported to have activity against herpes simplex virus and Newcastle disease *in vitro*.[9] The clinical significance of this is unknown.

MISCELLANEOUS

Peppermint oil has traditionally been used externally for a wide range of indications including headaches. One double-blind, placebo-controlled, randomized, cross-over clinical trial (n=32) reports that a combination of peppermint oil (10 g), eucalyptus oil (5 g) and ethanol (ad 100 g) significantly increased cognitive performance as well as produced mental and pericranial muscle relaxation. In addition, peppermint oil (10 g) in combination with ethanol (*ad* 100 g) produced a significant analgesic effect.[27]

ADVERSE EFFECTS

Regular consumption of peppermint leaf tea is considered safe; however, excessive use of the volatile oil (>0.3 g or 12 drops) may cause problems.[6] Clinical trials of enteric coated peppermint oil capsules for a variety of gastrointestinal complaints report few adverse effects. Heartburn and esophageal reflux can occur if the peppermint oil is accidentally released in the stomach.[16] In addition, a burning sensation during defecation (thought to be due to unabsorbed menthol reaching the rectum) has occasionally been observed when peppermint oil is taken in high doses. Reducing the dose reduces this adverse effect.

There have also been several reports of contact-sensitivity to the peppermint in a variety of oral products including toothpaste.[28-31] Symptoms include: burning sensation in the mouth, recurrent oral ulceration, stomatitis, glossitis, gingivitis, and perioral dermatitis.

One case report describes veno-occlusive disease in an 18-month old boy who had regularly consumed a tea believed to contain peppermint and coltsfoot (*Tussilago farfara* L., Asteraceae) for the previous 12 months. Analysis of the tea revealed that the tea contained *Adenosyles alliariae* (Gouan) Kern., Asteraceae, rather than the reported coltsfoot. The peppermint was not thought to play any role in the toxicity of the product.[32]

Cardiac fibrillation has been reported in patients whose condition was controlled with quinidine following the use of mentholated cigarettes or consumption of peppermint candy.[33]

CAUTIONS/CONTRAINDICATIONS

Peppermint should generally be given between meals and it should not be taken by patients with achlorhydria (i.e., patients with no hydrochloric acid in gastric juices).[16] Generally, peppermint (tea and topical application to nostrils) should be avoided in young children or infants because the menthol may cause a choking sensation.[6,31] In addition, oral consumption of peppermint oil should be avoided in situations of glucose-6 phosphate dehydrogenase deficiency since menthol may be implicated in this condition.[31]

DRUG INTERACTIONS

No known drug interactions.

DOSAGE REGIMENS

- Enteric coated peppermint oil capsules (0.2 mL peppermint oil/capsule): 1-2 capsules three times daily between meals[34]
- Tincture (1:5; 45% ethanol): 2-3 mL three times daily away from meals

Preparation of Peppermint Tea

Mix 160 mL (2/3 cup) of boiling water with 1.5 g (1 tablespoonful) of recently dried leaves and steep for 5 to 10 minutes. This amount is taken on an empty stomach three to four times daily to relieve upset stomach.[6]

REFERENCES

1. Wren R. *Potter's New Encyclopedia of Botanical Drugs and Preparations*. Saffron Walden: C.W. Daniel Company; 1988:362.
2. Murray MJ, Lincoln DE, Marble PM. Oil composition of *Mentha aquatica* x *M. sicata* F_1 hybrids in relation to the origin of *M.* x *piperita*. *Canadian Journal of Genetics and Cytology*. 1972;14:13-29.
3. Mills S. *Essential Book of Herbal Medicine.* London: Penguin Books Limited; 1991:677.
4. Foster S. Peppermint. *Mentha x piperita*. Austin, Texas: American Botanical Council; 1991:7
5. Evans W. *Trease and Evans' Pharmacognosy*. 13th ed. London: Bailliere Tindall; 1989:832.
6. Tyler VE. *Herbs of Choice. The Therapeutic Use of Phytomedicinals.* Binghamton, New York, NY: Pharmaceutical Products Press; 1994:209.
7. Sigmund CJ, McNally EF. The action of a carminitive on the lower esophageal sphincter. *Gastroenterology*. 1969;56(1):13-18.
8. Murray M. The clinical uses of peppermint. *The American Journal of Natural Medicine*. 1995;2(2):10-13.
9. Leung A, Foster S. *Encyclopedia of Common Natural Ingredients Used in Food, Drugs and Cosmetics.* 2nd ed. New York, NY: John Wiley and Sons; 1996:649.
10. Bauer K, Garbe D. *Common Fragrance and Flavor Materials: Preparation, Properties and Uses.* Deerfield Beach, FL: VCH Publishers; 1985.
11. Hoffmann D. *Holistic Herbal.* Rockport, CA: Element Books; 1996:256.
12. Weiss RF. *Herbal Medicine.* Gothenburg, Sweden: Ab Arcanum; 1988:362
13. Blumenthal M. Peppermint *Herbalgram*. 1990;49(23):32-3.
14. Blumenthal M, Brusse WR, Goldberg A, *et al. The Complete German Commission E Monographs*. Austin, TX: American Botanical Council; 1998:685
15. Somerville KW, Richmond CR, Bell GD. Delayed release of peppermint oil capsules (Colpermin) for the spastic colon syndrome: A pharmacokinetic study. *British Journal of Clinical Pharmacology*. 1984;18:638-40.
16. Rees WDW, Evans BK, Rhodes J. Treating irritable bowel syndrome with peppermint oil. *British Medical Journal*. 1979; October 6:835-6.
17. Dew MJ, Evans BK, Rhodes J. Peppermint oil for the irritable bowel syndrome: A multicentre trial. *British Journal of Clinical Practice*. 1984;38:394-8.
18. Hills JM, Aaronson PI. Mechanism of action of peppermint oil on GI smooth muscle. *Gastroenterology*. 1991;101:55-65.
19. Taylor BA, Luscombe DD, Duthie HL. Inhibitory effects of peppermint oil and menthol on isolated human coli. *Gut*. 1984;25:A1168-9.

20. Leicester RJ, Hunt RH. Peppermint oil to reduce colonic spasm during endoscopy. *Lancet*. 1982;30 October:989.
21. Jarvis LJ, Hogg JIC, Houghton CD. Topical peppermint oil for the relief of spasm at barium enema. *Clincial Radiology*. 1992;46:A435.
22. Sparks MJ, P OS, Herrington AA, Morcos SK. Does peppermint oil relieve spasm during barium enema? *British Journal of Radiology*. 1995;68(812):841-3.
23. Duthie HL. The effect of peppermint oil on colonic motility in man. [Abstract only]. *Surgical Research Society Abstracts*:820.
24. May B, Kuntz HD, Kieser M, Kohler S. Efficacy of a fixed peppermint oil/caraway oil combination in non-ulcer dyspepsia. *Arzneimittelforschung*. 1996;46(12):1149-53.
25. Pattnaik S, Subramanyam VR, Kole C. Antibacterial and antifungal activity of ten essential oils *in vitro*. *Microbios*. 1996;86(349):237-46.
26. Pattnaik S, Rath C, Subramanyam VR. Characterization of resistance to essential oils in a strain of *Pseudomonas aeruginosa* (VR-6). *Microbios*. 1995;81(326):29-31.
27. Gobel H, Schmidt G, Soyka D. Effect of peppermint and eucalyptus oil preparations on neurophysiological and experimental algesimetric headache parameters. *Cephalalgia*. 1994;14(3):228-34; discussion 182.
28. Morton CA, Garioch J, Todd P, *et al*. Contact sensitivity to menthol and peppermint in patients with intra-oral symptoms. *Contact Dermatitis*. 1995;32(5):281-4.
29. Wilkinson SM, Beck MH. Allergic contact dermatitis from menthol in peppermint. *Contact Dermatitis*. 1994;30(1):42-3.
30. Sainio EL, Kanerva L. Contact allergens in toothpastes and a review of their hypersensitivity. *Contact Dermatitis*. 1995;33(2):100-5.
31. Tisserand R, Balacs T. *Essential Oil Safety: A Guide for Health Care Professionals*. London: Churchill Livingstone; 1995:279.
32. Sperl W, Stuppner H, Gassner I, Judmaier W, Dietze O, Vogel W. Reversible hepatic veno-occlusive disease in an infant after consumption of pyrrolizidine-containing herbal tea. *European Journal of Pediatrics*. 1995;154(2):112-6.
33. Thomas J. Peppermint fibrillation. *Lancet*. 1962;27 Jan:222.
34. Murray MT. *The Healing Power of Herbs*. Rocklin, CA: Prima Publishing; 1992:246.

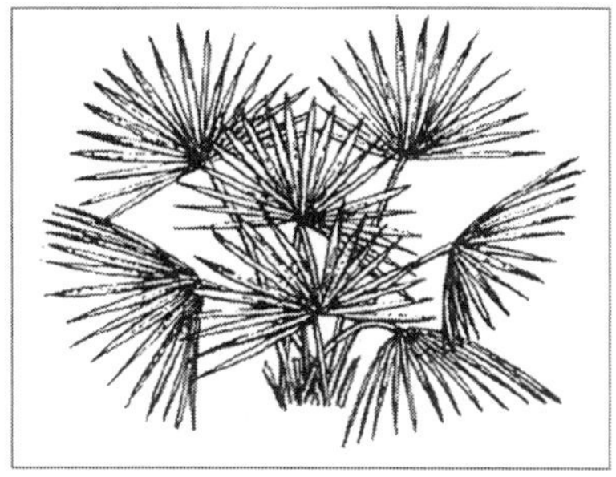

SAW PALMETTO

Serenoa repens (Bartram) Small

THUMBNAIL SKETCH

Active Constituents
- Fatty acids and sterols

Common Uses
- Benign prostatic hyperplasia (BPH)

Adverse Effects
- Rare, but gastro-intestinal upset can occur

Cautions/Contraindications
- Safety has not been established in pregnancy and lactation

Drug Interactions
- Theoretically may interact with existing hormonal therapy

Doses
- 160 mg liposterolic extract twice daily

INTRODUCTION

Family: Arecaceae (also known as Palmae)

Synonyms: *Serenoa serrulata* (Michx.) Nichols., *Sabal serrulata* (Michx.) Nutall ex. Schultes & Schultes, Sabal[1, 2]

The only surviving species of *Seronoa* is *Seronoa repens*, which can be found growing along the Atlantic coast of North America.[3] The shrub grows up to 3 m in height with a crown of palm-like leaves. The dark, wrinkled, oblong berries are the part used medicinally.[4]

Historically, the ripe fruit was partially dried and used for a variety of conditions of the bladder, urethra and prostate,[3] as well as a food source for early settlers in North America.[5] It was considered primarily a "male" remedy and was used to "improve flagging reproductive function" as well as "debility and senility in men."[6] Today, saw palmetto is best known for it use as a treatment for benign prostatic hyperplasia (BPH). Several excellent reviews have been written on this topic.[3, 7, 8]

Constituents [1-4]

- Fatty acids: lauric acid, linoleic acid, linolenic acid, capric acid, caproic acid, palmitic acid, oleic acid, caprylic acid, myristic acid, stearic acid
- Phytosterols: beta-sitosterol, stigmasterol, campesterol
- Alcohols: docosanol, hexacosanol, octacosanol, triacontanol
- Miscellaneous: carotenes, lipase, tannins

THERAPEUTIC USES & RELEVANT PHARMACOLOGY

PHARMACOLOGY

Currently most saw palmetto products are composed of 'liposterolic extracts' (i.e., containing the fatty acids and sterols) of the fruit.[3] There are three primary mechanisms by which these extracts appear to work against BPH:[3]

1. Androgen receptor blockade:[9-13] Dihydrotestosterone (DHT) is an active androgen (more active than testosterone) which has been implicated as a causative factor BPH.[11]

2. 5α-reductase inhibition:[13-18] 5α-reductase catalyzes the metabolism of testosterone to DHT. One recent study does not support this hypothesis; however, the researchers used half the usual dose of saw palmetto (80 mg BID) in their experiments.[19] Several recent *in vitro* studies which support this hypothesis suggest that the inhibition of saw palmetto extract is non-competitive in nature.[15, 17]

3. Disruption of the arachidonic cascade: Saw palmetto is reported to inhibit both the cyclooxygenase and lipoxygenase pathways,[20] which is believed to result in an anti-inflammatory effect which will provide added relief for the symptoms of BPH.

In addition, saw palmetto has a phytoestrogenic effect; it appears to compete with endogenous estrogen for receptor sites.[21, 22] One research team suggests that this may play a key role in its ability to decrease the symptoms of BPH.[22] It does not appear to affect plasma levels of testosterone, follicle-stimulating hormone (FSH) or luteinizing hormone (LH).[23] One study in rats demonstrated that saw palmetto extract was able to inhibit estradiol/testosterone-induced experimental prostate enlargement.[24]

BENIGN PROSTATIC HYPERPLASIA

A number of clinical studies including open trials;[25-30] double-blind, placebo-controlled trials;[31-35] and double-blind trials comparing saw palmetto with other treatments for BPH[36-38] have been completed to date. One multicenter open study involving 305 patients who took 160 mg of saw palmetto extract (Prostaserene®) twice daily for 3 months reports that 88% experienced improved symptoms, including: decreased prostate size and improved urinary flow rate.[29] Another study of 1,334 German outpatients found significant improvement in a variety of symptoms for those taking saw palmetto, including: decreased volume of residual urine, decreased urinary frequency, decreased nocturia, and decreased dysuria.[35] When saw palmetto (Permixon® 160 mg twice daily) was compared with finasteride (Proscar® 5 mg daily) in 1,098 patients in an international, multicentered trial, both treatments were found to decrease symptoms equally.[38] However, it should be noted that while saw palmetto appeared to be more effective in reducing the lower urinary tract symptoms of men with smaller prostate glands, those with more enlarged prostates had a greater reduction in size of prostate with finasteride. In addition, saw palmetto was associated with fewer side effects than finasteride.[38]

MISCELLANEOUS

Although no human clinical trials were available for review, saw palmetto has also been reported to be useful in the treatment of hirsutism.[8]

ADVERSE EFFECTS

Clinical trials report that saw palmetto is well-tolerated; however, the FDA in the United States lists saw palmetto as an herb of unknown safety.[1] Gastro-intestinal upset is rare, but possible.[34]

CAUTIONS/CONTRAINDICATIONS

Safety has not been established in pregnancy and lactation.[1]

DRUG INTERACTIONS

Theoretically, because of its anti-androgen and estrogenic activity, saw palmetto may interact with existing hormonal therapy, including hormone replacement therapy and contraceptive pills.[1]

DOSAGE REGIMENS

The majority of human clinical trials tested 160 mg of a liposterolic extract containing 85 to 95% fatty acids and sterols twice daily.[29, 39] This is equivalent to approximately 10 g crude berries twice daily. A liquid extract is also available: 0.6 to 1.5 mL daily.[1]

REFERENCES

1. Newall CA, Anderson LA, Phillipson JD. *Herbal Medicines: A Guide for Health Care Professionals*. London: The Pharmaceutical Press; 1996:296.
2. Leung A, Foster S. *Encyclopedia of Common Natural Ingredients Used in Food, Drugs and Cosmetics*. 2nd ed. New York, NY: John Wiley and Sons; 1996:649.
3. Awang DVC. Saw palmetto, African prune, and stinging nettle for benign prostatic hyperplasia (BPH). *Canadian Pharmaceutical Journal*. 1997; November:37-44,62.
4. Murray MT. *The Healing Power of Herbs*. Rocklin, CA: Prima Publishing; 1992:246.
5. Hutchens A. *Indian Herbology of North America*. Boston, MA: Shambhala; 1973:382.
6. Mills S. *Essential Book of Herbal Medicine*. London: Penguin Books Limited; 1991:677.
7. Brinker F. An overview of conventional, experimental and botanical treatments of non-malignant prostate conditions. *British Journal of Phytotherapy*. 1993/1994;3(4):154-76.
8. Snow JM. *Serenoa repens* Bartram (Palmae). *The Protocol Journal of Botanical Medicine*. 1996;1(3):15-16.
9. El-Sheikh MM, Dakkak MR, Saddique A. The effect of permixon on androgen receptors. *Acta Obstetrica et Gynecologica Scandinavica*. 1988;67:397-9.
10. Ravenna L, Di Silverio F, Russo MA, *et al.* Effects of the lipidosterolic extract of *Serenoa repens* (Permixon) on human prostatic cell lines. *Prostate*. 1996;29(4):219-30.
11. Wilson JD. The pathogenesis of benign prostatic hyperplasia. *American Journal of Medicine*. 1980;68:745-55.
12. Carilla E, Briley M, Fauran Fea. Binding of Permixon, a new treatment for prostatic benign hyperplasia, to cytosolic androgen receptor in rat prostate. *Journal of Steroid Biochemistry*. 1984;20:521-3.
13. Sultan C, Terrazza A, Devillier C, *et al.* Inhibition of androgen metabolism and binding by a liposterolic extract of *Serenoa repens* in human foreskin fibroblasts. *Journal of Steroid Biochemistry*. 1984;20(1):515-9.
14. Briley M, Carilla E, *et al.* Inhibitory effect of Permixon on testosterone 5α-reductase activity of rat ventral prostate. *British Journal of Pharmacology*. 1984;83(supplement):401.
15. Delos S, Iehle C, Martin PM, Raynaud JP. Inhibition of the activity of 'basic' 5α-reductase (type 1) detected in DU 145 cells and expressed in insect cells. *Journal of Steroid Biochemistry and Molecular Biology*. 1994;48(4):347-52.
16. Delos S, Carsol JL, Ghazarossian E, *et al* Testosterone metabolism in primary cultures of human prostate epithelial cells and fibroblasts. *Journal of Steroid Biochemistry and Molecular Biology*. 1995;55(3-4):375-83.
17. Iehle C, Delos S, Guirou O, *et al.* Human prostatic steroid 5 alpha-reductase isoforms—a comparative study of selective inhibitors. *Journal of Steroid Biochemistry and Molecular Biology*. 1995;54(5-6):273-9.
18. Rhodes L, Primka RL, Berman C, *et al.* Comparison of Finasteride (Proscar), a 5a reductase inhibitor, and various commercial plant extracts in *in vitro* and *in vivo* 5α reductase inhibition. *The Prostate*. 1993;22:43-51.
19. Strauch G, Perles P, Vergult G, *et al.* Comparison of finasteride (Proscar) and *Serenoa repens* (Permixon) in the inhibition of 5-alpha reductase in healthy male volunteers. *European Urology*. 1994;26(3):247-52.
20. Breu W, Hagenlocher M, Redl K, *et al.* Anti-inflammatory activity of Sabal fruit extracts prepared with supercritical carbon dioxide. *in vitro* antagonists of cyclooxygenase and 5-lipoxygenase metabolism. *Arzneimittelforschung*. 1992;42(4):547-51.
21. Elghamry MI, Hansel R. Activity and isolated phytoestrogen of shrub palmetto fruits (*Serenoa repens* Small), a new estrogenic plant. *Experientia*. 1969;25:828-9.
22. Di Silverio F, D'Eramo G, Lubrano C, *et al.* Evidence that *Serenoa repens* extract displays an antiestrogenic activity in prostatic tissue of benign prostatic hypertrophy patients. *European Urology*. 1992;21:309-14.
23. Casarosa C, Cosci di Coscio M, Fratta M. Lack of effects of a liposterolic extract of *Serenoa repens* on plasma levels of testosterone, FSH, and luteinizing hormone. *Clinical Therapeutics*. 1988;10:585-88.
24. Paubert-Braquet M, Richardson FO, Servent-Saez N, *et al.* Effect of *Serenoa repens* extract (Permixon) on estradiol/testosterone-induced experimental prostate enlargement in the rat. *Pharmacological Research*. 1996;34(3-4):171-9.
25. Cirillo-Marucco E, Pagliarulo A, Tritto G, *et al.* Extract of Serenoa repens (PermiconR) in the early treatment of prostatic hypertrophy. *Urologia*. 1983;5:1269-77.
26. Tripodi V, Giancaspro M, Pascarello M, *et al.* Treatment of prostatic hypertrophy with Seronoa repens extract. *Medical Praxis*. 1983;4:41-6.
27. Greca P, Volpi R. Experience with a new drug in the medical treatment of prostatic adenoma. *Urologia*. 1985;52:532-5.
28. Crimi A, Russo A. *Serenoa repens* for the treatment of the functional disturbances of prostate hypertrophy. *Medical Praxis*. 1983;4:47-51.
29. Braeckman J. The extract of *Seronoa repens* in the treatment of benign prostatic hyperplasia: A multicentre open study. *Current Therap. Research*. 1994;55(7):776-85.
30. Romics I, Schmitz H, Frang D. Experience in treating benign prostatic hypertrophy with *sabal serrulata* for one year. *International Urology and Nephrology*. 1993;25(6):565-69.

31. Boccafoschi, Annoscia S. Comparison of *Serenoa repens* extract with placebo by controlled clinical trial in patients with prostatic adenomatosis. *Urologia*. 1983;50:1257-68.
32. Emili E, Lo Cigno M, Petrone U. Clinical trial of a new drug for treating hypertrophy of the prostate (Permixon). *Urologia*. 1983;50:1042-8.
33. Champault G, Bonnard AM, Cauquil J, Patel JC. Medical treatment of prostatic adenoma. Controlled trial: PA 109 vs placebo in 110 patients. *Annales d'Urologie*. 1984;18:407-10.
34. Tasca A, Barulli M, Cavazzana A, *et al.* Treatment of obstruction in prostatic adenoma using an extract of Serenoa repens. Double-blind clinical test v. placebo. *Minerva Urologica E Nefrologica.* 1985;37:87-91.
35. Vahlensieck WJ, *et al.* Benign prostatic hyperplasia — Treatment with Sabal fruit extract. A treatment study of 1,334 patients. *Fortschritte der Medizin*. 1993;111:323-6.
36. Pannunzio E, *et al. Serenoa repens* in the treatment of human benign prostatic hypertrophy (BPH). *Journal of Urology.* 1987;137:226A.
37. Adriazola Semino M, *et al.* Symptomatic treatment of benign hypertrophy of the prostate. *Arch Esp Urol*. 1992;45:211-13.
38. Carraro JC, Raynaud JP, Koch G, *et al.* Comparison of phytotherapy (Permixon) with finasteride in the treatment of benign prostate hyperplasis: A randomized international study of 1,098 patients. *Prostate*. 1996;29:231-40.
39. Blumenthal M, Brusse WR, Goldberg A, *et al. The Complete German Commission E Monographs.* Austin, TX: American Botanical Council; 1998:685.

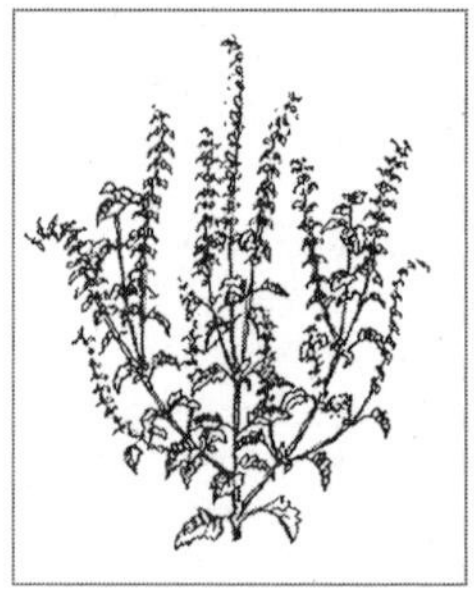

SCULLCAP

Scutellaria lateriflora L.

THUMBNAIL SKETCH

Active Constituents

- Flavonoids, volatile oils, iridoids and tannins

Common Uses

- Conditions of nervous tension, exhaustion, spasms and hysteria

Adverse Effects

- Drowsiness, giddiness, confusion and convulsions in large doses
- Scullcap has been implicated in cases of hepatotoxicity but this may be due to adulteration of products with germander

Cautions/Contraindications

- Pregnancy and lactation

Drug Interactions

- None known but caution is suggested in patients taking other centrally acting drugs.

Doses

- 0.5-2 g of dried herb/0.5-2 mL of liquid extract (1:1 in 25% alcohol) /2-4 mL of tincture (1:8 in 25% alcohol) up to 4 x daily

INTRODUCTION

Family: Laminaceae also known as Labiatae

Synonyms: Helmet flower, Hoodwort, Quaker bonnet, Scutellaria, Mad-dog scullcap, Skullcap, European or greater skullcap[1-3]

Many different species of the genus *Scutellaria* are used medicinally, although most texts identify *lateriflora* as the most common species.[2] In addition, *Scutellaria baicalensis* Georgi (Baikal Scullcap/Huang-qin) is a major medicinal herb used in Traditional Chinese Medicine.[3] In the western tradition the aerial parts of the plant are used medicinally, whereas the roots of Baikal Scullcap are used within the Traditional Chinese Medical model.[2, 3]

Constituents[1, 2, 4-6]

There is a lack of information specifically relating to *Scutellaria lateriflora* L.; thus, the information listed below refers to a number of species contained in the *Scutellaria* genus.

- Flavonoids including: apigenin, luteolin, scutellarin (baicalein, wogonin, baicalin are found in *S. baicalensis* Georgi)
- Volatile oils: primarily monoterpenes and sesquiterpenes.
- Iridoids: catalpol is found in both *S. lateriflora* and *S. galericulata* L.
- Miscellaneous including: tannins and resin

THERAPEUTIC USES & RELEVANT PHARMACOLOGY

COMMON USES

Scullcap is reputed to have sedative,[1, 7] nervine,[1, 7] anti-spasmodic,[1, 7] and anticonvulsant properties.[1, 7] Oral consumption is considered useful in the treatment of conditions related to nervous tension and exhaustion.[7] It is often used in patients with hysteria, spasms or convulsions.[1, 7]

PHARMACOLOGY[2, 4]

Little or no clinical information could be found relating to the pharmacology of *Scutellaria lateriflora* L., with most of the available work referring to *Scutellaria baicalensis* Georgi. Extracts of *Scutellaria baicalensis* Georgi and its constituents have been shown *in vivo* and *in vitro* to: inhibit lipid peroxidation,[8, 9] possess antibacterial and antiviral properties,[10] influence arachidonate metabolism,[11] influence lipolysis and lipogenesis,[12] decrease release of histamine from rat mast cells,[5] and decrease serum lipid levels.[13] Given the different species and the fact that the aerial parts rather than the root are used in Western herbalism, it is unknown how applicable the above information is to scullcap products used medicinally in North America.[14]

ADVERSE EFFECTS

Large doses of scullcap can cause giddiness, confusion, drowsiness and convulsions.[15] In addition, herbal products containing scullcap as one of the ingredients have been implicated in a number of cases of hepatotoxicity,[15,16] which has resulted in the removal of a number of herbal scullcap preparations from the market in the United Kingdom.[16] Instances of hepatotoxicity may have been due to adulteration or substitution of scullcap with any of several species of germander (*Teucrium canadense* L., *T. chamaedrys* L., etc.).[17]

CAUTIONS/CONTRAINDICATIONS

Given the lack of information and the cases of possible hepatotoxicity mentioned above, products containing scullcap should not be used in pregnancy or lactation.[2]

DRUG INTERACTIONS

While no clinical examples could be found, given scullcap's reputed sedative action it should be used with caution in patients taking conventional centrally acting medications.[18]

DOSAGE REGIMENS[19]

- 0.5-2 g of dried herb/0.5 –2 mL of liquid extract (1:1 in 25% alcohol)/2-4 mL of tincture (1:8 in 25% alcohol) up to 4 times daily.

REFERENCES

1. Wren R. *Potter's New Encyclopedia of Botanical Drugs and Preparations*. Saffron Walden: C.W. Daniel Company; 1988:362.
2. Newall C, Anderson L, Phillipson J. *Herbal Medicines: A Guide for Health Care Professionals*. London: The Pharmaceutical Press; 1996:296.
3. Foster S, Chongxi Y. *Herbal Emissaries*. 1st ed. Rochester, VT.: Healing Arts Press; 1992:356.
4. Leung A, Foster S. *Encyclopedia of Common Natural Ingredients Used in Food, Drugs and Cosmetics.* New York, NY: John Wiley and Sons; 1996:649.
5. Kubo M, Matsuda H, Kimura Y, *et al Scutellariae radix*. X. Inhibitory effects of various flavonoids on histamine release from rat peritoneal mast cells *in vitro*. *Chemical and Pharmaceutical Bulletin*. 1984;32(12):5051-4.
6. Tomimori T, Jin H, Miyaichi Y, *et al*. Studies on the constituents of Scutellaria species. VI. On the flavonoid constituents of theroot *Scutellaria baicalensis* Georgi (5). Quantitative analysis of flavonoids in Scutellaria roots by high-performance liquid chromatography. *Yakugaku Zasshi*. 1985;105(2):148-55.
7. Hoffmann D. *Holistic Herbal.* Rockport, CA: Element Books; 1996:256.
8. Kimura Y, Okuda H, Tani T, Arichi S. Studies on *Scutellaria radix*. VI. Effects of flavanone compounds on lipid peroxidation in rat liver. *Chemical and Pharmaceutical Bulletin*. 1982;30(5):1792-95.
9. Kimura Y, Okuda H, Taira Z, *et al*. Studies on *Scutellaria radix;* IX. New component inhibiting lipid peroxidation in rat liver. *Planta Medica*. 1984;50:290-5.
10. Kubo M, Kimura Y, Odani T, *et al* Studies on *Scutellaria radix*. Part II: The antibacterial substance. *Planta Medica*. 1981;43:194-201.
11. Kimura Y, Okuda H, Arichi S. Studies on *Scutellaria radix*; XIII. Effects of various flavonoids on arachidonate metabolism in leukocytes. *Planta Medica*. 1985;51:132-6.
12. Kimura Y, Kubo M, Kusaka K, *et al.* Studies on *Scutellaria radix*. V. Effects on ethanol-induced hyperlipemia and lipolysis in isolated fat cells. *Chemical and Pharmaceutical Bulletin*. 1982;30:219-22.
13. Kimura Y, Kubo M, Tani T, *et al*. Studies on *Scutellaria radix*. III. Effects on lipid metabolism in serum, liver and fat cells of rats. *Chemical and Pharmaceutical Bulletin*. 1981;29:2308-12.
14. Tyler VE. *The Honest Herbal.* 3rd ed. Philadelphia, PA: Pharmaceutical Products Press; 1993:375.

15. De Smet P. *Scutellaria* species. In: De Smet P, Keller K, Hansel R, Chandler R, eds. *Adverse Effects of Herbal Drugs* Heidelberg:Springer-Verlag; 1993:289-296.
16. Perharic L, Shaw D, Colbridge M, *et al*. Toxicological problems resulting from exposure to traditional remedies and food supplements. *Drug Safety*. 1994;11:284-94.
17. De Smet P. Notes added in proof. In: De Smet P, Keller K, Hansel R, Chandler R, eds. *Adverse Effects of Herbal Drugs.* Heidelberg: Springer-Verlag; 1996:229-240.
18. D'Arcy P. Adverse reactions and interactions with herbal medicines. Part 2-Drug Interactions. *Adverse Drug Reactions and Toxicological Reviews.*1993: 1293): 147-162.
19. Bradley P. *British Herbal Compendium*. Bournemouth: BHMA; 1992:239.

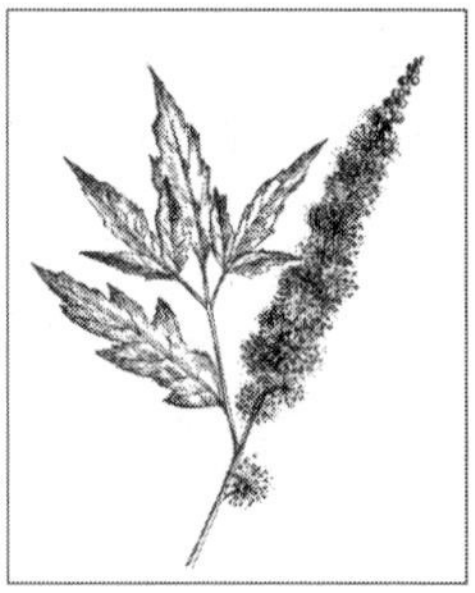

SLIPPERY ELM

Ulmus rubra Muhl.

THUMBNAIL SKETCH

Active Constituents

❖Mucilage, tannins

Common Uses

❖Internal: irritation of mucous membranes (including gastritis, peptic ulcer disease), coughs, sore throats and diarrhea.
❖Topical: sores, ulcers and abscesses

Adverse Effects

❖None known

Cautions/Contraindications

❖The whole bark may be abortifacient

Drug Interactions

❖None known

Doses

❖Usually taken as a gruel or lozenge. Review monograph for details.

INTRODUCTION

Family: Ulmaceae

Synonyms: *Ulmus fulva* Michx., Red elm, Moose elm, Indian elm, American elm [1-3]

Slippery elm is a deciduous tree standing 15 to 20m in height that is native to the United States and Canada.[4] The leaves are yellow/olive in color and the fruit produced is winged and round.[1] The part used medicinally is the inner part of the bark, which has a brownish yellow outer surface and inner yellow white color.[4] The bark has a distinctive 'fenugreek-like odor'.[4] Commercial harvesting of the bark often results in the death of the tree.[5]

Slippery elm gained favor amongst the First Nations because when the bark is mixed with water it produces a thick viscid mucilage.[6] This mucilage was used in conditions where the mucous membranes were inflamed and irritated, both externally and internally. It was also applied externally to sores, wounds and abscesses.[1]

Constituents [2, 3]

- Carbohydrates: complex mucilage containing a number of sugars
- Miscellaneous: tannins, sesquiterpenes and calcium oxalate

THERAPEUTIC USES & RELEVANT PHARMACOLOGY

COMMON USES

Slippery elm is reputed to have demulcent,[3-6] nutrient,[3, 5] emollient,[3, 5] astringent[5] and antitussive[3, 5, 6] properties. Oral consumption is considered useful in the treatment of any condition presenting with inflamed mucous membranes, including gastritis, peptic ulcer disease, enteritis and colitis.[3, 5, 7] Due to their astringent action, slippery elm products are also used within the herbal tradition to treat diarrhea and food poisoning.[5, 7] In addition, slippery elm is also often taken as a lozenge for the relief of coughs and minor throat irritation.[6] External application, usually as a poultice, is used for ulcers, boils, wounds and abscesses.[5]

No information regarding the pharmacology of slippery elm in particular could be found. Research on other plant species has shown that mucilage has a demulcent action and that tannins have astringent properties.[2, 7]

ADVERSE EFFECTS

No adverse effects could be found regarding the use of this medicinal herb.

CAUTIONS/CONTRAINDICATIONS

Products prepared from the whole bark were used as abortifacients. However, it appears that the same caution is *not* applicable to powdered slippery elm.[2]

DRUG INTERACTIONS

None could be found.

DOSAGE REGIMENS [2]

- 5 mL of liquid extract (1:1 in 60% alcohol) three times daily.
- 4-16 mL of a 1:8 decoction of powdered bark three times daily. The decoction should be made in the following manner: "Use 1 part of the powdered bark to 8 parts of water. Mix the powder in a little water initially to ensure it will mix. Bring to the boil and simmer gently for 10-15mins. Drink half a cup three times a day."[5]

As mentioned above, many proprietary lozenges containing slippery elm may be found on the North American market.

Slippery elm is often mixed with other demulcents notably marshmallow (*Althaea officinalis* L. Malvaceae).

REFERENCES

1. Hutchens A. *Indian Herbology of North America.* Boston, MA: Shambhala; 1973:382.
2. Newall C, Anderson L, Phillipson J. *Herbal Medicines. A Guide for Health Care Professionals.* London: The Pharmaceutical Press; 1996:296.
3. Wren R. *Potter's New Encyclopedia of Botanical Drugs and Preparations.* Saffron Walden: C.W. Daniel Company; 1988:362.
4. Evans W. *Trease and Evans' Pharmacognosy.* 13th Edition ed. London: Bailliere Tindall; 1989:832.
5. Hoffmann D. *Holistic Herbal.* Rockport, CA: Element Books; 1996:256.
6. Tyler V. *Herbs of Choice. The Therapeutic Use of Phytomedicinals.* Binghampton: Pharmaceutical Products Press; 1994:209.
7. Mills S. *The Essential Book of Herbal Medicine.* 2nd ed. London: Penguin; 1991:677.

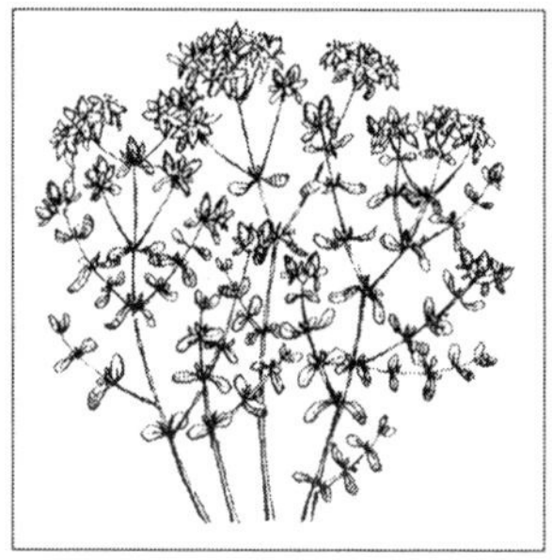

ST. JOHN'S WORT

Hypericum perforatum L.

THUMBNAIL SKETCH

Active Constituents

- Hypericin, isohypericin, protohypericin, flavinoids

Common Uses

- Mild to moderate depression

Adverse Effects

- Photosensitivity, GI upset, dizziness, sedation

Cautions/Contraindications

- Pregnancy and lactation

Drug Interactions

- Possibly similar to those of MAOI's; predicted interactions with conventional antidepressants

Doses

- 300-900mg of standardized St. John' wort extract (0.3% hypericin) per day, in divided doses

INTRODUCTION

Family: Clusiaceae (also known as Guttiferae, sometimes placed in Hypericaceae)

Synonyms: Hypericum, Millepertuis, Amber, Goatweed, Johnswort, Klamath weed, Tipton weed[1, 2]

St. John's wort is a shrub-like perennial plant that reaches a height of 60 cm. The leaves grow from cylindrical or oval stems, are irregular, oblong in shape, sessile, opposing and produce a red sap when crushed. The underside of the leaves are distinguished by pin-pricks and black spots. The five-petal yellow flowers bloom in the summer months. The plant has a turpentine-like odor and a bitter, acidic flavour. It is indigenous to all of Europe and Asia but now is also found in North America.[1, 3, 4] St. John's wort is listed as a noxious weed in many provinces and states due to its invasion of rangeland and photosensitization of livestock. This makes it necessary to take special precautions when the herb is being cultivated.[5]

St. John's wort has been recognized in the West as having medicinal properties since the classical period. The name itself has been associated with a colorful mythology involving Saint John the Baptist, and there are varied customs using the plant as a talisman to ward off misfortune. It was mentioned in the texts of Hippocrates, Pliny, and Galen as helpful for wound healing, pain, and as a diuretic. The use of this herb continued though the Renaissance and Victorian eras.[1, 3, 6] Its most recent historical and contemporary usage has been as an antidepressant, although its antiretroviral potential has received considerable attention since the emergence of the HIV strain viruses.

Constituents [2, 7-9]

- Anthraquinone derivatives: hypericin, isohypericin, protohypericin, pseudohypericin
- Flavonoids: quercetin, hyperoside, quercitrin, isoquercitrin, rutin, campherol, luteolin, I3-II8-biapigenin
- Procyanidines
- Phenols
- Phloroglucinols
- Tannins
- Volatile oils
- Xanthones
- Miscellaneous: organic acids, hydrocarbons and alcohols

THERAPEUTIC USES & RELEVANT PHARMACOLOGY

PHARMACOLOGY

Extracts of St. John's wort contain many constituents that vary depending on the strain.[10] The compounds responsible for the main putative therapeutic effects — antiretroviral and antidepressive — have not been identified definitively.[7] The red-pigmented hypericins were found to be absorbed in a dose-dependent manner within two hours, to be widely distributed, and to have a plasma half-life of approximately 24 hours, allowing steady-state concentrations to be reached within four days of thrice-daily dosing.[11, 12] Approximately 14-21% of the compounds were estimated to be systemically available.[12] *In vitro* experiments localize hypericin primarily in the cytoplasmic membrane and cytoplasm, with smaller amounts in the nucleus.[13]

ANTIRETROVIRAL

Relatively recent investigations into the potential antiretroviral activity of St. John's wort have paralleled the search for other effective treatments for HIV infection and AIDS. Antibacterial and antifungal effects of some constituents have been demonstrated *in vitro*.[9, 14] Antiviral activity against Sindbis, human poliovirus-1, and herpes simplex virus-1 has been found *in vitro*.[15] Murine cytomegalovirus, and human immunodefficiency virus-1 (HIV-1) were also inactivated *in vitro*. Light was found to potentiate the antiviral effects both on isolated virions and on virally infected cells. No damage to the cultured cells was observed.[16, 17] Although the mechanism of the antiviral effects are not known, researchers have found evidence for the hypericins' ability to inhibit protein kinase C.[18] A more detailed review of the potential mechanisms can be found in Diwu.[19]

The best data on the antiretroviral activity of hypericins come from a trio of papers from the Proceedings of the National Academy of Science (PNAS). Meruelo *et al.* reported in 1988, *in vitro* and *in vivo* antiretroviral activity with little toxicity.[20] The same group found increased survival in retrovirus infected animals treated with hypericin and pseudohypericin. These compounds were thought to affect retrovirus assembly and to inactivate mature viral particles.[21] Lenard *et al.* found that both hypericin and Rose Bengal (another pigmented compound) were able to photoinactivate enveloped viruses (human stomatits and HIV) at nanomolecular concentrations. Fusion or hemolysis of cells was inhibited in cells infected by these as well as Sendai and influenza viruses. In cells induced to express the HIV gp120 protein, sycytium formation with CD4+ cells was photoinhibited.[22]

ANTIDEPRESSANT EFFECTS

Although there is considerable evidence that St. John's wort has some antidepressant effects, clinical recommendations about its use at present must be tempered by the lack of long-term human data and studies in severe depression, uncertainty regarding mechanism of action, interaction with other medications and concerns regarding standardization and regulation of the content of commercial products in North America.[23-25] Extracts of *Hypericum perforatum* have reported affinities for a variety of neurotransmitter receptors including: adenosine, $GABA_A$, $GABA_B$, $5HT_1$, central benzodiazepine, forskolin, inositol triphosphate, and the monoamine oxidase A and B enzymes. However, based on the concentrations normally attained after oral administration, only GABA binding appears possible *in vivo*.[26] Non-clinical studies have found evidence for inhibition of serotonin uptake,[27, 28] decreased serotonin receptor expression,[29] inhibition of benzodiazepine binding,[30] changes on animal behavioural tests of antidepressant activity,[31] increased excretion of adrenergic metabolites,[32] modulation of cytokine expression,[33] and inhibition of monoamine oxidase.[34-36] Changes in behavioural test outcomes of animal studies caused by St. John's wort extracts are similar to those documented with other antidepressants.[31, 37, 38]

In humans, there is clear evidence of efficacy in mild to moderate depression.[39-47] In general there are few adverse effects associated with St. John's wort when used for depression.[41, 48] Characteristic EEG and sleep changes seen with tricyclic antidepressants are not observed with St. John's wort, [49] although there is some shortening of evoked potential latencies and enhancement of theta and beta-2 regions in the resting EEG.[50]

A comprehensive meta-analysis of 23 randomized clinical trials (and a total of 1757 patients) of St. John's wort for depression by Linde *et al.* was published in the *British Medical Journal*.[24] This meta-analysis reviewed studies in which St. John's wort alone (20 trials) or in combination with other herbs (3 trials) were tested against placebo (15 trials) or antidepressant drugs (8 trials). Overall, Linde concluded that St. John's wort was superior to placebo and comparable in efficacy to conventional drug treatment. In addition, there were fewer adverse effects and decreased drop-out rates in the St. John's wort group. Linde identified the heterogeneity of the patients, interventions, extract preparations and diagnostic classifications among the various trials as concerning.

St. John's wort extracts have been compared directly with several tricyclic antidepressants and found to be equally as effective as imipramine (25 mg three times daily),[44] maprotiline (25 mg three times daily)[40] or amitriptyline.[51] However, these studies have been heavily criticized due to the small numbers of patients and the low doses of conventional tricyclic antidepressants to which the St. John's wort was compared.[47] A more recent randomized, double-blind trial comparing 1800 mg daily of St. John's wort extract LI 160 to 150 mg daily of imipramine in 209 severely depressed patients from 20 psychiatric centers reported that both were equally effective (Hamilton Depression Scales) over the 6 week treatment period.[52] No comparisons with conventional selective serotonin reuptake inhibitors were found for this review.

ADVERSE EFFECTS[2, 24, 45, 48, 52, 53]

In general, St. John's wort is associated with fewer adverse effects than conventional antidepressants, but they may include: photodermatitis; delayed hypersensitivity; gastrointestinal irritation; dizziness; dry mouth; sedation; restlessness; and constipation.

CAUTIONS/CONTRAINDICATIONS[2]

St. John's wort should be used with caution in pregnant or lactating women, patients with cardiovascular disease, or phaeochromocytoma. Prolonged or intense exposure to sunlight should be avoided by patients ingesting St. John's wort.

DRUG INTERACTIONS[2, 54]

Given the antidepressant activity of St. John's wort, and the lack of consistent data about its mechanism of action, there are potentially dangerous interactions (including hypertensive crises) with other medications similar to those with monoamine oxidase inhibitors such as tranylcypromine and phenelzine, and with selective serotonin reuptake inhibitors:

The following drugs should not be used in combination with St. John's wort or preparations containing derivatives of Hypericum:

- Monoamine Oxidase Inhibitors (MAOIs) including phenelzine, tranylcypromine, isocarboxazid
- Selective Serotonin Reuptake Inhibitors (SSRIs) including fluoxetine, paroxetine
- Dibenzazepine Derivatives including amitriptyline, protriptyline, nortriptyline, desipramine, amoxapine, imipramine, doxepine, perphenazine, carbamazepine, cyclobenzapine, clomipramine, maprotiline, trimipramine

- Sympathomimetics including amphetamines, ephedrine (found in many cold and hay fever remedies), methyldopa, dopamine, levodopa, trytophan
- Others including morphine, meperidine, dextromethorphan, foods high in tyramine

DOSAGE REGIMENS

- 300-900 mg of standardized St. John's wort extract (0.3% hypericin) per day, in divided doses[24]
- 2-4 g of dried herb, three times per day[2]

REFERENCES

1. Unknown. *Hypericum perforatum* (St. John's wort). *The Canadian Journal of Herbalism.* 1990;11(11):3-7.
2. Newall C, Anderson L, Phillipson J. *Herbal Medicines: A Guide for Health Care Professionals.* London: The Pharmaceutical Press; 1996:296.
3. Upton R. St. John's wort (*Hypericum perforatum*). In: Upton R, ed. *American Herbal Pharmacopoeia and Therapeutic Compendium:* American Herbal Pharmacopoeia; 1997.
4. Tyler V. *Herbs of Choice. The Therapeutic Use of Phytomedicinals*. Binghamton, NY: Pharmaceutical Products Press; 1994:209.
5. Marles RJ, Associate Professor, Department of Botany, Brandon University, Brandon, Manitoba. Review of Medicinal Plant Modules for CCNM; 1997.
6. Murray MT. *The Healing Power of Herbs*. Rocklin, CA: Prima Publishing; 1992:246.
7. Wagner H, Bladt S. Pharmaceutical quality of hypericum extracts. *Journal of Geriatric Psychiatry and Neurology.* 1994;7 (Suppl 1):S65-8.
8. Rath G, Potterat O, Mavi S, Hostettmann K. Xanthones from *Hypericum roeperanum. Phytochemistry*. 1996;43(2):513-20.
9. Rocha L, Marston A, Potterat O, *et al* Antibacterial phloroglucinols and flavonoids rom *Hypericum brasiliense*. *Phytochemistry*. 1995;40(5):1447-52.
10. Kartnig T, Gobel I, Heydel B. Production of hypericin, pseudohypericin and flavonoids in cell cultures of various Hypericum species and their chemotypes. *Planta Medica*. 1996;62(1):51-3.
11. Staffeldt B, Kerb R, Brockmoller J, *et al*. Pharmacokinetics of hypericin and pseudohypericin after oral intake of the *Hypericum perforatum* extract LI 160 in healthy volunteers. *Journal of Geriatric Psychiatry and Neurology.* 1994;7 (Suppl 1):S47-53.
12. Kerb R, Brockmoller J, Staffeldt B, *et al*. Single-dose and steady-state pharmacokinetics of hypericin and pseudohypericin. *Antimicrobial Agents and Chemotherapy*. 1996;40(9):2087-93.
13. Miskovsky P, Sureau F, Chinsky L, *et al*. Subcellular distribution of hypericin in human cancer cells. *Photochemistry and Photobiology.* 1995; 62(3):546-549.
14. Rocha L, Marston A, Kaplan MA, *et al.* An antifungal gamma-pyrone and xanthones with monoamine oxidase inhibitory activity from *Hypericum brasiliense. Phytochemistry*. 1994;36(6):1381-5.
15. Taylor RS, Manandhar NP, Hudson JB, Towers GH. Antiviral activities of Nepalese medicinal plants. *Journal of Ethnopharmacology.* 1996;52(3):157-63.
16. Hudson JB, Lopez-Bazzocchi I, Towers G. Antiviral activities of hypericin. *Antiviral Research.* 1991;15:101-112.
17. Lopez-Bazzocchi I, Hudson JB, Towers G. Antiviral activity of the photoactive plant pigment hypericin. *Photochemistry and Photobiology.* 1991;54(1):95-98.
18. Takahashi I, Nakanishi S, Kobayashi E, *et al.* Hypericin and pseudohypericin specifically inhibit protein kinase C: Possible relation to their antiretroviral activity. *Biochemical and Biophysical Research Communications.* 1989;165(3):1207-1212.
19. Diwu Z. Novel therapeutic and diagnostic applications of hypocrellins and hypericins. *Photochemistry and Photobiology.* 1995;61(6):529-39.
20. Meruelo D, Lavie G, Lavie D. Therapeutic agents with dramatic antiretroviral activity and little toxicity at

effective doses: Aromatic polycyclic diones hypericin and pseudohypericin. *Proceedings of the National Academy of Science.* 1988;85:5230-5234.

21. Lavie G, Valentine F, Levin B, *et al.* Studies of the mechanisms of action of the antiretroviral agents hypericin and pseudohypericin. *Proceedings of the National Academy of Science.* 1989;86:5963-5967.
22. Lenard J, Rabson A. Photodynamic inactivation of infectivity of human immunodeficiency virus and other enveloped viruses using hypericin and rose bengal: Inhibition of fusion and sycytia formation. *Proceedings of the National Academy of Science.* 1993;90:158-162.
23. De Smet PA, Nolen WA. St John's wort as an antidepressant. [Editorial; see comments]. *British Medical Journal.* 1996;313(7052):241-2.
24. Linde K, Ramirez G, Mulrow C, *et al.* St John's wort for depression — an overview and meta-analysis of randomised clinical trials. *British Medical Journal.* 1996;313:253-258.
25. Jenike MA. Editorial. *Journal of Geriatric Psychiatry and Neurology.* 1994; 7(Suppl 1):S1.
26. Cott JM. *in vitro* receptor binding and enzyme inhibition by *Hypericum perforatum* extract. *Pharmacopsychiatry.* 1997; 30 (Supplement 2):108-112.
27. Perovic S, Muller WE. Pharmacological profile of hypericum extract. Effect on serotonin uptake by postsynaptic receptors. *Arzneimittelforschung.* 1995;45(11):1145-8.
28. Muller WE, Rolli M, Schafer C, Hafner U. Effects of hypericum extract (LI 160) in biochemical models of antidepressant activity. *Pharmacopsychiatry.* 1997;30 (Suppl 2):102-107.
29. Muller WE, Rossol R. Effects of hypericum extract on the expression of serotonin receptors. *Journal of Geriatric Psychiatry and Neurology.* 1994;7(Suppl 1):S63-4.
30. Baureithel KH, Buter KB, Engesser A, *et al.* Inhibition of benzodiazepine binding *in vitro* by amentoflavone, a constituent of various species of hypericum. *Pharmaceutica Acta Helvetiae.* 1997;72(3):153-7.
31. Von SNO, Weischer ML. Experimental animal studies of the psychotropic activity of a hypericum extract. *Drug Research.* 1987;37(1):10-13.
32. Von HM, Zoller M. Antidepressive effect of a hypericum extract. *Drug Research.* 1984;34(2):918-920.
33. Thiele B, Brink I, Ploch M. Modulation of cytokine expression by hypericum extract. *Journal of Geriatric Psychiatry and Neurology.* 1994;7(Suppl 1):S60-2.
34. Suzuki H, Ohta Y, Takino T, Fugisawa Kea. Effects of glycyrrhizin on biochemical tests in patients with chronic hepatitis — Double blind trial. *Asian Medical Journal.* 1984;26:423-38.
35. Bladt S, Wagner H. Inhibition of MAO by fractions and constituents of hypericum extract. *Journal of Geriatric Psychiatry and Neurology.* 1994; 7(Suppl 1): S57-9.
36. Thiede HM, Walper A. Inhibition of MAO and COMT by hypericum extracts and hypericin. *Journal of Geriatric Psychiatry and Neurology.* 1994;7(Suppl 1):S54-6.
37. Ozturk Y. Testing the antidepressant effects of hypericum species on animal models. *Pharmacopsychiatry.* 1997; 30 (Suppl 2): 125-128.
38. Butterwick V, Wall A, Lieflander-Wulf U, *et al.* Effects of the total extract and fractions of *Hypericum perforatum* in animal assays for antidepressant activity. *Pharmacopsychiatry.* 1997; 30: 117-124.
39. Payk TR. Treatment of depression. *Journal of Geriatric Psychiatry and Neurology.* 1994;7(Suppl 1):S3-5.
40. Harrer G, Schulz V. Clinical investigation of the antidepressant effectiveness of hypericum. *Journal of Geriatric Psychiatry and Neurology.* 1994;7(Suppl 1):S6-8.
41. Sommer H, Harrer G. Placebo-controlled double-blind study examining the effectiveness of an hypericum preparation in 105 mildly depressed patients. *Journal of Geriatric Psychiatry and Neurology.* 1994; 7 (Suppl 1): S9-11.
42. Hubner WD, Lande S, Podzuweit H. Hypericum treatment of mild depressions with somatic symptoms. *Journal of Geriatric Psychiatry and Neurology.* 1994;7(Suppl 1):S12-4.
43. Hansgen KD, Vesper J, Ploch M. Multicenter double-blind study examining the antidepressant effectiveness of the hypericum extract LI 160. *Journal of Geriatric Psychiatry and Neurology.* 1994; 7 (Suppl 1): S15-8.
44. Vorbach EU, Hubner WD, Arnoldt KH. Effectiveness and tolerance of the hypericum extract LI 160 in comparison with imipramine: Randomized double-blind study with 135 outpatients. *Journal of Geriatric Psychiatry and Neurology.* 1994; 7(Suppl 1): S19-23.
45. Harrer G, Hubner WD, Podzuweit H. Effectiveness and tolerance of the hypericum extract LI 160 compared to maprotiline: a multicenter double-blind study. *Journal of Geriatric Psychiatry and Neurology.* 1994; 7(Suppl 1): S24-8.
46. Martinez B, Kasper S, Ruhrmann S, Moller HJ. Hypericum in the treatment of seasonal affective disorders. *Journal of Geriatric Psychiatry and Neurology.* 1994; 7(Suppl 1): S29-33.

47. Volz H-P. Controlled clinical trials of hypericum extracts in depressed patients — an overview. *Pharmacopsychiatry.* 1997; 30 (Suppl 2): 72-76.
48. Woelk H, Burkard G, Grunwald J. Benefits and risks of the hypericum extract LI 160: drug monitoring study with 3250 patients. *Journal of Geriatric Psychiatry and Neurology*. 1994; 7 (Suppl 1): S34-8.
49. Schulz H, Jobert M. Effects of hypericum extract on the sleep EEG in older volunteers. *Journal of Geriatric Psychiatry and Neurology.* 1994; 7 (Suppl 1): S39-43.
50. Johnson D, Ksciuk H, Woelk H, *et al*. Effects of hypericum extract LI 160 compared with maprotiline on resting EEG and evoked potentials in 24 volunteers. *J Geriatr Psychiatry Neurol.* 1994; 7 (Suppl 1): S44-6.
51. Bergmann RJ, Nubner J, Demling J. Behandlung leichter bis mittelschwerer depressionen. Vergleich von *Hypericum perforatum* mit amitriptylin. *TW Neurologie Psychiatrie.* 1993; 7: 135-240.
52. Vorbach EU, Arnoldt KH, Hubner W-D. Efficacy and tolerability of St. John's wort extract LI 160 versus imipramine in patients with severe depressive episodes according to ICD-10. *Pharmacopsychiatry*. 1997; 30 (Suppl 2): 81-85.
53. Brockmoller J, Reum T, Bauer S, *et al*, Roots I. Hypericin and pseudohypericin: Pharmacokinetics and effects on photosensitivity in humans. *Pharmacopsychiatry*. 1997; 30(Suppl 2): 94-101.
54. Gillis MC. (ed.) *Compendium of Pharmaceuticals and Specialties*. 31 ed. Ottawa: Canadian Pharmaceutical Association; 1998.

The authors would like to acknowledge the contribution of Dr. Albert H. Wong to this monograph.

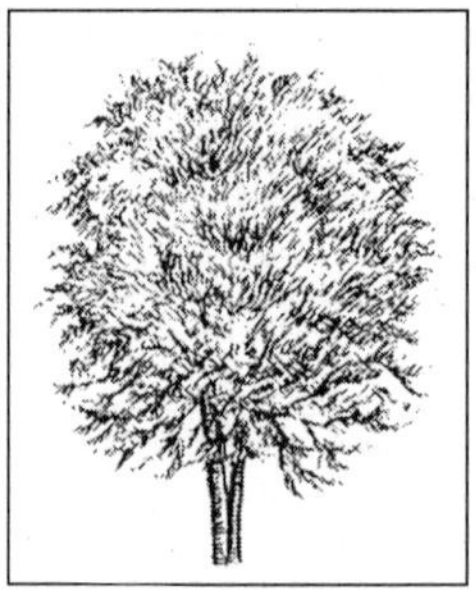

TEA TREE OIL

Melaleuca alternifolia (Maiden & Betche) Cheel

THUMBNAIL SKETCH

Active Constituents

- Terpinen-4-ol

Common Uses

- Fungal infections

Adverse Effects

- Skin irritation

Cautions/Contraindications

- Oral administration

Drug Interactions

- None found

Doses

- No guidelines could be found

INTRODUCTION

Family: Myrtaceae

Synonyms: None found

Tea tree is a member of the myrtle family and is found only in Southeastern Australia. The indigenous people have long prized the aromatic leaves both for medicinal and religious purposes. Its name comes from the fact that a 'tea' was made from it by the early European settlers.[1]

Due to increased popular demand, the commercial production of Australian tea tree oil increased in the early 1990s from 20 tonnes/annum to 140 tonnes/annum. In addition to its medicinal applications, it is now used extensively in the cosmetic and skin-care industry.[2]

The essential oil produced from steam distillation of the leaves is the part used medicinally.

Constituents [3, 4]

- Volatile oil contains various terpenes, including: terpinen-4-ol, pinene, terpinene, cymene and cineole.

In 1985, an 'Australian Standard, *Oil of Melaleuca*' was established, suggesting that the essential oil should contain 30% or more terpinen-4-ol and less than 15% cineole.[1, 3] Tyler cautions, "it is important that the commercial product not be derived from other *Melaleuca* species, some of which contain high concentrations of cineole, a skin irritant that also reduces the antiseptic effectiveness of terpinen-4-ol." [5]

THERAPEUTIC USES & RELEVANT PHARMACOLOGY

COMMON USES

The essential oil is considered to be both an antiseptic and antimicrobial. It is reputed to be useful in the management of many conditions including acne, fungal infections (tinea pedis, onychomycosis, ringworm), vaginal yeast infections, oral thrush and a number of skin conditions.[1, 6]

PHARMACOLOGY

Tea tree oil has been reported to act against a number of bacteria, fungi and yeasts, most notably *Candida* sp., *Trichophyton rubrum* and *Staphylococcus aureus in vivo.*[1, 2, 6] It appears that *Staphylococcus aureus* is less susceptible to tea tree oil than *Candida albicans.*[2]

CLINICAL TRIALS

Acne Vulgaris

In a clinical trial of patients (n=124) suffering from acne vulgaris, the effectiveness of a 5% tea tree oil gel was compared to that of a 5% benzoyl peroxide lotion after 3 months. While the tea tree oil product was considered effective, it had a longer onset of action and it was found to be less active on the inflamed lesions than the benzoyl peroxide product. However, the tea tree oil treatment resulted in an appreciably lower incidence of adverse effects including skin dryness, pruritis and skin scaling than the benzoyl peroxide.[7]

Topical Fungal Infections

In a randomized, double blind trial of patients (n=104) suffering from tinea pedis, the effectiveness of a tea tree oil cream (10%) was compared to 1% tolnaftate cream or placebo. Outcome measures included culture and clinical symptoms (skin scaling, inflammation, itching and burning). While the tea tree oil was shown to be as effective as tolnaftate and superior to placebo in causing relief of symptoms, it was no better than placebo with respect to the culture samples. The study was carried out over a five-week period.[8]

Another randomized, multi-center, controlled trial in patients (n=117) suffering from onychomycosis, compared the effectiveness of tea tree oil (100%) to a conventional treatment of 1% clotrimazole cream over 6 months. Comparable improvement (cure, clinical assessment and subjective improvement) was seen in both groups. The two preparations were also comparable in cost and shared the same incidence of adverse effects (7%).

ADVERSE EFFECTS

Tea tree oil is considered 'very mildly irritating' on topical application but 'strongly irritant' following oral administration. It is not considered to result in either sensitization or phototoxicity;[9] however it is recommended that care should be taken when using very concentrated tea tree oil products in children and fair skinned individuals.[10]

CAUTIONS/CONTRAINDICATIONS

Given the lack of guidelines available, tea tree oil should not be administered orally.

DRUG INTERACTIONS

No cases of interactions between conventional therapy and tea tree oil could be found.

DOSAGE REGIMENS

No dosage guidelines for tea tree oil could be found. Preparations used in the above clinical trials range from 5 to 100%. It should be noted that in general, the concentrations of tea tree oil used in the clinical trials described above are considerably lower than those often seen in clinical practice.[10, 11] Many 'tea tree oil products' used in the cosmetic and toiletries industry contain only small amounts of active substance and the medicinal efficacy is often questionable.[2] The Australian guidelines for terpinen-4-ol/cineole content should be considered when using a tea tree oil product therapeutically.

REFERENCES

1. Altman P. Australian tea tree oil. *Australian Journal of Pharmacy*. 1988;69:276-278.
2. Williams L, Home V. A comparative study of some essential oils for potential use in topical applications for the treatment of the yeast *Candida albicans. Australian Journal of Medical Herbalism*. 1995;7(3):57-62.
3. Leung A, Foster S. *Encylopedia of Common Natural Ingredients Used in Food, Drugs and Cosmetics.* New York, NY: John Wiley and Sons; 1996:649.
4. Tyler V. *Herbs of Choice. The Therapeutic Use of Phytomedicinals.* Binghampton, NY: Pharmaceutical Products Press; 1994:209.
5. Tyler VE. *The Honest Herbal.* 3rd ed. Philadelphia: Pharmaceutical Products Press; 1993:375.
6. Buck D, Midorf D, Addino J. Comparison of two topical preparations for the treatment of onychomycosis: *Melaleuca alternifolia*(tea tree) oil and clotrimazole. *Journal of Family Practice*. 1994;38:601-605.
7. Bassett IB, Pannowitz DL, Barnetson RS. A comparative study of tea-tree oil versus benzoyl peroxide in the treatment of acne. *Medical Journal of Australia.* 1990;153:455-8.
8. Tong M, Altmann P, Barnetson R. Tea tree oil in the treatment of tinea pedis. *Australian Journal of Dermatology*. 1992;33:145-9.
9. Tisserand R, Balacs T. *Essential Oil Safety: A Guide for Health Care Professionals.* London: Churchill Livingstone; 1995:279.
10. Brown D. Topical tea tree oil for onychomycosis. *Quarterly Review of Natural Medicine*. 1995;Spring:11.
11. Brown D. Tea tree oil for athlete's foot. *Quarterly Review of Natural Medicine*. 1993;Winter:15.

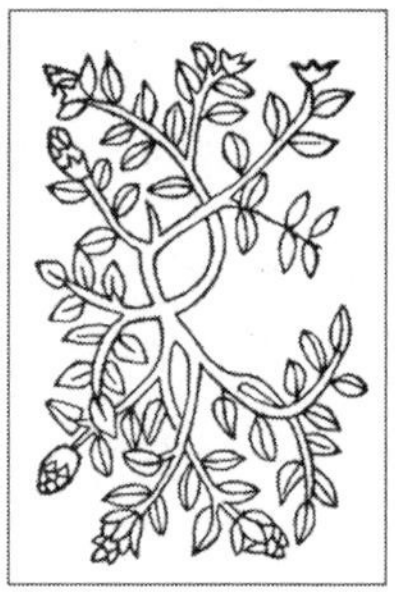

THYME

Thymus vulgaris L.

THUMBNAIL SKETCH

Active Constituents
- Volatile oil (thymol and carvacrol), flavonoids

Common Uses
- Spasmodic respiratory conditions, dyspepsia, parasites and fungal infections

Adverse Effects (volatile oil portion)

Oral:
- Nausea, vomiting, gastric distress, headache, dizziness, convulsions, coma, cardiac and respiratory collapse.

Topical:
- Considered to be moderately irritating

Cautions/Contraindications
- Pregnancy

Drug Interactions
- None known

Doses

Oral:
- 1-4 g of dried herb (often taken as an infusion) or 2-6 mL (1:5 in 45% alcohol) three times daily

Topical:
- Thyme oil should only be used after diluting with a suitable carrier oil

INTRODUCTION

Family: Laminaceae (also know as mint or Labiatae)

Synonyms: Common thyme, French thyme, Garden thyme, Rubbed thyme [1, 2]

Thyme is a shrub native to Mediterranean Europe but is also cultivated in the United States. Like other members of the mint family, it is rich in volatile oils producing a characteristic aromatic scent. It is an evergreen standing up to 45 cm in height with multiple hairy stems arising from a single woody fibrous root. The part used medicinally is the oil, which is extracted from the leaves and flowering tops by steam distillation.[2] Two oils exist, the red and white oil. The red oil is made by redistilling the white oil and has often been seen to be adulterated.[2] Many subspecies exist and this can result in differences in medicinal action and composition of the volatile oil, primarily due to differences in the proportion of phenols.[3-5]

Constituents[1, 2, 5-7]

- Volatile oils containing monoterpenoids, predominately the phenols thymol and carvacrol, as well as unsubstituted cymene and terpinene and the alcohols alpha-terpineol, linalool, and thujan-4-ol
- Phenylpropanoids including eugenol, caffeic acid, and rosmarinic acid
- Triterpenes including ursolic acid and oleanolic acid
- Miscellaneous including flavonoids, dimethylbiphenyl and tannins.

THERAPEUTIC USES & RELEVANT PHARMACOLOGY

COMMON USES

Thyme is reputed to have many therapeutic actions including: carminative,[4, 8, 9] antimicrobial/antiseptic,[8, 9] expectorant,[3, 4, 8, 9] antitussive,[3, 9] and diaphoretic actions.[8] Oral consumption is considered to be useful in the treatment of conditions associated with spasm including: upper respiratory tract conditions (e.g., bronchitis, pertussis and asthma)[4, 8] and digestive upset.[4, 8] It is also used both orally and topically for a number of parasitic and fungal infections.[4, 8]

PHARMACOLOGY

General antispasmodic activity and specific bronchospasmolytic action has been demonstrated *in vitro*.[6, 10] The flavonoid and phenolic components are thought to be responsible for this property with a proposed mechanism of action being calcium channel antagonism.[1, 11]

The volatile oil has been shown to possess antibacterial and antifungal activity *in vitro*.[2, 12] The anti-bacterial action against *Staphylococcus aureus* was shown to be decreased by agents known to inhibit the action of the phenolic components.[13] An aqueous extract of thyme has been reported to inhibit *Helicobacter pylori in vitro*.[14] In addition, antimutagenic properties have been demonstrated *in vitro*.[15]

Thyme oil has been shown to increase respiration and exert a hypotensive action in a number of animal models.[1, 2] Rosmarinic acid has also been shown to exert an anti-inflammatory action in both *in vivo* and *in vitro* models.[6, 16] Dimethylbiphenyl and a flavonoid, eriodictyol, have been shown to exert profound antioxidant action possibly by inhibiting superoxide generation.[17]

ADVERSE EFFECTS

Thyme oil is considered to be a moderate dermal irritant and strong mucous membrane irritant.[5] Adverse effects of the volatile oil include: nausea, vomiting, digestive distress, headache, dizziness, sweating, convulsions, coma and respiratory/cardiac collapse.[1, 2, 18] Local irritation has resulted from the use of toothpaste containing thyme extracts.[1] In addition, a case of occupational asthma was noted in an individual in contact with a number of aromatic herbs including thyme. A sensitivity to thyme was confirmed later by skin prick test.[19]

CAUTIONS/CONTRAINDICATIONS

Thyme is reputed to be an emmenagogue and so should be used with caution in pregnancy especially if given in high doses.[1, 4, 18] Experimentally cross-sensitivity with other members of the mint (Laminaceae) has been noted.[20]

DRUG INTERACTIONS

No cases of drug interaction could be found.

DOSAGE REGIMENS

- 1-4 g of dried herb (often taken as an infusion) or 2-6 mL (1:5 in 45% alcohol) three times daily.[1]
- 1-2 g (0.5-1 g in children under 1 year of age) of the dried herb as an infusion several times a day. [6]
- 40 drops (tincture, 1:10, 70% alcohol) up to three times daily.[6]

Thyme oil should only be applied topically after it has been diluted with a suitable carrier oil.[1]

REFERENCES

1. Newall C, Anderson L, Phillipson J. *Herbal Medicines: A Guide for Health Care Professionals.* London: The Pharmaceutical Press; 1996:296.
2. Leung A, Foster S. *Encylopedia of Common Natural Ingredients Used in Food, Drugs and Cosmetics.* New York, NY: John Wiley and Sons; 1996:649.
3. Tyler V. *Herbs of Choice. The Therapeutic Use of Phytomedicinals.* Binghampton, NY: Pharmaceutical Products Press; 1994:209.
4. Mills S. *The Essential Book of Herbal Medicine*. 2nd ed. London: Penguin 1991:677.
5. Tisserand R, Balacs T. *Essential Oil Safety: A Guide for Health Care Professionals*. London: Churchill Livingstone; 1995:279.
6. ESCOP. Thymi Herba/Thyme. In: *ESCOP Monographs (Fascicule 1)* Exeter: ESCOP; 1996:62.
7. Marles RJ, Associate Professor, Department of Botany, Brandon University, Brandon, Manitoba. Review of Medicinal Plant Modules for CCNM; 1998.

8. Hoffmann D. *Holistic Herbal.* Rockport, CA: Element Books; 1996:256.
9. Wren R. Potter's *New Encyclopedia of Botanical Drugs and Preparations.* Saffron Walden: C.W. Daniel Company; 1988:362.
10. Van Den Broucke CO, Lernli JA. Pharmacological and chemical investigation of thyme liquid extracts. *Planta Medica*. 1981;41:129-35.
11. Van Den Broucke CO. The therapeutic value of Thymus species. *Fitoterapia*. 1983;4:171-4.
12. Agnihotri S, Vaidya AD. A novel approach to study antibacterial properties of volatile components of selected Indian medicinal herbs. *Indian Journal of Experimental Biology*. 1996;34(7):712-5.
13. Juven BJ, Kanner J, Schved F, Weisslowicz H. Factors that interact with the antibacterial action of thyme essential oil and its active constituents. *Journal of Applied Bacteriology*. 1994;76(6):626-31.
14. Tabak M, Armon R, Potasman I, Neeman I. *In vitro* inhibition of *Helicobacter pylori* by extracts of thyme. *Journal of Applied Bacteriology*. 1996;80(6):667-72.
15. Vukovic-Gacic B, Simic D. Identification of natural antimutagens with modulating effects on DNA repair. *Basic Life Sciences*. 1993;61:269-77.
16. Englberger W, Hadding U, Etschenberg E, *et al.* Rosmarinic acid: A new inhibitor of complement C3-convertase with anti-inflammatory activity. *International Journal of Immunopharmacology*. 1988;10:729-37.
17. Haraguchi H, Saito T, Ishikawa H, *et al.* Antiperoxidative components in *Thymus vulgaris*. *Planta Medica*. 1996;62(3):217-21.
18. Brinker F. *The Toxicology of Botanical Medicines*. 2nd ed. Portland, OR: National College of Naturopathic Medicine; 1983:141.
19. Lemiere C, Cartier A, Lehrer SB, Malo JL. Occupational asthma caused by aromatic herbs. *Allergy*. 1996;51(9):647-9.
20. Benito M, Jorro G, Morales C, *et al.* Labiatae allergy: systemic reactions due to ingestion of oregano and thyme. *Annals of Allergy Asthma and Immunology*. 1996;76(5):416-8.

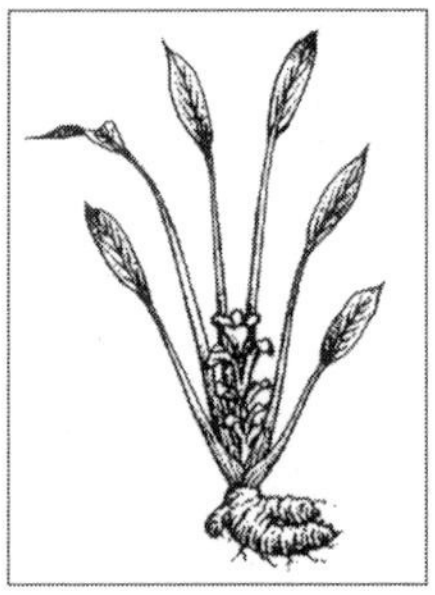

TURMERIC

Curcuma longa Linn.

THUMBNAIL SKETCH

Active Constituents
- Curcumin

Common Uses
- Inflammation (e.g., arthritis)
- Liver disorders

Adverse Effects
- None known

Cautions/Contraindications
- Blockage of the bile duct; gallstones; safety in pregnancy and lactation has not been established

Drug Interactions
- None known

Doses
- 250 to 500 mg curcumin daily in divided doses
- 1.5 to 3 g turmeric three times daily

INTRODUCTION

Family: Zingiberaceae

Synonyms:[1, 2] *Curcuma domestica* Val., Curcuma, Indian saffron

This perennial herb is native to Southern Asia and cultivated throughout the tropics, including many parts of the Carribean.[2] It is a member of the ginger family and produces large oblong leaves which arise from a tuberous rhizome.[2] It has been used historically for both its flavor (i.e., it is a major ingredient in curry powder) and its color (i.e., it is used in the preparation of mustard). The parts used medicinally are the primary and secondary rhizomes which are usually cured (i.e., boiled, cleaned, and sundried) and polished.[3] Turmeric is used medicinally in both Traditional Chinese Medicine and in the traditional medicine of India for a variety of inflammatory conditions as well as flatulence, jaundice, menstrual difficulties, bruises and colic.[2]

Constituents[2-4]

- Volatile oil: turmerone, zingiberene, bisabolane, guaiane, curlone
- Curcumin
- Miscellaneous: sugars including glucose, fructose, arabinose; resins, protein, vitamins and minerals

Note: curcumin is a phenylpropanoid derivative responsible for the characteristic yellow color as well as the main pharmacological activity.[4]

THERAPEUTIC USES & RELEVANT PHARMACOLOGY

PHARMACOLOGY

Curcumin is reported to be a potent anti-inflammatory component – its action is reported to be comparable to hydrocortisone and phenylbutazone.[3] Several hypotheses have been offered regarding its mechanism of action, including: 1) it has an indirect action via the adrenal cortex;[3] 2) it inhibits cortisone metabolism in the liver, thus increasing the amount of circulating cortisone;[3] 3) it inhibits 5-lipoxygenase;[5, 6] and 4) it inhibits lipopolysaccharide (LPS) -induced production of tumor necrosis factor (TNF) and interleukin-1beta (IL-1).[7]

In addition, curcumin has been shown to have a variety of other direct effects, including inhibition of leukotriene formation, and platelet aggregation, as well as increasing the breakdown of fibrin and promoting liver function in a variety of ways.[6, 8-10] Turmeric has been reported to increase bile secretion and bile flow.[3, 11] It has also been shown to have a significant anti-oxidant activity.[12, 13]

ANTI-INFLAMMATORY ACTIVITY

Several experimental models have demonstrated the anti-inflammatory activity of the volatile oil component of turmeric,[14, 15] as well as curcumin and its analogs.[6, 8, 9, 16]

Rheumatoid Arthritis

Several clinical studies have reported curcumin's effectiveness in the treatment of rheumatoid arthritis.[17, 18] One study found that symptoms such as joint swelling, walking speed and morning stiffness were improved to the same degree in patients taking either curcumin (1200 mg daily) or phenylbutazone (300 mg daily).[17] Another used the postoperative inflammation model for evaluating non-steroidal anti-inflammatory drugs (NSAIDs) and found 400 mg of curcumin to be as effective as 100 mg of phenylbutazone.[18]

GASTROINTESTINAL ACTIVITY

Turmeric has a long history of use in the management of ulcerative conditions; however the evidence supporting its use not consistently positive.[19] Despite this, the German Commission E has approved turmeric as an effective cholagogue and digestive aid.[20] Duke reviews a study in which turmeric given at a dose of 250 mg three times daily relieved ulcer pain.[21] However, another randomized, double-blind, placebo-controlled trial of patients newly diagnosed with duodenal ulcers (n=130) reported no significant difference in the symptom relief of those receiving turmeric (6 g daily in three divided doses) when compared with those taking a placebo after the 8-week study period.[22]

HEPATOPROTECTIVE ACTIVITY

Historically turmeric was used for a variety of liver conditions. Experimental evidence from animal studies confirms that it appears to increase bile flow and may play a role in protecting the liver from toxins.[8, 23] In addition, a related species, *Curcuma xanthorrhiza* Roxb., has been shown in animal experiments to provide protection from hepatotoxin-induced liver damage.[24] However, our literature review did not find any human studies which investigated turmeric's efficacy for these indications.

ANTI-CANCER ACTIVITY

Animal studies suggest that curcumin may have an inhibitory effect on a variety of experimentally-induced cancers including: carcinogen-induced cancers of the duodenum, colon and forestomach in mice;[25, 26] Ehrlich ascites tumor in mice;[27] carcinogen-induced skin tumor formation in mice;[28] aflatoxin-induced hepatocarcinogenicity in rats;[29] and carcinogen-induced cancer of the oral mucosa in hamsters.[26] *In vitro* experiments have shown that curcumin may inhibit the growth of estragen-positive human breast MCF-7 cells induced by a variety of carcinogens[30] and that it is phototoxic to rat basophilic leukemia cells in the presence of oxygen.[31] Researchers hypothesize that these effects are due in part to curcumin's antioxidant action (it appears to inhibit superoxide production).[27] The clinical significance of these findings remains unknown.

ANTIMICROBIAL ACTION

Several studies have reported that curcumin has the ability to inhibit the replication of human immunodeficiency virus.[32-34] Researchers suggest that this activity is due in part to its inhibition of HIV-1 integrase.[32] Clinical trials of curcumin in AIDS patients are reportedly scheduled.[32]

Turmeric has been shown to have some nematocidal,[35] anti-fungal activity,[36] and anti-bacterial activity.[37-39]

MISCELLANEOUS

Curcumin has been reported to decrease cholesterol and lipid levels in animal studies.[40, 41] Antioxidant properties have also been reported in animal studies.[2]

ADVERSE EFFECTS

Turmeric and curcumin appear to have no adverse effects.[3, 42] Prolonged use may occasionally result in gastrointestinal upset.[1]

CAUTIONS/CONTRAINDICATIONS

Individuals with blockage of the common bile duct or gallstones should avoid consuming turmeric due to its reputed ability to increase bile flow.[1] An animal study has demonstrated that the active constituents of turmeric are transferred translactationally.[43] Safety in pregnancy and lactation has not yet been established.

DRUG INTERACTIONS

- No known drug interactions.

DOSAGE REGIMENS

- The clinical trials reviewed used 400 mg curcumin three times daily.[17, 18]
- 1.5-3 g turmeric daily[1]

REFERENCES

1. Tyler VE. *Herbs of Choice. The Therapeutic Use of Phytomedicinals.* Binghamton, NY: Pharmaceutical Products Press; 1994:209.
2. Leung AY. *Encyclopedia of Common Natural Ingredients Used in Food, Drugs and Cosmetics*. New York, NY: John Wiley and Sons; 1980.
3. Murray MT. *The Healing Power of Herbs.* Rocklin, CA: Prima Publishing; 1992:246.
4. Marles RJ, Associate Professor, Department of Botany, Brandon University, Brandon, Manitoba. Review of Medicinal Plant Modules for CCNM; 1998.
5. Srivastava R. Inhibition of neutrophil response by curcumin. *Agents and Actions*. 1989;28:298-303.
6. Ammon HP, Safayhi H, Mack T, Sabieraj J. Mechanism of antiinflammatory actions of curcumine and boswellic acids. *Journal of Ethnopharmacology*. 1993;38(2-3):113-9.
7. Chan MM. Inhibition of tumor necrosis factor by curcumin, a phytochemical. *Biochemical Pharmacology*. 1995;49(11):1551-6.
8. Srimal R, Dhawan B. Pharmacology of diferuloyl methane (curcumin), a non-steroidal anti-inflammatory agent. *Journal of Pharmacy and Pharmacology*. 1973;25:447-52.
9. Mukhopadhyay A, Basu N, Ghatak N, Gujral P. Anti-inflammatory and irritant activities of curcumin analogues in rats. *Agents and Actions*. 1982;12:508-15.
10. Srivastava R, Srimal RC. Modification of certain inflammation-induced biochemical changes by curcumin. *Indian Journal of Medical Research*. 1985;81:215-23.
11. Ramprasad C, Sirsi M. *Curcuma longa* and bile secretion: quantitative changes in the bile constituents induced by sodium curcuminate. *J Sci Ind Res*. 1957;16C:108-10.
12. Selvam R, Subramanian L, Gayathri R, Angayarkanni N. The anti-oxidant activity of turmeric (*Curcuma longa*). *Journal of Ethnopharmacology*. 1995;47(2):59-67.

13. Osawa T, Sugiyama Y, Inayoshi M, Kawakishi S. Antioxidative activity of tetrahydrocurcuminoids. *Bioscience Biotechnology and Biochemistry*. 1995;59(9):1609-12.
14. Chandra D, Gupta S. Anti-inflammatory and anti-arthritic activity of volatile oil of *Curcuma longa* (Haldi). *Indian Journal of Medical Research*. 1972;60:138-42.
15. Arora R, Basu N, Kapoor V, Jain A. Anti-inflammatory studies on *Curcuma longa* (turmeric). *Indian Journal of Medical Research*. 1971;60:138-42.
16. Ghatak N, Basu N. Sodium curcuminate as an effective anti-inflammatory agent. *Indian Journal of Experimental Biology*. 1972;10:235-6.
17. Deodhar SD, Sethi R, Srimal RC. Preliminary studies on antirheumatic activity of curcumin (di-feruloyl methane). *Indian Journal of Medical Research*. 1980;71:632-4.
18. Satoskar RR, Shah SJ, Shenony SG. Evaluation of anti-inflammatory property of curcumin (di-feruloyl methane) in patients with postoperative inflammation. *International Journal of Clinical Pharmacology Therapy and Toxicology*. 1986;24:651-4.
19. Rafatullah S, *et al.* Evaluation of turmeric (*Curcuma longa*) for gastric and duodenal antiulcer activity in rats. *Journal of Ethnopharmacology*. 1990;29(1):25-34.
20. Blumenthal M, Brusse WR, Goldberg A, *et al. The Complete German Commission E Monographs.* Austin, TX: American botanical Council; 1998: 685.
21. Duke J. *The Green Pharmacy.* New York, NY: Rodale Press Inc.; 1997:617
22. van Dau N, Ngoc Ham N, Huy Khac D, *et al.* The effects of a traditional drug, turmeric (*Curcuma longa*), and placebo on the healing of duodenal ulcer. *Phytomedicine*. 1998;5:29-34.
23. Kiso Y, Suzuki Y, Watanabe N, *et al.* Antihepatotoxic principles of *Curcuma longa* rhizomes. *Planta Medica*. 1983;49:185-7.
24. Lin SC, Lin CC, Lin YH, Supriyatna S, Teng CW. Protective and therapeutic effects of *Curcuma xanthorrhiza* on hepatotoxin-induced liver damage. *American Journal of Chinese Medicine*. 1995;23(3-4):243-54.
25. Huang MT, Lou YR, Ma W, Newmark HL, *et al.* Inhibitory effects of dietary curcumin on forestomach, duodenal, and colon carcinogenesis in mice. *Cancer Research*. 1994;54(22):5841-7.
26. Azuine MA, Bhide SV. Adjuvant chemoprevention of experimental cancer: catechin and dietary turmeric in forestomach and oral cancer models. *Journal of Ethnopharmacology*. 1994;44(3):211-7.
27. Ruby AJ, Kuttan G, Babu KD, *et al.* Anti-tumour and antioxidant activity of natural curcuminoids. *Cancer Letters*. 1995;94(1):79-83.
28. Limtrakul P, Lipigorngoson S, Namwong O, *et al.* Inhibitory effect of dietary curcumin on skin carcinogenesis in mice. *Cancer Letters*. 1997;116(2):197-203.
29. Soni KB, Lahiri M, Chackradeo P, *et al.* Protective effect of food additives on aflatoxin-induced mutagenicity and hepatocarcinogenicity. *Cancer Letters*. 1997;115(2):129-33.
30. Verma SP, Salamone E, Goldin B. Curcumin and genistein, plant natural products, show synergistic inhibitory effects on the growth of human breast cancer MCF-7 cells induced by estrogenic pesticides. *Biochemical and Biophysical Research Communications*. 1997;233(3):692-6.
31. Dahl TA, Bilski P, Reszka KJ, Chignell CF. Photocytotoxicity of curcumin. *Photochemistry and Photobiology*. 1994;59(3):290-4.
32. Mazumder A, Raghavan K, Weinstein J, *et al.* Inhibition of human immunodeficiency virus type-1 integrase by curcumin. *Biochemical Pharmacology*. 1995;49(8):1165-70.
33. Sui Z, Salto R, Li J, Craik C, Ortiz de Montellano PR. Inhibition of the HIV-1 and HIV-2 proteases by curcumin and curcumin boron complexes. *Bioorganic and Medicinal Chemistry*. 1993;1(6):415-22.
34. Li CJ, Zhang LJ, Dezube BJ, Crumpacker CS, *et al.* Three inhibitors of type 1 human immunodeficiency virus long terminal repeat-directed gene expression and virus replication. *Proceedings of the National Academy of Sciences of the USA*. 1993;90:1839-42.
35. Kiuchi F, Goto Y, Sugimoto N, *et al.* Nematocidal activity of turmeric: synergistic action of curcuminoids. *Chemical and Pharmaceutical Bulletin (Tokyo)*. 1993;41(9):1640-3.
36. Apisariyakul A, Vanittanakom N, Buddhasukh D. Antifungal activity of turmeric oil extracted from *Curcuma longa* (Zingiberaceae). *Journal of Ethnopharmacology*. 1995;49(3):163-9.
37. Shankar TNB, Muthy IAS. Effect of tumeric *Curcuma longa* fractions on the growth of some intestinal and pathogenic bacteria *in vitro*. *Indian Journal of Experimental Biology*. 1978;17:1363-6.
38. Tonnesen HH, de Vries H, Karlsen J, van Hengouwen GB. Studies on curcumin and curcuminoids IX: Investigation of the photo biological activity of curcumin using bacterial indicator systems. *Journal of Pharmaceutical Sciences.* 1987;76:371-3.

39. Dahl TA, McGowan WM, Shand MA, Srinivasan VS. Photokilling of bacteria by the natural dye curcumin. *Archives of Microbiology*. 1989;151:183-5.
40. Roa SD, Chandrashekhera N, Satyanarayana N, Srinivasan M. Effect of curcumin on serum and liver cholesterol levels in the rat. *Journal of Nutrition*. 1970;100:1307-16.
41. Dixit VP, Jain P, Joshi SC. Hypolipidaemic effect of *Curcuma longa* L. and *Nardostachys jatamansi* DC in triton-induced hyper lipidaemic rats. *Indian Journal of Physiology and Pharmacology*. 1988;32:299-304.
42. Shankar TNB, Shantha NV, Ramesh HP, *et al.* Toxicity studies on tumeric (*Curcuma longa*): Acute toxicity studies in rats, guinea pigs, and monkeys. *Indian Journal of Experimental Biology*. 1980;18:73-5.
43. Singh A, Singh SP, Bamezai R. Postnatal modulation of hepatic biotransformation system enzymes via translactational exposure of F1 mouse pups to turmeric and curcumin. *Cancer Letters*. 1995;96(1):87-93.

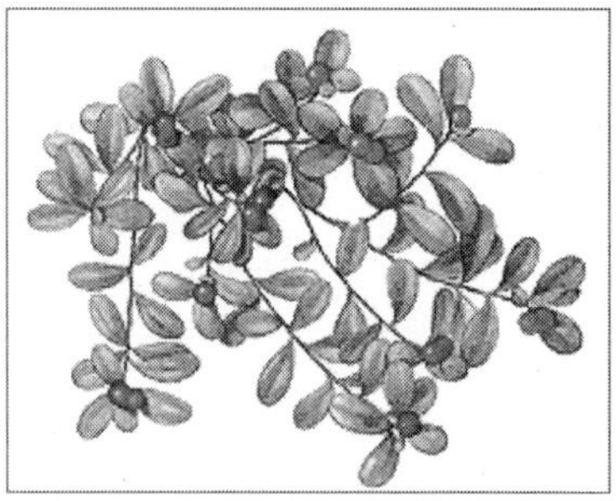

UVA-URSI

Arctostaphylos uva-ursi (L.) Spreng.

THUMBNAIL SKETCH

Active Constituents

- Phenolic glycosides (arbutin, methylarbutin).

Common Uses

- Uncomplicated infections of the lower urinary tract

Adverse Effects

- Nausea and vomiting
- Consumption of large doses may result in symptoms of hydroquinone toxicity (details mentioned in the monograph)

Cautions/Contraindications

- Pregnancy, lactation, kidney disease

Drug Interactions

- None known

Doses

- 1.5-4 g of dried leaves or 1.5-4.0 mL fluid extract (1:1 in 25% alcohol) three times a day for a maximum of 2 weeks

INTRODUCTION

Family: Ericaceae

Synonyms: Bearberry, Common bearberry, Beargrape, Hogberry, Rockberry, Sandberry, Mountain cranberry [1-3]

Uva-ursi is a trailing evergreen shrub native to many regions of the Northern Hemisphere including Canada. It produces small leathery oblong leaves and small pale pink flowers.[2] Bears are thought to like the sour red berries, giving rise to the popular name of bearberry.[3] This also gave rise to its Latin binomial name, *Arctostaphylos,* meaning bearberry in Greek and *uva-ursi* meaning the same in Latin.[4] The leaves, which are the part used medicinally, have an astringent and bitter taste.[5]

Constituents [1, 2, 6-10]

- Phenolic glycosides: arbutin (hydroquinone beta-glucoside), methylarbutin, piceoside and para-methoxyphenol.
- Flavonoids including glycosides of quercetin, kaempferol and myricetin
- Iridoids: monotropein, unedoside (root)
- Miscellaneous including hydrolysable tannins, ursolic acid, terpenoids and allantoin.

THERAPEUTIC USES & RELEVANT PHARMACOLOGY

COMMON USES

Uva-ursi is used primarily for its action as a urinary antiseptic, often in the management of uncomplicated infections of the lower urinary tract (e.g., cystitis, urethritis and prostatitis).[3, 11, 12] While it has been reported to be a diuretic[2, 13], other research suggests that this is probably not the case.[11, 12, 14] As a result of its astringent properties, uva-ursi has also been used in conditions of the lower digestive tract (e.g., diarrhea) and for enuresis.[3, 13] It is also reputed to be useful in bronchitis and urinary stones.[2, 13, 15]

PHARMACOLOGY

The phenolic glycosides, especially arbutin, appear to be the primary active agents. However, the therapeutic effectiveness of uva-ursi is dependent on the conversion of these phenolic glycosides to a known antimicrobial agent, hydroquinone. Arbutin appears to be absorbed intact, undergoing hydrolysis in the urine to hydroquinone.[1, 16] It has been suggested that other agents in the whole extract may protect the arbutin from degradation in the gastrointestinal tract.[1] Other researchers have argued that this conversion occurs in the gastrointestinal tract with the hydroquinone being transported as a conjugate systemically and free hydroquinone being liberated in the urine.[12] Antimicrobial action is noted only when the urine is alkaline with a pH of 8 or greater.[10, 12] Since uva-ursi exerts an antibacterial action in the genitourinary tract, it has been suggested that the resultant uroepithelial protection may prevent the retention of microcalculi.[17] Antimicrobial properties have been demonstrated *in vitro* for uva-ursi against a number of organisms, including *Staphylococcus aureus, Bacillus subtilis, Escherichia coli and Shigella sp.*[18]

ADVERSE EFFECTS

Consumption of large doses of uva-ursi have resulted in nausea and vomiting. In addition, hydroquinone is known to have a toxic potential causing tinnitus, nausea, vomiting, shortness of breath, cyanosis, convulsions, delirium and collapse.[19]

CAUTIONS/CONTRAINDICATIONS

Uva-ursi should be considered contraindicated in kidney disorders,[10, 14] pregnancy and lactation.[10, 14] Due to the presence of hydroquinone and the large amount of tannins, prolonged use or the consumption of large amounts of uva-ursi should be avoided.[1]

DRUG INTERACTIONS

No cases of interactions with conventional medications could be found. Theoretically, caution should be exercised with drugs known to interact with hydroquinone.

DOSAGE REGIMENS

- 1.5-4 g of dried leaves or 1.5-4.0 mL fluid extract (1:1 in 25% alcohol) three times daily[1]
- The ESCOP monograph recommends "cold water infusions of the crude drug equivalent to 400-800 mg arbutin per day in divided doses." [10]
- The duration of treatment should be limited to 2 weeks and medical attention sought if there is a worsening of symptoms.[10]
- Cold water infusions are preferable to hot ones because they contain fewer tannins.
- Uva-ursi is often given with an alkalinizing agent such as sodium bicarbonate.

REFERENCES

1. Newall C, Anderson L, Phillipson J. *Herbal Medicines: A Guide for Health Care Professionals*. London: The Pharmaceutical Press; 1996:296.
2. Leung A, Foster S. *Encylopedia of Common Natural Ingredients Used in Food, Drugs and Cosmetics*. New York, NY: John Wiley and Sons; 1996:649.
3. Mills S. *The Essential Book of Herbal Medicine*. 2nd ed. London: Penguin Publishing; 1991:677.
4. Tyler VE. *The Honest Herbal*. 3rd ed. Philadelphia, PA: Pharmaceutical Products Press;1993:375.
5. Evans W. *Trease and Evans' Pharmacognosy*. 13th ed. London: Bailliere Tindall; 1989:832.
6. Jahodar L, Leifertova I. The evaluation of p-methoxyphenol in the leaves of *Arctostaphylos uva-ursi*. *Pharmazie*. 1979;34:188-9.
7. Karikas GA, Euerby M, Waigh R. Isolation of piceoside from *Arctostaphylos uva-ursi*. *Planta Medica*. 1987;53: 307-8.
8. Jahodar L, Kolb I, Leifertova I. Unedoside in *Arctostaphylos uva-ursi* roots. *Pharmazie*. 1981;36:294-6.
9. Jahodar L, Leifertova I, Lisa M, *et al.* Investigation of iridoid substances in *Arctostaphylos uva-ursi*. *Pharmazie*. 1978;33:536-7.
10. ESCOP. Uvae Ursi Folium/Bearberry. In: *ESCOP Monographs (Fascicule 5)*.Exeter: ESCOP; 1997:65pp.
11. Weiss RF. *Herbal Medicine*. Beaconsfield, England: Beaconsfield Publishers Ltd.; 1988.

12. Tyler V. *Herbs of Choice. The Therapeutic Use of Phytomedicinals*. Binghampton, NY: Pharmaceutical Products Press; 1994:209.
13. Hoffmann D. *Holistic Herbal*. Rockport, CA: Element Books; 1996:256.
14. Houghton P. Bearberry, Dandelion and Celery. *Pharmaceutical Journal*. 1995;255:272-273.
15. Bradley P. *British Herbal Compendium*. Bournemouth: BHMA; 1992:239.
16. Frohne D. Untersuchungen zur Frage der Harndesinfizierenden Wirkungen von Barentraubenblatt-Extrakten. *Planta Medica*. 1970;18:23-5.
17. Grases F, Melero G, Costa-Bauza A, *et al* Urolithiasis and phytotherapy. *International Urology and Nephrology*. 1994;26(5):507-11.
18. Moskalenko SA. Preliminary screening of far-Eastern ethnomedicinal plants for antibacterial activity. *Journal of Ethnopharmacology*. 1986;15:231-59.
19. Merck. *Merck Index*. 10th ed. Rahway, NJ: Merck and Company; 1983:1156.

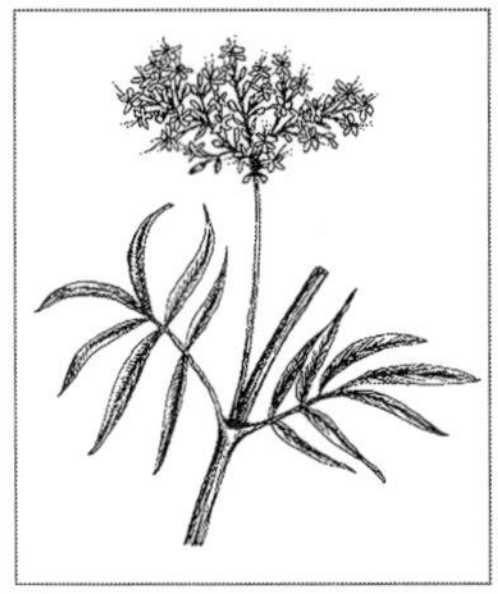

VALERIAN

Valeriana officinalis L. and other species of *Valeriana*

THUMBNAIL SKETCH

Active Constituents

- Gamma-aminobutyric acid (GABA), alkaloids, valepotriates, volatile oils

Common Uses

- Sedative-hypnotic

Adverse Effects

- Sedation

Cautions/Contraindications

- May impair driving and operation of hazardous machinery; contraindicated in pregnancy and lactation

Drug Interactions

- May potentiate the sedative effects of other CNS depressants

Doses

- 2-3 g of dried root orally three times daily or at bedtime

INTRODUCTION

Family: Valerianaceae

Synonyms: Belgian valerian, Common valerian, Fragrant valerian, Garden valerian[1-3]

There are over 200 valerian species and variants found in Australia, China, Europe, India, Japan, and North America (including Mexico). The perennial plant grows up to four feet in height, with pairs of opposing, almond-shaped, serrated-edge leaves arising from a grooved, hollow stem. Small, rose-colored flowers bloom from the top of the stem in the summer months. The tuberous root and dried rhizome of three species, *V. officinalis* L., *V. jatamansi* Jones (Indian Valerian) and *V. edulis* Nutt. ex. Torr. & Gray spp. *procera* F.G. Meyer (Mexican Valerian), are most often used as for medicinal purposes.[2-6] The root produces an odor variously described as offensive, distinctive, and penetrating.[4, 7]

Although not specifically mentioned in classical Greek or Roman medical writings, the use of valerian has been attributed to Hippocrates as early as 425 B.C.[8] Valerian's medicinal usage in Asia, Australia, Europe, the Middle East and North America has been documented in Greek, Anglo-Saxon, Medieval and Renaissance texts. It has been used as a sedative, an anti-nauseant, and for gastrointestinal and urinary symptoms.[3]

Constituents [1, 6, 9-12]

- Amino Acids: gamma-aminobutyric acid (GABA)
- Alkaloids: actinidine, chatinine, skyanthine, valerianine, valerine
- Iridoids (valepotriates): valerate(s), dihydrovalerate(s), valerosidate
- Volatile oils: monoterpenes, sesquiterpenes (e.g. valerenic acid), valerenyl esters
- Phenylpropanoids: caffeic and chlorogenic acids
- Sesquiterpenoids: valerenolic acid and acetylvalerenolic acid

THERAPEUTIC USES & RELEVANT PHARMACOLOGY

COMMON USES

Valerian is most often used as a sedative-hypnotic agent. Due to its reputed muscle relaxing properties it is often used, alone or in combination with other herbs, in the management of musculoskeletal conditions.

PHARMACOLOGY

Because of valerian's historical use as a sedative, anticonvulsant, migraine treatment and pain reliever, most basic science research has been directed at the interaction of valerian constituents with the GABA neurotransmitter receptor system. These studies remain inconclusive and all require independent replication. The mechanism of action of valerian in general, and as a mild sedative in particular, remains unknown. Valerian extracts appear to have some affinity for the $GABA_A$

(benzodiazepine) receptor,[13, 14] but this activity does not appear to be mediated by valerenic acid, but rather by the relatively high content of GABA itself.[15, 16] The amount of GABA present in aqueous extracts of valerian is sufficient to account for the release of GABA from synaptosomes, and also may inhibit reuptake.[17, 18] However, GABA does not cross the blood-brain barrier efficiently at low concentrations, so these *in vitro* results cannot account for the clinical data. Catabolism of GABA may be inhibited by valerenolic acid and acetylvalerenolic acid.[19]

Interactions with the serotonin neurotransmitter system have also been investigated and hydroxypinoresinol was found to have high affinity for the 5-HT_{1A} receptor.[12, 20] One paper reports an interaction with the adenosine receptor but not with the benzodiazepine receptor.[21]

Valerian has been reported to decrease gastrointestinal motility.[22] There is also some suggestion of an antipyretic or anti-inflammatory effect of valerian extracts.[23-25]

Animal Studies

Behavioral studies on rodents have demonstrated that valerian has some sedative properties. Valerian extracts produce changes in behavioral tests such as rotorod performance, activity, and augmentation of barbiturate-induced sleep similar to changes observed with benzodiazepines.[12, 26-35] Only weak anticonvulsive effects were found.[36] In contrast, Hiller *et al.* found no sedative effects in mice but did report some anticonvulsant effects.[37] One study reported that *Valeriana coreana* Briq. methanol extracts were able to decrease immobility in the forced swimming test in mice,[38] and reversed resperpine-induced hypothermia,[32] which suggests potential antidepressant activity. EEG changes in rats have also been found,[39] but these effects were not confirmed in cats.[40] Cerebral nuclear medicine imaging in rats using radiolabelled glucose showed central nervous system (CNS) depressant effects for a dichloromethane extract of valerian but not for the essential oil, valerenic acid, valeranone, valtrate, didrovaltrate, nor homobaldrinal.[12, 41, 42]

Human Clinical Studies

The human clinical studies of valerian have concentrated on evaluating its hypnotic effects. As would be expected from the basic science and animal data, valerian appears to have a mild sedative effect making it suitable as a sleep aid.[43] Its precise effects on the components of sleep are not consistent in the small number of studies reviewed here. There are reports that an aqueous extract of valerian root improves sleep quality[7, 44] and produces a decrease in the latency of sleep onset.[45] Leathwood *et al.* have also found that subjective measures of sleep quality, latency, and awakening were improved with valerian, in the absence of side-effects.[46-48] Objective EEG measurements confirmed the trend but did not reach statistical significance. Others confirm a subjective reduction in sleep latency and night-time awakening.[49] Objective laboratory sleep observations showed no significant difference between placebo and valerian. No change was observed in sleep stages or EEG patterns. Schultz *et al.*[50] report increased slow wave sleep, decreased stage I sleep, and increased density of K-complexes. There was no change in sleep latency, awakening or subjective sleep quality.

Only one English-language report of a subjective anxiolytic effect under experimental conditions was found for this review.[51]

ADVERSE EFFECTS

Data on the toxicity associated with valerian preparations is sparse, but there is some evidence of cytotoxicity.[6] Braun *et al.*[52] found no *in vivo* toxicity of valerian derivatives on hematopoietic precursor cells in contrast to *in vitro* data.[53, 54] Hepatotoxicity has been reported with herbal sleep remedies but these contained other ingredients in combination with valerian.[55, 56] Bounthanh *et al.*[57] report that valepotriates significantly inhibit both DNA and protein synthesis. Potential teratogenicity has been investigated in rats with no adverse effects identified.[58] However, this single study does not establish that valerian is safe to use in pregnancy, and therefore its use should be avoided until further data are available even though some authors have suggested that valerian is safe to use in pregnancy.[59, 60] Large doses (400mg/kg) of valerenic acid were found to be fatal in mice.[26]

CAUTIONS/CONTRAINDICATIONS

Valerian should be used with caution in children under 3 years of age and in pregnant or lactating women. Individuals taking valerian should be cautious when operating a motor vehicle or hazardous machinery.[12]

DRUG INTERACTIONS

Little data on specific drug interactions exists at present. However, given the evidence of hypnotic-sedative effects, the use of valerian preparations in conjunction with other CNS depressants should be avoided or approached with caution. Valerian may potentiate the effects of other CNS depressants including ethanol.[23, 26, 32, 61]

DOSAGE REGIMENS

- 2-3 g of root or rhizome (or equivalent dry extracts) orally three times daily or at bedtime.[12]
- 1-3 mL of tincture (20% concentration by volume in a 70% ethanol solution) three times daily or at bedtime.[12]

REFERENCES

1. Newall C, Anderson L, Phillipson J. *Herbal Medicines: A Guide for Health Care Professionals.* London: The Pharmaceutical Press; 1996:296.
2. Houghton PJ. The biological activity of valerian and related plants. *Journal of Ethnopharmacology*. 1988;22:121-42.
3. Hobbs C. Valerian and other anti-hysterics in European and American medicine (1733-1936). *Pharmacy in History*. 1990;32(3):132-137.
4. Tyler V. *Herbs of Choice. The Therapeutic Use of Phytomedicinals.* Binghamton, NY: Pharmaceutical Products Press; 1994:209.
5. Murray MT. *The Healing Power of Herbs*. Rocklin, CA: Prima Publishing; 1992:246.
6. Bos R, Woerdenbag HJ, De Smet PAGM, Scheffer JJC. Valeriana Species. In: De Smet PAGM, Keller K, Hansel R, Chandler RF, eds. *Adverse Effects of Herbal Drugs.* Berlin, Heidelberg: Springer-Verlag; 1997:165-180.
7. Leathwood PD, Chauffard F, Heck E, Munoz-Box R. Aqueous extract of Valerian Root (*Valeriana officinalis* L.) improves sleep quality in man. *Pharmacology, Biochemistry and Behavior*. 1982;17:65-71.
8. Fuchs R. Samtliche Werke (Collected Works). Munich; 1895-1908.
9. Hendriks H, Smith D, Hazelhoff B. Eugenyl isovalerate and isoeugenyl isovalerate in the essential oil of Valerian root. *Phytochemistry*. 1977;16:1853-54.
10. Bos R, Hendriks H, Kloosterman J, Sipma G. Isolation of the sesquiterpene alcohol (-)-Pacifigorgiol from *Valeriana officinalis*. *Phytochemistry*. 1986;25(5):1234-35.
11. Bos R, Hendriks H, Bruins AP, *et al*. Isolation and identification of Valerenane sesquiterpenoids from *Valeriana officinalis*. *Phytochemistry*. 1986;25(1):133-35.
12. European Scientific Cooperative on Phytotherapy (ESCOP) . *Valerianae Radix/Valerian Root*. In: *ESCOP Monographs* (Fascicule 4) Exeter: ESCOP; 1997:58.

13. Holzl J, Godau P. Receptor binding studies with *Valeriana officinalis* on the benzodiazepine receptor. *Planta Medica*. 1989;55:642.
14. Mennini T, Bernasconi P, Bombardelli E, Morazzoni P. *In vitro* study on the interaction of extracts and pure com pounds form *Valeriana officinalis* roots with GABA, benzodiazepine and barbiturate receptors in rat brain. *Fitoterapia*. 1993;64:291-300.
15. Cavadas C, Araujo I, Cotrim MD, *et al. In vitro* study on the interaction of *Valeriana officinalis* L. extracts and their amino acids on GABAA receptor in rat brain. *Arzneimittelforschung*. 1995;45(7):753-5.
16. Bodesheim U, Holzl J. Isolation and receptor binding properties of alkaloids and lignans from *V. officinalis* L. *Pharmazie*. 1997;52(5):386-391.
17. Santos MS, Ferreira F, Cunha AP, *et al*. An aqueous extract of valerian influences the transport of GABA in synaptosomes. [Letter]. *Planta Medica*. 1994;60(3):278-9.
18. Santos MS, Ferreira F, Faro C, *et al.* The amount of GABA present in aqueous extracts of valerian is sufficient to account for [3H]GABA release in synaptosomes. [Letter]. *Planta Medica*. 1994;60(5):475-6.
19. Riedel E, Hansel R, Ehrke G. Inhibition of GABA catabolism by Valerenic acid derivatives. *Planta Medica*. 1982;46:219-220.
20. Holzl J. Baldrian - Ein mittel gegen Schlafstorungen und Nervositat. *Deutsch Apotheker Zeitung*. 1996;136:751-9.
21. Balduini W, Cattabeni F. Displacement of [^{3}H]-N^6-cyclohexyladenosine binding to rat cortical membranes by an hydroalcoholic extract of *Valeriana officinalis*. *Medical Science Research* 1989;17:639-40.
22. Hazelhoff B, *et al*. Antispasmodic effects of *Valeriana* compounds: an *in vivo* and *in vitro* study on the guinea-pig ileum. *Archives Internationales de Pharmacodynamie et de Therapie*. 1982;257:274-287.
23. Shrivastava SC, Sisodia CS. Analgesic studies on *Vitax Negundo* and *Valeriana wallichii*. *Indian Veterinary Journal*. 1970;47:170-75.
24. Girgune JB, Jain NK, Grag BD. Antimicrobial activity of the essential oil from *Valeriana wallichii* D.C. (Valerianaceae). *Indian Journal of Microbiology*. 1980;20:142-143.
25. Chen S, Xie X, Du B, *et al*. Infantile rotavirus enteritis treated with herbal *Valeriana jatamansi* (VJ). *Journal of Traditional Chinese Medicine*. 1984;4:297-300.
26. Hendriks H, Bos R, Woerdenbag HJ, Koster AS. Central nervous system depressant activity of valerenic acid in the mouse. *Planta Medica*. 1985:28-31.
27. Hendriks H, Bos R, Allersma DP, Malingre TM, Koster AS. Pharmacological screening of valerenal and some other components of essential oil of *Valeriana officinalis*. *Planta Medica*. 1981;42:62-68.
28. Veith J, Schneider G, Lemmer B, Willems M. The influence of some degredation products of valepotriates on the motor activity of light-dark synchronized mice. *Planta Medica*. 1986:179-183.
29. Wagner H, Jurcic K, Schaette R. Comparative studies on the sedative action of Valeriana extracts, valepotriates and their degradation products. *Planta Medica*. 1980;36:358-365.
30. Hansel R, Keller K, Rimpler H, Schneider G. Valeriana. *Hagers Handbuch der Parmzeutischen Praxis.* 5th ed. Berlin: Springer-Verlag; 1994:1067-95.
31. Torrent MT, Iglesias J, Adzet T. Valoracion experimental de la actividad sedante de la tinctura de *Valeriana officinalis* L. *Circular Farmaceutica*. 1972;30:107-12.
32. Sakamoto T, Mitana Y, Nakajima K. Psychotropic effects of Japanese valerian root extracts. *Chemical and Pharmaceutical Bulletin*. 1992;40:758-61.
33. Hikino H, Hikino Y, Kobinata H, Aizawa A. Sedative properties of valeriana roots. *Shoyakugako Zasshi*. 1980;34:19-24.
34. Takamura K, Kawaguchi M, Nabata H. The preparation and pharmacological screening of kessoglycol derivative. *Yakugaku Zasshi*. 1975;95:1198-1204.
35. Takamura K, Nabata H, Kawaguchi M. The pharmacological action on the kessoglycol-8-monoacetate. *Yakugaku Zasshi*. 1975;95(1205-1209).
36. Leuschner J, Muller J, Rudmann M. Characterisation of the central nervous depressant activity of a commercially available valerian root extract. *Arzneimittelforschung*. 1993;43(6):638-41.
37. Hiller K-O, Zetler G. Neuropharmacological studies on ethanol extracts of *Valeriana officinalis* L. behavioural and anticonvulsant properties. *Phytotherapy Research*. 1996;10:145-51.
38. Oshima Y, Matsuoka S, Ohizumi Y. Antidepressant principles of *Valeriana fauriei* roots. *Chemical and Pharmaceutical Bulletin (Tokyo)*. 1995;43(1):169-70.
39. Brattstrom A. Evidence of efficacy for herbal remedies exemplified for a fixed combination of hops and valerian. *Forsch Komplementarmed*. 1996;3(4):188-195.

40. Holm E, Kowollik H, Reinecke A, von Henning GE, *et al*. Vergeichende neurophysiologische Untersuchungen mit Valtratum/Isovaltratum und Extractum Valerianae an Katzen. *Medizinische Welt*. 1980;31:982-90.
41. Krieglstein J, Grusla D. Zentral dampfende Inhaltsstoffe im Baldrian. Valpotriate, Valerensaure, Valeranon and atherisches Ol sind jedoch unwirksam. *Deutsch Apotheker Zeitung*. 1988;128:2041-6.
42. Grusla D, Holzl J, J. K. Baldrianwirkungen im Gehirn der Ratte. *Deutsch Apotheker Zeitung*. 1986;126:2249-53.
43. Houghton P. Valerian. *The Pharmaceutical Journal*. 1994;253:95-96.
44. Lindahl O, Lindwall L. Double blind study of a valerian preparation. *Pharmacology Biochemistry and Behavior*. 1989;32:1065-6.
45. Leathwood PD, Chauffard F. Aqueous extract of valerian reduces latency to fall asleep in man. *Planta Medica*. 1985;51:144-148.
46. Leathwood PD, Chauffard F. Quantifying the effects of mild sedatives. *Journal of Psychiatric Research*. 1982;17(2):115-122.
47. Leathwood PD, Chauffard F, Munoz-Box R. Effect of *Valeriana officinalis* L. on subjective and objective sleep parameters. *6th European Congress on Sleep Research*. Zurich: Basel-Karger; 1983:402-405.
48. Chauffard F, Heck E, Leathwood PD. Detection of mild sedative effects: valerian and sleep in man. [ABS] *Biochemistry*.622:37:622.
49. Balderer G, Borbely AA. Effect of valerian on human sleep. *Psychopharmacology*. 1985;87:406-409.
50. Schulz H, Stolz C, Muller J. The effect of valerian extract on sleep polygraphy in poor sleepers: a pilot study. *Pharmacopsychiatry*. 1994;27(4):147-51.
51. Kohnen R, Oswald W. The effects of valerian, propranolol, and their combination on activation, performance, and mood of healthy volunteers under social stress conditions. *Pharmacopsychiatry*. 1988;21:447-8.
52. Braun R, Dittmar W, Hubner GE, Maurer HR. *In vivo* effect of valtrate/isovaltrate on the bone marrow cells and the metabolic activity of the liver in mice. *Planta Medica*. 1984:1:1-4.
53. Keochanthala-Bounthanh C, Haag-Berrurier M, Beck JP, Anton R. Effects of thiol compounds versus cytotoxicity of valepotriates on cultured hepatoma cells. *Planta Medica*. 1990;56:190-192.
54. Keochanthala-Bounthanh C, Beck JP, Haag-Berrurier M, Anton R. Effects of two monoterpene esters, valtrate and didrovaltrate, isolated from *valeriana wallichii*, on the ultrastructure of hepatoma cells in culture. *Phytotherapy Research*. 1993;7:124-127.
55. McGregor FB, Abernethy VE, Dahabra S, *et al*. Hepatotoxicity of herbal remedies. *British Medical Journal*. 1989;299:1156-1157.
56. Shepherd C. Sleep Disorders. Liver damage warning with insomnia remedy. *British Medical Journal*. 1993;306:1472.
57. Bounthanh C, Richert L, Beck JP, Haag-Berrurier M, Anton R. The action of valepotriates on the synthesis of DNA and proteins of cultured hepatoma cells. *Journal of Medicinal Plant Research*. 1983;49:138-142.
58. Tufik S, Fujita K, Seabra ML, Lobo LL. Effects of a prolonged administration of valepotriates in rats on the mothers and their offspring. *Journal of Ethnopharmacology*. 1994;41(1-2):39-44.
59. Berglund F, Flodh H, Lundborg P, *et al*. Drug use during pregnancy and lactation. A classification for drug information. *Acta Obstetricia et Gynecologica Scandinavica Supplement*. 1984;126:1-55.
60. Committee ADE. Medicines in pregnancy. An Australian categorization of risk. Canberra: Australian Government Publishing Service; 1989.
61. Takamura K, Kakimoto M, Kawaguchi M, Iwasaki T. Pharmacological studies on the constituents of crude drugs and plants. I: Pharmacological action of. *Yakugaku Zasshi – Journal of the Pharmaceutical Society of Japan*. 1973;93: 599-606.

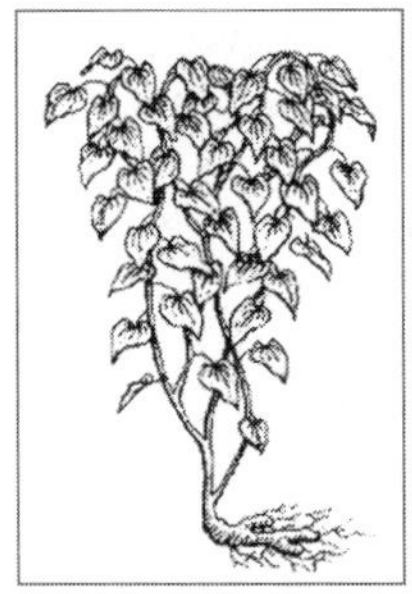

WILD YAM

Dioscorea villosa L.

THUMBNAIL SKETCH

Active Constituents

❖Steroidal glycosides based on the sapogenin diosgenin

Common Uses

❖Abdominal colic, diverticulitis, irritable bowel syndrome, arthritis, rheumatism, and gynecological problems (dysmennorhoea and ovarian pains)

Adverse Effects

❖None could be found for the plant itself but consumption of the sapogenins may result in bruising

Cautions/Contraindications

❖Avoid in pregnancy

Drug Interactions

❖None could be found

Doses

❖2-4mL of tincture three times daily

INTRODUCTION

Family: Dioscoreaceae

Synonyms: Colic root, Rheumatism root[1]

Many different species of the genus *Dioscorea* exist but within the complementary medical model, *Dioscorea villosa* is the one most often used. *Dioscorea villosa* is a perennial plant producing a large fibrous root stock and is native to the Eastern United States and Central America.[2] It has a characteristic taste which has often been described as insipid.[3,4] The roots are the part used medicinally. The therapeutic actions disappear on storage and it is best harvested annually.[4] Wild yam was used extensively by eclectic physicians in the United States during the mid to latter part of last century.[5] Wild yam (*Dioscorea villosa*) is distinct from the vegetable often referred to as yam (*Ipomoea batatas* (L.) Lam., Convolvulaceae).[5]

Constituents[1,3]

- Steroidal saponins (based on the sapogenin diosgenin) including dioscin and dioscorin.
- Dioscorein is not an actual constituent but refers to a dried solid extract.[5]

THERAPEUTIC USES & RELEVANT PHARMACOLOGY

COMMON USES

Wild yam is reputed to have antispasmodic,[2,4,6] anti-inflammatory,[2,6] diuretic,[2] hepatic,[2,6] and anti-rhuematic properties.[2,6] Oral consumption is considered useful in the treatment of digestive conditions such as intestinal colic, diverticulitis, irritable bowel syndrome and bilious indigestion.[2,6] As a traditional 'anti-rheumatic' it is used in situations of arthritis and joint inflammation.[2,5,6] It is also considered a 'relaxing remedy' and is used to treat a number of gynecological problems such as ovarian pain, painful menstruation and in labor.[2,5,6]

PHARMACOLOGY

No details regarding the mode of action of *Dioscorea villosa* itself could be found for this monograph. Diosgenin, isolated from Mexican yam, was originally considered of prime importance in the pharmaceutical manufacture of a number of steroidal substances, including early oral contraceptives.[2,3]

Confusion has arisen because of claims made that diosgenin can be converted into a number of steroidal substances, including dehydroepiandrosterone (DHEA) and progesterone, following oral or topical administration. Some products have been marketed as 'hormonal precursors'. No evidence could be found to substantiate these claims. Araghiniknam *et al.* demonstrated that oral administration of a compound containing 90% 'wild yam extract' did not increase serum dehydroepiandrosterone sulfate (DHEA-S) levels in a group of elderly patients (over 65 years of age, n=7).[7] The results of this study were supported by a similar investigation in which saliva specimens were analyzed in a group of women taking products containing Mexican yam.[8]

ADVERSE EFFECTS

No situations of adverse reactions could be found for the plant itself.

Cases of 'hormonal effects' (early menopause symptoms, masculinization of females and hypertension) have been attributed to one commercial product.[9] No details were given with respect to the exact composition of this product and therefore the clinical relevance to the use of *Dioscorea villosa* in general cannot really be ascertained.

CAUTIONS/CONTRAINDICATIONS

Concerns have been raised regarding the effect of products referred to as 'Mexican Wild Yam' and conditions with a strong hormonal element such as breast and prostate cancer.[9] A case of occupational allergy caused by frequent exposure to Sanyak / Chinese yam (*Dioscorea oppositifolia* L.) has been reported in a 25-year-old male who worked in a herbal pharmacy.[10] Given the lack of information and the fact that the herb acts as on smooth muscle, wild yam should be avoided in pregnancy.

DRUG INTERACTIONS

No cases of drug interaction could be found.

DOSAGE REGIMENS

- 2-4mL of tincture three times daily.[6]

As mentioned above, concerns have been made regarding the use and marketing of 'wild yam' extracts as 'hormonal precursors'. There appears to be no evidence to support this claim. This confusion seems to be particularly important regarding the use of natural progesterone products.[5]

REFERENCES

1. Wren R. *Potter's New Encyclopedia of Botanical Drugs and Preparations.* Saffron Walden: C.W. Daniel Company; 1988:362.
2. Chevalier A. *The Encyclopedia of Medicinal Plants.* London: Reader's Digest; 1996:336.
3. Evans W. *Trease and Evans' Pharmacognosy*. 13th ed. London: Bailliere Tindall; 1989:832.
4. Grieve M. *A Modern Herbal.* London: Penguin ; 1984:912.
5. Hudson T. Wild Yam, Natural Progesterone, Unraveling the Confusion. *Townsend Letter for Doctors and Patients*. 1996; July:125-127.
6. Hoffmann D. *Holistic Herbal.* Rockport, CA: Element Books; 1996:256.
7. Araghiniknam M, Chung S, Nelson-White T, Eskelson C, Watson RR. Antioxidant activity of dioscorea and dehydroepian drosterone (DHEA) in older humans. *Life Sciences*. 1996;59(11):147-57.
8. Dollbaum C. Lab analyses of salivary DHEA and progesterone following ingestion of yam-containing products. *Townsend Newsletter for Doctors*. 1996;159:104.
9. Craddick J. Potential hazards of Mexican Yam. *Townsend Letter for Doctors and Patients*. 1996;August/September:101.
10. Park HS, Kim MJ, Moon HB. Occupational asthma caused by two herb materials, *Dioscorea batatas* and *Pinellia ternata*. *Clinical and Experimental Allergy*. 1994;24(6):575-81.

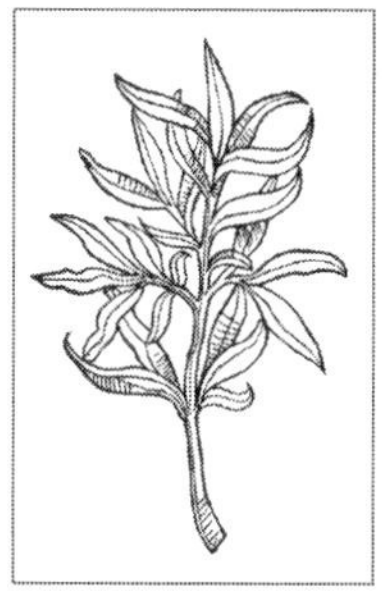

WILLOW

Salix spp

THUMBNAIL SKETCH

Active Constituents

- Phenolic glycosides (including salicin and salicortin)

Common Uses

- Arthritic conditions and as an analgesic

Adverse Effects

- Rare nausea, headache and digestive upset

Cautions/Contraindications

- Classic ones applicable to salicylates in general

Drug Interactions

- Classic ones applicable to salicylates in general

Doses

- Oral: 20-40 mg of salicin three times daily or maximum of 240 mg of salicin daily
- 1-2 mL of liquid extract (1:1, 25% ethanol) three times daily
- 5-8 mL of tincture (1:5, 25% ethanol) three times daily
- 5-10 g of raw herb three times daily

INTRODUCTION

Family: Salicaeae

Members of the salix genus commonly used medicinally include: *S. fragilis* L. (Crack willow), *S. nigra* Marsh. (Black willow), *S. alba* L. (White willow), *S. purpurea* L.(Purple osier willow), *S. daphnoides* Villars (European daphne willow) and *S. cinerea* L. (Large gray willow).[1, 2]

Willow has a long history in many different healing traditions. It was especially popular in the treatment of rheumatism and ague (i.e, fever, chills).[3] While in North America white willow and black willow are most often used, [3, 4] pharmacologically these may not be the most active since other members of the genus (e.g., *S. fragilis* L., *S. purpurea* and *S. daphnoides* Villars) are richer in the medicinally active phenolic glycosides.[4] The bark of young branches is the part most commonly used medicinally. However, it has been shown that the leaves of some species may contain as much, and maybe more, of the phenolic glycosides than the bark. Accordingly, it has been argued that there is no reason why these parts cannot be used therapeutically.[5]

Constituents [1, 5-8]

- Phenolic glycosides including salicin, salicortin, tremulacin and salireposide
- Miscellaneous including condensed tannins, flavonoids and catechins

There is great variability between species of the salix genus, of particular importance are the phenolic glycoside components. While *Salix purpurea* L. can contain up to 8% salicin and *Salix fragilis* L. up to 10%[4, 7], *S. alba* L. often has less than 1% salicin.[4]

THERAPEUTIC USES AND RELEVANT PHARMACOLOGY

COMMON USES

Preparations of white willow bark have been used in the treatment of feverish conditions, rheumatism and as mild pain-killers in such conditions as headache.[7, 9] Given the relatively low amount of phenolic glycosides (notably salicin), compared to conventional salicylate medications, it has been argued that in pharmacological terms, it is unlikely that any willow preparation will be effective in the management of these conditions.[4]

PHARMACOLOGY

The pharmacological action of willow appears to be determined not only by salicin content. The other phenolic glycosides also have therapeutic properties.[4] It is hypothesized that the phenolic glycosides do not act directly but rather act as pro-drugs. They are converted in multiple stages, primarily in the liver and intestines, to the active moieties (most notably salicylic acid).[7] The action is therefore slower in onset than conventional salicylic acid but has a longer duration of action.[4] It should be noted that salicin does not irreversibly inhibit platelet aggregation, as is the case with acetylsalicylic acid.[7]

Limited *in vivo* studies demonstrate that a number of the phenolic glycosides have anti-inflammatory properties.[7] Little research has been conducted on the salicylates and salicylic acid obtained from plant sources such as willow.

ADVERSE EFFECTS

Adverse effects seem to be rare and mild, limited to nausea, digestive upset and headache.[7] A case of hemorrhage in a 64 year old women with glucose-6-phosphate dehydrogenase (G6PD) deficiency has been documented following the consumption of an ayurvedic product containing *Salix caprea* L.. No information is given in the case report with regards to other ingredients present in the preparation.[10]

CAUTIONS/CONTRAINDICATIONS

The contraindications applicable to the use of conventional salicylate preparations are believed to be applicable to the consumption of willow products. Consequently, use should be avoided in individuals with conditions such as asthma, diabetes, gout, haemophilia, hyperthrombinaemia, hepatic/renal disease, active peptic ulcer disease, glucose-6-phosphate dehydrogenase (G6PD) deficiency and individuals sensitive to aspirin.[1] Until more detailed information is available, preparations containing willow should not be administered during pregnancy or lactation. No information could be found regarding the use of willow products in children given that salicylate-containing products are normally restricted to individuals over 12 years of age.

DRUG INTERACTIONS

No cases could be found but drug interactions common to conventional salicylates appear applicable.[1]

DOSAGE REGIMENS

- Daily doses of preparations (dried, hydroalcoholic or aqueous extracts, tinctures or fluid extracts) equivalent to 60-120 mg (up to 240mg) of salicin daily.[7]
- 20-40 mg of salicin, 1-2 mL of liquid extract (1:1, 25% ethanol), 5-8 mL of hydro alcoholic tincture (1:5, 25% ethanol) or 5-10 g of raw herb three times daily.[11]

REFERENCES

1. Newall C, Anderson L, Phillipson J. *Herbal Medicines: A Guide for Health Care Professionals.* London: The Pharmaceutical Press; 1996:296.
2. Marles RJ, Associate Professor, Department of Botany, Brandon University, Brandon, Manitoba. Review of Medicinal Plant Modules for CCNM ; 1998.
3. Hutchens A. *Indian Herbology of North America.* Boston, MA: Shambhala; 1973:382.
4. Tyler V. *Herbs of Choice. The Therapeutic Use of Phytomedicinals.* Binghampton, NY: Pharmaceutical Products Press; 1994:209.
5. Meier B. Pharmaceutical aspects of the use of willows in herbal remedies. *Planta Medica.* 1988;54:559-60.
6. Karl C. Flavonoide aus *Salix alba*, die Struktur des terniflorins und eines Weiteren Acylflavonoides.

Phytochemistry. 1976;15:1084-5.
7. ESCOP. Salicis Cortex/Willow Bark. In: *ESCOP Monograph Fascicule 4.* Exeter: ESCOP; 1997:58pp.
8. Meier B, Lehman D, Sticher O, *et al*. Identifikation und Bestimmung von je acht Phenolglykosiden in *Salix purpurea* und Salix daphnoides mit moderner HPLC. *Pharmaceutica Acta Helvetica*. 1985;60:269-74.
9. Hoffmann D. *Holistic Herbal.* Rockport, CA: Element Books; 1996:256.
10. Baker S, Thomas PS. Herbal medicine precipitating massive haemolysis. *Lancet*. 1987(i):1039-40.
11. Bradley P. *British Herbal Compendium*. Bournemouth: BHMA; 1992:239.